Motorcycle Accident Reconstruction

Motorcycle Accident Reconstruction

NATHAN A. ROSE

Principal and Director
Kineticorp, LLC
nrose@kineticorp.com

WILLIAM T.C. NEALE

Director of Visualization
Motorcycle Safety Instructor
wneale@kineticorp.com

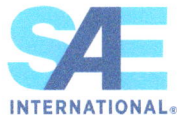

SAE INTERNATIONAL®

Warrendale, Pennsylvania, USA

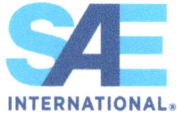

400 Commonwealth Drive
Warrendale, PA 15096-0001 USA
E-mail: CustomerService@sae.org
Phone: 877-606-7323 (inside USA and Canada)
                724-776-4970 (outside USA)
Fax: 724-776-0790

Library of Congress Catalog Number 2018949732
SAE Order Number R-483
http://dx.doi.org/10.4271/R-483

Information contained in this work has been obtained by SAE International from sources believed to be reliable. However, neither SAE International nor its authors guarantee the accuracy or completeness of any information published herein and neither SAE International nor its authors shall be responsible for any errors, omissions, or damages arising out of use of this information. This work is published with the understanding that SAE International and its authors are supplying information, but are not attempting to render engineering or other professional services. If such services are required, the assistance of an appropriate professional should be sought.

ISBN-Print 978-0-7680-9507-4
ISBN-PDF 978-0-7680-9508-1
ISBN-ePUB 978-0-7680-9510-4
ISBN-PRC 978-0-7680-9509-8
ISBN-HTML 978-0-7680-9511-1

To purchase bulk quantities, please contact: SAE Customer Service

E-mail: CustomerService@sae.org
Phone: 877-606-7323 *(inside USA and Canada)*
                724-776-4970 *(outside USA)*
Fax: 724-776-0790

Visit the SAE International Bookstore at books.sae.org

dedication

This book is dedicated to Ray Brach, whose research and writing I cut my teeth on and whose critique of my own work when I was a young accident reconstructionist helped me tremendously.

I still return to your articles and books on a regular basis.

*—**Nathan A. Rose***

contents

CHAPTER 6

Sliding and Tumbling of the Motorcycle and Rider   133

CHAPTER 7

Motorcycle Falls   145

author bios

Nathan Rose is a partner, director, and principal accident reconstructionist at Kineticorp, LLC, a Denver-based accident reconstruction, forensic engineering, and forensic visualization firm that he helped found in 2005. Prior to that, he held positions as an engineer (1998 to 2003) and a senior engineer (2003 to 2005) at Knott Laboratory, another Denver-based forensic engineering firm. He holds a bachelor's degree in engineering with a civil specialty from the Colorado School of Mines (1998) and a master's degree in mechanical engineering from the University of Colorado at Denver (2003). Nathan is accredited as a traffic accident reconstructionist by the Accreditation Commission for Traffic Accident Reconstruction (ACTAR), and he has offered expert testimony as a reconstructionist in courts around the United States. During his graduate studies, he specialized in dynamics and impact mechanics and he has published numerous technical articles and reports related to vehicular accident reconstruction. These articles have covered many topics, including rollover accident reconstruction, motorcycle accident reconstruction, crash simulation, video analysis, crush analysis, restitution, and crash test sensor analysis. Nathan is a past organizer for the Rollover, Rear Impact, and Accident Reconstruction Sessions held annually at the Society of Automotive Engineers (SAE) World Congress. He used to teach a 1-day course for SAE on rollover accident reconstruction, and he currently teaches a 3-day accident reconstruction course for SAE. Nathan holds a motorcycle endorsement in the State of Colorado. You can find additional articles, research, and blog posts authored by Nathan at www.nathanarose.com.

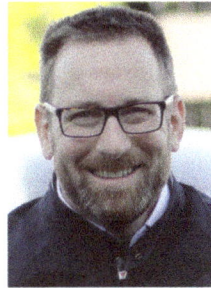

William Neale is a partner and director at Kineticorp, a firm that he also helped found in 2005. He is certified as a motorcycle safety instructor by the Motorcycle Safety Foundation. For many years, William taught, licensed, and trained riders in the safe operation and handling of motorcycles, teaching both the Basic RiderCourse and the Advanced RiderCourse. He has also been certified in Level I and Level II Motorcycle Accident Scene Management and has taken Motorcycle Reconstruction coursework at Northwestern University School for Public Safety. He is an accredited traffic accident reconstructionist through ACTAR, and he has offered testimony as an accident reconstructionist and a motorcycle safety instructor in courts across the United States. From 2013 to 2015, William served a 2-year term on Colorado's Motorcycle Safety Operation Advisory Board. William has also published extensively about the forensic evaluation of nighttime lighting and visibility and has applied that in analyzing motorcycle accidents that occur at night.

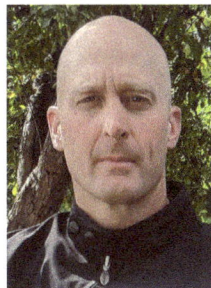

acknowledgments

We would like to thank Andrew O'Donnell and Jordan Dickinson for their contributions to the illustrations and graphics in this book. Also, Neal Carter, Connor Smith, Tilo Voitel, Nathan McKelvey, David Pentecost, Alireza Hashemian, Tomas Owens, Sean McDonough, Martin Randolph, and Daniel Koch all made helpful contributions to the testing and analysis reported in this book. Neal Carter has been a valuable and insightful sounding board throughout this project. His efforts were integral to many sections in this book, including the cornering and physical evidence documentation sections. Louis Peck has also been an integral part of this project, making helpful and much appreciated contributions by providing data related to motorcycle braking and motorcycle EDRs and reading and commenting on portions of the book. Ken Strohmeyer of the Scottsdale Police Department provided a helpful reading and editing of a draft version of this book. He also provided me with the notes from a presentation he gave in 2018 on motorcycle accident reconstruction. Jarrod Carter made much needed corrections to the grammar, reminding me that acceleration is already a rate. Shaun Helman of the Transportation Research Laboratory directed me to research he conducted related to motorcycle conspicuity, which significantly improved the chapter on human factors. Much thanks to these individuals. Any errors or omissions, of course, remain ours.

preface

In this book, our aim is a treatment of motorcycle accident reconstruction for engineers and reconstructionists that is thorough, systematic, and scientific. Oddly, such a book does not currently exist. The most widely used accident reconstruction text for engineers does not contain a chapter on motorcycle crashes (*Vehicle Accident Analysis and Reconstruction Methods*, Raymond M. Brach and R. Matthew Brach, SAE International, ISBN 0768007763, 2005). The motorcycle crash reconstruction course offered by SAE has no book associated with it. The two motorcycle accident reconstruction texts that currently exist fall short of the rigor and depth demanded by engineers practicing as accident reconstructionists, as does the single chapter on motorcycle crashes in Lynne Fricke's *Crash Reconstruction*. The engineer has so far been left to their own efforts at pulling together the vast literature on motorcycle accident reconstruction.

Speaking of vast literature, it is worth mentioning what this book is not. This is not a book about motorcycle dynamics. Even in 1978, Roy Rice of Calspan could state "the analysis of two-wheel vehicle dynamics has been the subject of many a research treatise over the last several decades. Some 200 papers were identified in preparing the bibliography which has been assembled for this meeting." Since then, the number of papers and articles related to motorcycle dynamics has increased significantly. While certainly we have made efforts to write a text that is consistent with principles of motorcycle dynamics, the focus here is on physical evidence from motorcycle crashes and the specific methods that practicing accident reconstructionists would employ in analyzing that physical evidence. Readers interested in delving into motorcycle dynamics are referred to the text *Motorcycle Dynamics* by Vittore Cossalter (ISBN:978-1-4303-0861-4).

Here in this book, we have attempted to pull together as much of the relevant accident reconstruction literature and science as possible. I am by nature a curator and I learn by writing. I bring to this book a love for studying physical evidence and understanding what it means, along with a love for bringing math and physics to bear on analysis of physical evidence. William Neale comes at this from the perspective of a motorcycle safety instructor, and his research and professional interests often take him into the realm of evaluating rider behavior and performance. He also has extensive expertise in nighttime lighting, photography, and visibility and he has brought that expertise to this book. William and I have been friends and business partners for many years, and the old-married-couple kind of arguments we regularly have make me better and have hopefully made this book better.

A word about terminology: There is sometimes controversy surrounding the use of words such as *accident*, *crash*, *collision*, and *impact*. For example, the British Medical Journal has banned the use of the word *accident*, stating that "an accident is often understood to be unpredictable – a chance occurrence or an 'act of God' – and therefore unavoidable. However, most injuries and their precipitating events are predictable and preventable."* While I certainly agree that most of the *crashes* that lead to injuries are preventable, rejecting the word *accident* seems needlessly pedantic. Many *crashes*, while caused by human errors, are also *accidents*, at least in the sense that they were not intentional or premeditated. The word *accident* is still widely used and we use it here.

---

* Davis, R.M. and Pless, B., "BMJ Bans 'Accidents,'" *British Medical Journal* 322 (June 2001).

We also use the word *crash*. To me, the words *collision* and *impact* are synonyms, but their scope is more limited than the words *accident* or *crash*. When we use the words *collision* or *impact*, it will refer to the actual contact between two vehicles or a vehicle and another object. We typically will not use terms like *collision reconstruction* or *impact reconstruction* because these terms are narrower than we will usually intend.

I hope you enjoy and benefit from this book!

Nathan A. Rose
Greenwood Village, Colorado
April 2018

Introduction to Accident Reconstruction

Accident reconstruction utilizes principles of physics and empirical data to analyze the physical, electronic, video, audio, and testimonial evidence from a crash, to determine how and why the crash occurred or to determine whose description of the crash is most accurate. Crash reconstructionists may also analyze how a crash could have been avoided. Crash reconstruction draws together aspects of mathematics, physics, engineering, materials science, and psychology and combines analytical models with empirical test data. Different types of crashes—vehicle-to-vehicle collisions, single-vehicle rollover crashes, pedestrian and bicycle crashes, motorcycle crashes, or heavy truck crashes, for instance—produce different types of evidence and call for different analysis methods. Still, the basic philosophical approach of the reconstructionist is the same from crash type to crash type, as are the physical principles that are brought to bear on the analysis. This introductory chapter covers a basic approach to crash reconstruction along with the underlying physical principles employed. The chapters that follow address how this approach and these physical principles are applied specifically to motorcycle crashes.

1.1 The Approach Used in Accident Reconstruction

1.1.1 The Context of Reconstruction

Accident reconstruction is carried out in several contexts. For instance, reconstruction in a research context can evaluate or improve safety systems for vehicles and drivers. In this context, reconstruction seeks to understand and characterize the real-world conditions under which vehicle occupants are injured. Defining these conditions could include quantifying the severity of an impact, determining speeds and accelerations, analyzing accident avoidance scenarios, and analyzing the real-world performance of vehicle restraint and safety systems and structures.

In other instances, crash reconstruction is carried out in a forensic setting and is aimed at answering technical questions relevant to litigation. In this context, crash reconstruction aims at assisting lawyers, judges, and juries in their roles of assessing responsibility for a crash and the injuries that result. Rule 702 of the Federal Rules of Evidence states that "a witness who is qualified as an expert by knowledge, skill, experience, training, or education may testify in the form of an opinion or otherwise if: (a) the expert's scientific, technical, or other specialized knowledge will help the trier of fact to understand the evidence or to determine a fact at issue; (b) the testimony is based on sufficient facts or data; (c) the testimony is the product of reliable principles and methods; and (d) the expert has reliably applied the principles and methods to the facts of the case." The notes of the Advisory Committee on this rule state that "an intelligent evaluation of facts is often difficult or impossible without the application of some scientific, technical, or other specialized knowledge. The most common source of this knowledge is the expert witness, although there are other techniques for supplying it." Thus, in a forensic setting, the reconstructionist steps into the role of teacher, instructing the trier of fact and helping them to understand the technical issues relevant to the facts of the crash that is the subject of litigation.

1.1.2 Investigation and Analysis

Reconstruction is a scientific activity that employs an understanding of physical principles obtained through study, testing, and observation, as well as an intellectual understanding through reason and logic. Reconstruction typically involves both investigation and analysis. The goal of the *investigation* phase is to gather all the available evidence relevant to the analysis (physical, electronic, video, audio, and testimonial). This will often include: (1) Documenting, mapping, and diagramming geometrical conditions of the crash location like slope, cross-slope, lane widths, shoulder width, roadway surface type, and off-road surface types. (2) Documenting, mapping, and diagraming the physical evidence deposited at the scene. Some of this evidence may still be present during a crash site inspection. Other evidence locations may need to be reconstructed during the analysis phase based on measurements taken by police or using methods of photogrammetry. (3) Documenting, mapping, and diagramming the pre-crash geometry of the vehicle. At times, this involves obtaining manufacturer specifications for the vehicle or equipment involved in the crash, or inspecting an exemplar. (4) Documenting and diagraming the physical evidence deposited on the vehicle. This often involves physically inspecting the vehicle but could also rely on photogrammetric analysis and analysis of photographs or video.

The *analysis* phase typically follows the investigation phase and includes: (1) photographic or photogrammetric analysis to locate physical evidence that was no longer present during the site and vehicle or equipment inspections; (2) determining the motion that accounts for the physical evidence identified at the scene or damage identified on components, vehicles, or equipment involved in the crash; (3) applying principles of physics to interpret the physical evidence and add the quantitative elements to the reconstruction—speeds, times, and distances; (4) applying scientific principles to incorporate any electronic, video, audio, or testimonial evidence into the analysis;

(5) analyzing the pre-collision motion and scenarios under which drivers, riders, or pedestrians could have avoided a crash; and (6) evaluating factors that may have contributed to the crash.

1.1.3 Analysis by Phases

Reconstruction typically involves analyzing a crash in phases. For example, vehicle-to-vehicle collisions can be segmented into the pre-impact, impact, and post-impact phases. Single-vehicle rollover crashes can be segmented into the loss-of-control, trip, and roll phases. Single-vehicle motorcycle crashes can be segmented into the loss-of-control, impact, capsizing, and sliding phases. Pedestrian crashes can be segmented into the pre-impact, impact, airborne, and sliding or tumbling phases. For each of these crash types, the analysis of each phase will draw on different evidence and analysis techniques. In each of these instances, there will also be a human factors phase preceding the other phases of the crash. In this phase, a hazard (or some other stimulus) appears that may initiate a response by a driver, motorcycle rider, or pedestrian. Human factors may also be relevant to the other phases. Crash reconstruction often involves analyzing human factors—evaluating the driver or rider's perception, response, decision-making, and behavior. This analysis will lead the reconstructionist to an understanding of what the driver or rider's response was and if that response was typical, appropriate, or within the normal range of expected human driver responses.

1.1.4 Theoretical and Empirical Modeling

Crash reconstruction utilizes both theoretical and empirical modeling. As an example, the reconstruction of vehicle-pedestrian collisions has historically drawn on both theoretical models and empirical models [1]. On the theoretical side, researchers have developed projectile models describing the motion of pedestrians following a collision. Searle's models are, perhaps, the best known of these theoretical models [2, 3], but others have been derived by Aronberg [4], Eubanks [5], Han and Brach [6], and others. On the empirical side, several authors have generated equations relating vehicle impact speed to pedestrian throw distance by fitting curves to experimental data [7, 8]. This area of reconstruction benefits from empirical models because, as Toor notes, the theoretical models "are very difficult to apply to real world collisions, because the data necessary to solve the mathematical equations is only partly available from the real-world collisions." This difficulty largely arises from the complex interaction that can occur between the pedestrian and the striking vehicle. Theoretical projection models have continued to be successfully applied to various areas of reconstruction, though, including occupant ejection modeling for rollover crashes [9, 10] and motorcycle rider projection analysis. Beyond that, even for pedestrian crash reconstruction, the theoretical models are helpful for identifying which parameters are significant to a model and to a reconstruction, and thus which parameters should be considered in the empirical modeling or in setting up an experiment.

1.1.5 Uncertainty Analysis

Accident reconstruction calculations will often involve taking measurements or selecting reasonable inputs for a formula. For example, calculating a vehicle speed from skid marks will require the analyst to measure the length of the skid marks and to select a reasonable value, or range of values, for the coefficient of friction. The coefficient of friction could be selected based on test data in the literature, or testing could be conducted at a specific site. Either way, there will be uncertainty in the skid mark distance and the coefficient of friction. This uncertainty propagates to uncertainty in the calculated speed.

Various authors have discussed methods for quantifying the uncertainty in accident reconstruction calculations. Brach and Dunn [11], for instance, published a treatise covering analytical methods of uncertainty analysis in a forensic science setting. In a 1994 article, Brach covered some of the same techniques of uncertainty analysis specifically in a crash reconstruction context [12]. Several other treatments have appeared in the accident reconstruction literature, including Kost and Werner [13], Wood and O'Riordain [14], Tubergen [15], and Rose [16].

Between these sources, three methods of uncertainty analysis are often mentioned. First, a simple high-low approach can be used, where the analyst combines the high and low ends of the input ranges to produce the highest and lowest results from the formula. This approach yields an overestimate of the uncertainty since it is improbable that the actual values of the inputs would all fall at an extreme of the ranges simultaneously. Second, an analytical approach that utilize differential calculus can be utilized. This approach involves first taking partial derivatives of the formula with respect to each of the variables. Then, the uncertainty in the dependent variable can be calculated using the following formula [12]:

$$dy = \frac{\partial y}{\partial u} du + \frac{\partial y}{\partial v} dv + \ldots \tag{1.1}$$

In this equation,
dy is the uncertainty in the dependent variable y
du and dv are the uncertainties in the independent variables u and v

This equation can be extended to accommodate any number of independent variables. When calculating the uncertainty with this equation, the partial derivatives are evaluated at a nominal or reference set of values, typically the values at the middle of the range for each variable. This approach has been applied in an accident reconstruction setting—see Reference [17], for instance—but it can become cumbersome with many of the formulas employed by crash reconstructionists. One advantage of this approach, though, is that it allows for comparison of the relative contributions of uncertainty in each independent variable to the overall uncertainty in the dependent variable.

Third, reconstructionists have often employed a statistical technique called Monte Carlo analysis [16, 18]. Brach [12] referred to this technique as "a brute force randomized simulation on a computer of a mathematical model using appropriate statistical distributions for each of the variables." Kost and Werner [13] noted that, in Monte Carlo simulation, "appropriate probability distributions are assigned to the desired input parameters, and the analyses are repeatedly performed with values of the input parameters selected in accordance with the probability distributions. The results are expressed in the form of probability distributions of each of the desired output parameters, which then allows the analyst to determine the probability of the results falling within selected ranges." Wood and O'Riordain [14] noted that "Monte Carlo simulation methods are well established in many fields and are successfully used where non-linear relationships between variables occur. With the advent of higher computing speeds for microcomputers, it is now possible to carry out sizeable Monte Carlo simulations in realistic time scales." Several software packages for performing Monte Carlo simulation are commercially available.

Bartlett et al. [19] published a study quantifying the uncertainty in various measurements that are commonly used in crash reconstruction. Much of the data for their study was collected through measurements taken by participants at the World Reconstruction Exposition in 2000 (WREX2000) in College Station, Texas. As an example, this study included distance measurements utilizing a 25-foot carpenter's tape measure, a flexible measuring tape, and a roller wheel. Using the flexible measuring tape, two "short" measurements of 36.06 and 38.50 ft had standard deviations of 0.017 and 0.025 ft (0.2 and 0.3 in.). Two "long" measurements of 90.60 and 91.60 ft had standard deviations of 0.061 and 0.060 (0.73 and 0.72 in.). The distribution of measurements was found to be normal with a mean that coincided closely with the actual measurement. Using a single-wheel roller wheel, a "short" measurement had a standard deviation of 0.081 ft (0.97 in.) and a "long" measurement had a standard deviation of 0.116 ft (1.39 in.). Using a dual-wheel roller wheel, a "short" measurement had a standard deviation of 0.076 ft (0.91 in.) and a "long" measurement had a standard deviation of 0.160 ft (1.92 in.). This study also quantified uncertainties for measurements of the radius of an arced tire mark, for angle measurements, for frictional drag measurements, and for vehicle crush measurements.

In addition to the choice of methods for quantifying uncertainty, how a reconstructionist addresses uncertainty in their analysis will also be influenced by the context in which they are carrying out a reconstruction. In a civil litigation context, the criteria for the reconstruction will typically be what is most probable—perhaps stating conclusions on a more-probable-than-not basis or to a reasonable degree of certainty or probability. In a criminal context, on the other hand, the criteria for the reconstruction is an analysis that reaches conclusions beyond a reasonable doubt. In a civil litigation context, ranges on inputs can be considered, and the reconstructionist can state that the speed of the vehicle is within some range that represents reasonable consideration of the input uncertainties. The reconstructionist could state, for example: "The speed of the vehicle was between 52 and 62 mph." In a criminal context, on the other hand, the question may be something like, "Was the driver speeding?" If the range on speeds in this context was 52 to 62 mph and the speed limit was 55 mph, then the reconstructionist would not be able to say, beyond a reasonable doubt, that the driver was speeding since part of the range falls below the speed limit.

1.1.6 Incorporating Witness Statements and Testimony

Robins [20] and others have noted that witnesses often provide poor estimates of crash variables such as speed, time, and distances. However, that witness estimates are not always reliable is not grounds for dismissing or ignoring what a witness says. Witness testimony is not likely to be all right or all wrong. Witness statements provide information, some of which may be important, particularly related to the events leading up to a crash for which there may be no physical evidence. For those practicing crash reconstruction in a legal context, their role is often to bring physics and physical evidence into the conversation and to inform our clients or a jury what the physics and physical evidence say about how a crash occurred. In this regard, eyewitnesses and involved drivers sometimes make *testable statements*—a statement where the veracity of what they say can be tested against physics, physical evidence, or logic and reasoning. One valuable role a crash reconstructionist can play is to test statements from witnesses and involved drivers and to reach a conclusion about which of the stories is more consistent with scientific principles and physical evidence.

A few additional points are worth considering when a reconstructionist is evaluating witness statements. First, the reconstructionist should consider what first alerted a witness to something unusual and how much time the witness had to observe the events they are describing. As Robins has noted: "You cannot remember what you never consciously processed in the first place." If a witness's attention was drawn to a crash by the sound of collision itself, this witness may not have much first-hand knowledge about what occurred prior to the collision. When recounting the events, though, this witness may still talk about what happened prior to the collision, for as Robins has also observed, "witnesses are exposed to a variety of postimpact sources of information which are for the most part uncontrolled. Witnesses may be questioned by police and other investigators, they may talk with and share information with other participants and witnesses, they may be exposed to a variety of reports of the original events provided by radio, television, and print media." Second, a witness who is driving will be allocating at least part of their attention to their own driving. This will distract from their focus from the events related to a crash. Third, a witness's position and vantage point will also influence what they can see and when they see it. Accident reconstructionists can often evaluate the vantage point of a witness and determine based on geometric considerations if there is any reason to doubt their description.

Loftus [21] notes that there are three stages that an eyewitness progresses through in giving a description of the event they witnessed—acquisition, retention, and retrieval. The acquisition phase is the witness's original perception of the event during which information is stored in memory. The retention phase is the period between the event and the eventual recollection and recounting of information about that event. The retrieval phase is the witness's actual recalling and recounting of information about the event. The level of accuracy present in a witness statement depends on factors that play out in each of these phases, factors related to the event itself and factors related to the witness. For instance, according to Loftus, the following factors *related to the event* influence the success of the **acquisition** stage: (1) the duration of the event ("…the less time a witness has to look at something, the less accurate the perception…an eyewitness should be better able to recall an event when the event transpired and was observed over a longer period of time" (p. 23).), (2) the number of times the event occurs, (3) the detail salience ("Some things just catch our attention more readily than others" (p. 25).), and (4) the type of fact being acquired ("Is the witness being asked to remember the height or weight of a criminal, the amount of time an incident lasted, the speed of a car before an accident, the details of a conversation, or the color of the traffic signal? These different types of facts are not equally easy to perceive and recall" (p. 27).). Similarly, the following factors *related to the witness* can influence the success of the **acquisition** stage: (1) stress, (2) expectations, (3) distraction, and (4) what the witness knows before the event.

An older article by Loftus and Palmer [22] raised an additional concern. They conducted two experiments in which the test subjects watched films of automobile accidents and then answered questions related to these accidents. For example, some subjects were asked "About how fast were the cars going when they *smashed* into each other?" This question resulted in higher estimates of speed from test subjects than the estimates from subjects that were asked the same question using the words *collided, bumped, contacted,* or *hit*, rather than *smashed*. Even on a retest, a week later, those who were originally asked this question with the word *smashed* were more likely to say they had seen broken glass, even though the film did not depict any glass breaking. Loftus and Palmer observe that "these results are consistent with the view that the questions asked subsequent to an event can cause a reconstruction in one's memory of that event."

1.1.7 Causation

Fricke [23] observed that "reconstruction does not try to explain why a collision happened. That would require describing the entire combination of conditions that would produce another collision." Harris [24], on the other hand, stated that "the ultimate goal of a traffic accident investigation or reconstruction is to determine the events of the accident or what caused the accident." Fricke states elsewhere that "a *cause* is whatever is required to produce a *result*," and so his point seems to be that describing the *entire* set of factors that make up the cause of a crash is beyond the scope of most crash reconstructions. Harris agrees, observing that "determining all the factors that were present in any single accident would be a monumental undertaking…there are simply too many variables, factors, modifiers and circumstances present that may have disappeared long before the investigator becomes involved. Other circumstances may simply never be revealed, or realized, by the parties involved."

Still, though, many reconstructionists and those that hire them would not consider their work complete until they had at least examined the actions of the involved drivers to determine how those actions contributed to the crash. In many instances, the reconstructionist will also evaluate factors related to the involved vehicles and the environment [25]. Along these lines, Harris argues that "cause in law is different from cause in the rest of the world. In the eyes of the courts, cause is an issue of policy and not an instrument of factual analysis. The issue for the court is whether, as a policy decision, a defendant should be held liable for a plaintiff's injuries and the resolution of that issue in an accident case depends on whether the crash was a reasonably foreseeable result of the defendant's negligence…the essential test for proximate cause under the law is the accident must be the natural and probable result of the negligent act or omission and be of such a character as an ordinarily prudent person ought to have foreseen as likely to occur as a result of negligence…This definition makes the work of the reconstructionist easier in that not all the factors present in an accident may be sufficiently relevant to the cause for consideration. Mere presence is insufficient, it must have in some significant way contributed to the result…With a good understanding of the relationships of accident factors, circumstances and modifiers, and sufficient data, an accident can be analyzed, causation determined and the conclusions effectively presented."

Harris goes on to note that, when accident reconstruction is practiced in a legal setting, "the work of the reconstructionist is preliminary to the analysis performed by the jury. The jury is bound to consider the evidence and will consider the quality and completeness of the investigator's presentation in coming to a conclusion." Thus, the reconstructionist's role in a legal setting is to inform the jury as they make their determination about the degree to which a defendant will be held responsible for a plaintiff's injuries. This may involve the reconstructionist testifying about factors they have identified which contributed to or caused a crash.

Within the context of crash reconstruction, epidemiological studies are useful in illuminating factors that have contributed to crashes in the past, and thus may have contributed to a crash under consideration. However, these studies cannot reveal which factors *actually* contributed to any particular crash. Determining which factors contributed to a particular crash will involve evaluating the evidence and facts specific to that crash. For example, epidemiological studies related to motorcycle crashes have demonstrated that, after being involved in a crash with a motorcycle, passenger car drivers sometimes report not having "seen" the motorcycle. Researchers have identified many factors that could contribute to the motorcycle not being seen—the small and narrow profile of motorcycles, the passenger car driver not expecting to see a motorcyclist, the motorcycle being occluded by other traffic or some geometric feature of the site, a lack of lighting to make the motorcycle detectable, or a lack of contrast between the rider and surrounding environment, for instance. Researchers have also proposed modifications to design features of motorcycles and the operator's clothing to increase the probability of passenger car drivers recognizing the presence of motorcyclists.

For a particular crash, though, it must be determined through reconstruction what specific factors contributed to the crash. The reconstructionist will need to evaluate the evidence, perform testing, or engage in some other scientific process to determine if a common explanation for many crashes happens to also be the correct explanation for a specific crash. It is possible that none of the common factors contributed to a crash and that the physical evidence will show that the driver did see the motorcyclist (there may be pre-impact skid marks, for instance, even though the driver reported not having seen the motorcyclist). It is also possible that some common factors were present, but that the actual cause was an inattentive or distracted driver. The principle here is that a reconstructionist's conclusions related to any crash should be driven by the evidence and facts related to that case, not by the findings of epidemiological studies.

A study conducted by the Association of European Motorcycle Manufacturers (ACEM) and referred to as the Motorcycle Accidents in Depth Study (MAIDS) examined the causes of motorcycle accidents in five European countries (France, Germany, Netherlands, Spain, and Italy) [26]. This study utilized a well-defined methodology for evaluating accident causation for specific motorcycle accidents, which included classifying each potential contributing factor into one of the following categories:

1. The factor was present, but did not contribute.
2. The factor was the precipitating event that initiated the accident sequence.
3. The factor was the primary contributing factor in causing the accident.
4. The factor was a contributing factor that was present in addition to other contributing factors.
5. The factor was not present.

The MAIDS report notes that "the last portion of the investigative process was to determine the contribution of a given factor (e.g., human, vehicle or environmental factor) in the causation of the accident. Typically, this was done at a team meeting, where all the investigative specialists were able to provide input on the accident's causation." The MAIDS researchers defined the following categories of *human* factors:

a. <u>Perception Failure</u>: One of the drivers failed to detect a dangerous condition.
b. <u>Comprehension Failure</u>: One of the drivers detected a condition but failed to comprehend the danger associated with that condition.
c. <u>Decision Failure</u>: The dangerous condition was detected and comprehended, but a driver or motorcycle operator failed to make the correct decision to avoid the dangerous condition.

These researchers also included a category for "reaction failure," which they defined as a driver or motorcycle operator "failed to react to the dangerous condition, resulting in a continuation or faulty collision avoidance." This seems closely related and potentially indistinguishable from the comprehension and decision failure categories. Any of these four types of human factors could be also be an indication of an <u>attention failure</u>, which was defined as "any activity of the vehicle operator that distracted him or her from the normal operation of the vehicle…including the normal observation of traffic both in front of and behind the vehicle operator." These researchers further noted that "a proper assessment of the presence of an attention failure depends upon the interview skills of the investigator, since in most cases, the rider or…driver must admit to being distracted…." The MAIDS researchers also mentioned other human failure types, including traffic-scan errors and failing to account for visual obstructions. The MAIDS researchers defined the following categories of *environmental factors*: roadway design or maintenance defects, traffic hazards present from maintenance or construction, and weather. They also noted that *vehicle* component failures could contribute to the occurrence of an accident.

1.1.8 Analyzing Avoidance Scenarios

As a related issue to causation, a reconstruction often culminates in an evaluation of how a crash could have been avoided. In conducting this analysis, several principles should be considered. First, the reconstructionist will need to demonstrate that any proposed alternative course of action was feasible for a typical driver in the subject scenario. This will often involve evaluating a reasonable range of perception-response times for a driver, rider, or pedestrian, determining what level of deceleration the driver or rider could reasonably produce with braking, or what lateral acceleration level the driver or rider could produce with swerving. Second, to ensure that they are imposing reasonable expectations on a driver or rider, the reconstructionist will need to consider human variability.

As Olson [27] has observed: "There are great differences in raw ability from one individual to the next, and great differences in how a given individual will respond to an identical situation on different occasions. Human variability is a recognized fact that is, sadly, often ignored by crash investigators when offering opinions concerning the performance of a particular individual…it is important to remember that the average is but a single point in a distribution. The average tells us nothing about the scatter in performance, the shape of the distribution, or how that distribution relates to other distributions that may be of interest. In addition, the average is of virtually no help in predicting what can be expected from one randomly-selected individual… Reconstructionists are generally interested in assessing the performance of a given individual, who is drawn from an unknown part of the distribution of interest. In such cases the average is virtually useless as a guide and may be seriously misleading…An individual interested in offering an opinion concerning the reasonableness of a person's behavior must compare what is known of that person's behavior with the range of 'reasonable' behavior for the dimension of concern [perception-response time, for instance]." Thus, in evaluating a driver's or motorcyclist's ability to avoid a collision, the reconstructionist should not simply assume a 50th-percentile perception-response time for the driver or motorcyclist. This amounts to expecting the driver or operator to be faster than 50% of the population. It would be more reasonable to assume an 85th-percentile perception-response time or some other percentile that effectively considers the variability of the larger group of people.

Another issue in evaluating a driver or operator's ability to avoid a collision is that the reconstructionist will need to decide where in space and time to invoke a hypothetical change in driver behavior, essentially drawing a control volume around the scenario to mark out the relevant time frame or area. For example, consider an intersection collision where a vehicle accelerates away from a stop sign and is struck by an oncoming motorcycle traveling through the intersection at a 90° angle to the left turning vehicle. Even if the oncoming motorcycle had the right-of-way through the intersection, there may still be questions of how the speed of that motorcycle contributed to the occurrence of the crash.

In running a hypothetical scenario where the speed of the oncoming motorcycle is different than what it was in the real crash, one option is to invoke that change at the time the other vehicle begins to pull away from the stop sign or stop bar. Another option would be to invoke the change at the time the driver of the turning vehicle begins making their decision to turn. This decision-making process is described in References [28] and [29]. Some scenarios will not have a clear physical event that can define the control volume, and the reconstructionist will need to give careful thought to how to define the scenario and how the boundaries of the control volume will influence the outcome of the scenario.

1.2 Physical Principles Used in Accident Reconstruction

1.2.1 Conservation of Energy

One physical principle that is used frequently in accident reconstruction is *conservation of energy* [30]. Application of this principle to determine the initial speed of a car or motorcycle in a single-vehicle crash involves identifying the mechanisms by which the vehicle's initial kinetic energy was dissipated, quantifying how much kinetic energy was dissipated by each mechanism, and then adding those dissipated energies up to arrive at an estimate of the vehicle's initial kinetic energy. The initial speed of the vehicle can then be calculated from this initial kinetic energy. Conceptually, this process can be illustrated with Equation (1.2). In this equation, the initial kinetic energy of the vehicle is determined by adding up the energy dissipated by various mechanisms. These mechanisms could include crushing of the structure of the car or motorcycle or frictional-type energy losses that occur during braking, yawing, sliding, tripping, or tumbling and rolling:

$$KE_{initial} = \Delta E_{crushing} + \Delta E_{braking} + \Delta E_{yawing} + \Delta E_{sliding} + \Delta E_{tripping} + \Delta E_{rolling} \tag{1.2}$$

For analysis of the impact phase of a two-vehicle collision, the energies of the two vehicles need to be considered together, as illustrated in Equation (1.3). This equation indicates that the total kinetic energy that the two vehicles bring to the collision is equal to the energy dissipated by crushing of the vehicle structures plus the total kinetic energy of the two vehicles following the collision. These kinetic energies can include both translational and rotational motion. The post-collision kinetic energies for each vehicle would be calculated with an expression like Equation (1.2):

$$KE_{initial,1} + KE_{initial,2} = \Delta E_{crushing,1} + \Delta E_{crushing,1} + KE_{final,1} + KE_{final,2} \tag{1.3}$$

1.2.2 Newton's Second Law and the Principle of Work and Energy

The process of determining how much energy was dissipated by each mechanism typically utilizes the *principle of work and energy* [31], which equates a change in kinetic energy to the work performed by the force that accomplishes the change in kinetic energy. *Work* is defined as the action of a force through a distance. This principle can be derived from *Newton's second law*, another physical principle utilized by accident reconstructionists. Newton's second law is given by Equation (1.4). It states that a body will be accelerated in proportion to the sum of the forces applied to the body. The acceleration will occur along the line of action of the vector sum of the forces and the mass of the body, m, acts as the proportionality constant:

$$\sum \vec{F} = m\vec{a} \tag{1.4}$$

As a side note, Newton's second law is also one of the underlying physical principles utilized in crash simulation packages, such as PC-Crash and HVE. If one can determine the forces applied to a vehicle at any instant in time, then one can calculate the acceleration the vehicle is experiencing. Thus, reconstructionists have developed models to calculate instantaneous tire forces, suspension forces, and collision forces.

The *principle of work and energy* can be derived from Newton's second law, by first considering Equation (1.4) along one coordinate axis, as follows:

$$F_i = ma_i \tag{1.5}$$

In this equation, i designates the coordinate direction being considered—x, y, or z in a Cartesian coordinate system. Since acceleration is equal to a differential change in velocity (dv_i) over a differential change in time (dt) and velocity is equal to a differential change in position (ds_i) over a differential change in time, Equation (1.4) can be rewritten as follows:

$$F_i = m\frac{dv_i}{dt} = m\frac{dv_i}{ds_i}\frac{ds_i}{dt} = mv_i\frac{dv_i}{ds_i} \tag{1.6}$$

Equation (1.6) can be rewritten as follows:

$$F_i ds_i = mv_i dv_i \tag{1.7}$$

Equation (1.7) can be integrated along the coordinate direction i along a distance from Point 1 to Point 2, as follows:

$$\int_1^2 F_i ds_i = \int_1^2 mv_i dv_i = \frac{1}{2}m\left(v_{i,2}^2 - v_{i,1}^2\right) \tag{1.8}$$

The left side of Equation (1.8) is the work performed by the force acting through the distance from 1 to 2 and the right side is the change in kinetic energy experienced by the body. This means that the ΔE terms in Equations (1.2) and (1.3) will take the form of forces acting through a distance. For example, for a frictional-type energy loss, the change in energy will be calculated as follows:

$$\Delta E_{frictional} = \mu W d \tag{1.9}$$

In this equation,
    μ is the coefficient of friction
    W is the vehicle weight

The coefficient of friction multiplied by the weight is the frictional force that act through the distance, d.

FIGURE 1.1 Video frame from motorcycle-to-car crash test conducted at WREX2016.

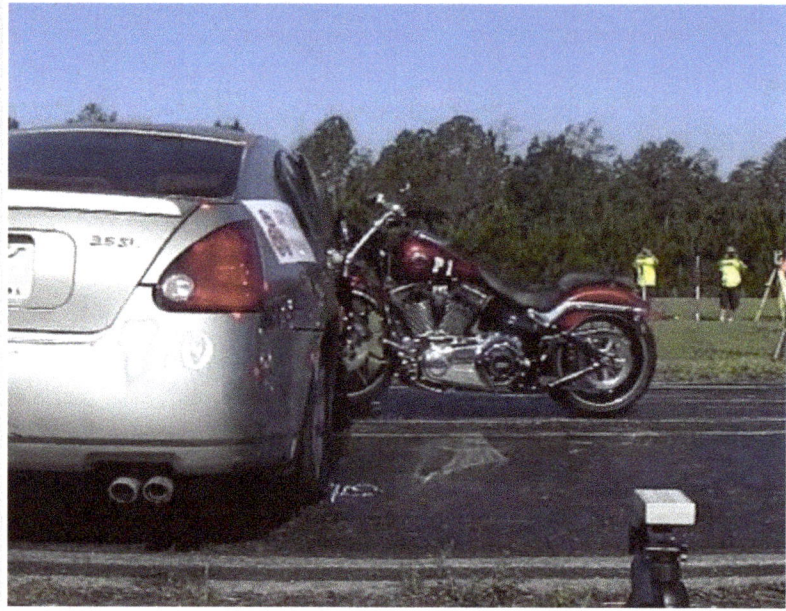

Another example is the work done in compressing a spring, an analogy that is used by crash reconstructionists to model the crushing behavior of vehicle structures. The energy expended in compressing a spring from its undeformed position through a distance, Δx, is given by the following equation:

$$E_{spring} = k \cdot \Delta x^2 \qquad (1.10)$$

Figure 1.1 contains a frame of video from a motorcycle-to-vehicle collision conducted at the World Reconstruction Exposition (WREX) in 2016. This frame shows the motorcycle impacting the side of the passenger car and the motorcycle forks and front wheel deforming, along with the side of the passenger car. The deformation to both vehicles in this collision could be modeled with the spring analogy.

FIGURE 1.2 Absorbed, restored, and dissipated energies.

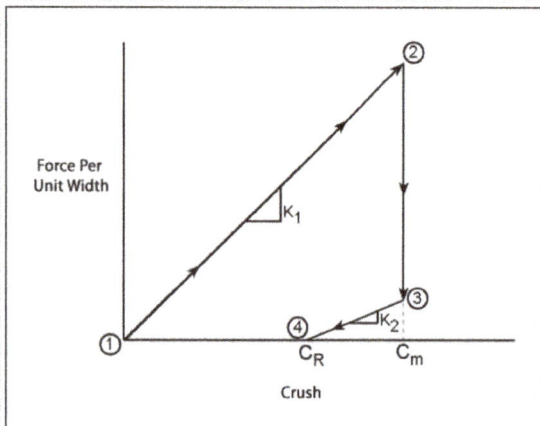

In this collision, the motorcycle impacted the car with an initial velocity, V_A, and thus with an initial kinetic energy. All or most of this kinetic energy is absorbed through the crushing of the motorcycle and vehicle structures. During the first phase of the impact—the approach or compression phase—the deformations of both the car and the motorcycle reach a maximum level. Figure 1.2 depicts an idealized force-crush curve that could be used to model the force that builds up as each vehicle deforms [32]. This idealized force-crush curve begins where there is no crush and no force. The curve ascends in a linear fashion (constant stiffness, K_1) to the maximum dynamic force, which is achieved coincident with the maximum dynamic crush (C_m). Per Newton's third law, the collision force applied to first vehicle will be equal in magnitude to the collision force applied to the other vehicle, although each vehicle will likely have a unique stiffness, and thus the collision partners will experience different levels of crush.

The absorbed energy (E_A) for each vehicle is equal to the area under the portion of the force-crush curve from Points 1 to 2.

After the approach phase is complete, the impact force drops quickly as the structure of each vehicle experiences a partial rebound from the maximum crush (Points 2 to 3). This structural rebound has the effect of imparting a velocity to each vehicle that leads to separation. Some kinetic energy is restored to each vehicle. When the vehicles separate, the collision force drops to zero and the vehicle structures finish their rebound, settling in on the final residual crush (C_R) from Points 3 to 4 (wheelbase reduction and wheel deformation for the motorcycle). The phase during which the vehicles rebound from the collision and experience partial structural restoration is referred to as the *restitution or rebound phase* of the collision. Again, this is assumed to occur with a constant stiffness (K_2) for each vehicle. The energy imparted to the vehicle during the restitution phase is referred to as the restored energy, E_R. This energy is the area under the line from Points 3 to 4.

The coefficient of restitution for the impact characterizes this restoration of energy and can be calculated with the following equation:

$$\varepsilon = \sqrt{\frac{E_R}{E_A}} \tag{1.11}$$

In addition to the absorbed and restored energies, the idealized force-crush curve of Figure 1.2 can be used to illustrate an additional energy value—the dissipated energy (energy loss). This is the difference between the absorbed and restored energies, or the area between the line for the approach phase and the line for the rebound phase.

Crash reconstructionists have developed methods for calculating the energies delineated in Figure 1.2. These methods typically utilize measurement of the post-crash crush to each of the vehicles along with application of stiffness characteristics of those vehicles determined from crash tests. These together enable the reconstructionists to calculate both the collision force and the absorbed energy. Equation (1.12) can then be used to calculate the relative speed of impact between the vehicles, along the line of action of the collision force. In this equation, $E_{A,total}$ is the total absorbed energy for the two vehicles involved in the collision and γ_1 and γ_2 are the effective mass multipliers, which account for collision forces that do not pass through the center of mass of the vehicles (non-central collisions) [33, 34, 35]:

$$V_A = (1+\varepsilon) \cdot \sqrt{\frac{\gamma_1 m_1 + \gamma_2 m_2}{\gamma_1 m_1 \cdot \gamma_2 m_2} \cdot 2 E_{A,total}} \tag{1.12}$$

The effective mass multipliers are defined as follows, where k_i is the radius of gyration of the vehicle under consideration and h_i is the moment arm of the collision force about the center of gravity of the vehicle under consideration:

$$\gamma_i = \frac{k_i^2}{k_i^2 + h_i^2} \tag{1.13}$$

McHenry developed a method for quantifying the absorbed energy based on vehicle crush and implemented it in a software package called CRASH computer program (Computer Reconstruction of Automobile Speeds on the Highway) [36]. The CRASH program was created in conjunction with the SMAC program

FIGURE 1.3 Linear force-crush characteristics used in CRASH.

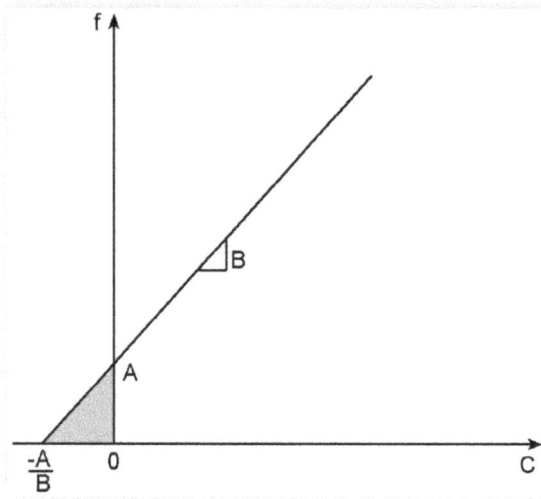

(Simulation Model of Automobile Collisions), an accident simulation program that required the user to input an estimate of the initial speeds of the vehicles and then to iteratively change those speeds to achieve a match with physical evidence. The CRASH program was originally intended to be a pre-processor for SMAC, providing initial estimates of the vehicle impact speeds for use with the SMAC program. However, the CRASH program has often been used within the field of accident reconstruction as a stand-alone method.

The CRASH method assumed that the crushing vehicle structure could be represented as a series of springs, each with a linear force-crush relationship. McHenry represented the stiffness properties for these linear springs by the two parameters, A and B. The graphic of Figure 1.3 depicts how the A and B values define the linear force-crush relationship in CRASH. The horizontal axis in the figure represents the residual crush depth, and the vertical axis represents the force per unit width of damage. The B value, the slope of the linear force-crush relationship, governs the proportionality between residual crush and impact force. The A value, the force intercept on the force-crush plot, represents the force that can be applied to the vehicle structure before the onset of permanent crush.

The force-crush line intersects the crush axis at a value of $-A/B$. This negative intercept on the crush axis has traditionally been interpreted as the elastic recovery of the vehicle structure, which is the difference between the dynamic crush and the residual crush. With this interpretation, the A value rises because of the use of residual crush in the model and shifting the force-residual crush line over a distance of A/B would yield the dynamic force-crush line. This interpretation of the A value is sound, if the difference between the dynamic maximum crush and the residual maximum crush is constant and independent of the severity of the impact.

Equation (1.14) describes the force-crush curve of Figure 1.3:

$$f = A + BC_R \tag{1.14}$$

Using Equation (1.14) to describe the force, McHenry integrated over the crush depth and damage width to determine the deformation energy and obtained the following equation:

$$E_A = \left(\frac{B}{2}C_R^2 + AC_R + \frac{A^2}{2B} \right) \cdot w_0 \tag{1.15}$$

While, in general, a crush profile will not have a constant crush depth, a general crush profile can be represented by an equivalent damage width and average crush depth value. Woolley has discussed methods for calculating a representative damage width and crush depth for a general crush profile [37].

CRASH originally included default stiffness values for six vehicle categories, delineated by wheelbase. Within each vehicle category, CRASH contained stiffness parameters for the front, rear, and side structures. These default stiffness values have been updated several times through the years, and government-sponsored crash research still utilizes them. However, in general, there is no reason why vehicles with similar wheelbases would necessarily exhibit similar crush stiffness. Thus, on any single case, the use of the CRASH default stiffness parameters can introduce significant error. For this reason, most commercially available CRASH-derivative programs allow the user to enter vehicle-specific stiffness data.

A method for obtaining the A and B stiffness coefficients for CRASH can be developed by recognizing that Equation (1.15) is quadratic in the residual crush depth, C_R. Application of the quadratic formula to Equation (1.15) yields the following equation:

$$\sqrt{\frac{2E_A}{w_0}} = \sqrt{B}C_R + \frac{A}{\sqrt{B}} \tag{1.16}$$

The left side of Equation (1.16) is a normalized energy term, which has been referred to as the Energy of Approach Factor (EAF). For a barrier impact, the damage energy in Equation (1.16) would be set equal to the initial kinetic energy of the vehicle. For other impact types, say a vehicle-to-vehicle frontal impact, the damage energy in Equation (1.16) would be set equal to the damage energy absorbed by the vehicle of interest during the impact. Each crash test will provide one point for constructing an EAF versus residual crush plot. With multiple points, a line can be fit to the data. The slope and the intercept of this line will yield the A and B coefficients.

When residual crush measurements are taken perpendicular to the original shape of the impacted vehicle side, the damage energy that results from Equation (1.15) will only include the work done by the component of the collision force that acted normal to the vehicle side. In many cases, the collision force will not have acted perpendicular to one of the vehicle sides and, therefore, crush measured perpendicular to the original vehicle surface will not represent the crush along the actual collision force direction. The absorbed damage energy, thus, may need to be adjusted to include the work done by the component of the collision force that acted tangential to the vehicle surface.

One approach for adjusting the damage energy is to adjust the residual crush depth so that it represents the distance the structure was displaced along the direction of the collision force. This approach is used in CRASH3, and it results in the calculated damage energy being multiplied by the following multiplier:

$$1 + \tan^2 \alpha \tag{1.17}$$

In Equation (1.17), α is the angle between the normal to the vehicle side and the actual direction of the collision force. Fonda [39] and Woolley [38] proposed that the width of the damaged region should also be adjusted to reflect the direction of the collision force. When both the crush depth and the crush width are adjusted, the crush energy of Equation (1.15) would be adjusted using the following multiplier:

$$\frac{1}{\cos \alpha} \tag{1.18}$$

1.2.3 Principle of Impulse and Momentum (Conservation of Momentum)

In addition to the principle of work and energy, crash reconstructionists also utilize the *principle of impulse and momentum*, which can be utilized to relate the initial (immediately prior to the collision) and final (immediately after separation) velocities. Brach's

FIGURE 1.4   Two-dimensional particle impact model.

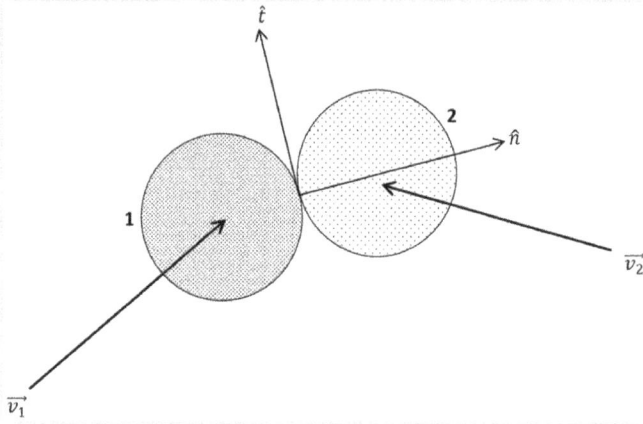

book *Mechanical Impact Dynamics* contains a thorough treatment of the application of the principle of impulse and momentum to collision analysis [40]. The application of this principle will be illustrated here with the two-dimensional (planar) particle impact model of Figure 1.4. This figure depicts two particles colliding, with velocities $\vec{v_1}$ and $\vec{v_2}$. A normal axis and a tangential axis are depicted, and the velocities of the particles are assumed to lie entirely in the plane defined by these axes. The force generated by deformation occurs on the normal axis, and frictional-type forces occur along the tangential axis. Often, when a particle impact model is introduced, collision forces along the tangential axis are assumed negligible, but that assumption is not invoked here. The following assumptions will be invoked: (1) the duration of contact is assumed short enough to be approximated as instantaneous (this equates to no change in position or orientation of the particles during the collision); (2) the deforming region is assumed to be small relative to the size of the particle; (3) angular velocities are assumed negligible, both before and after the collision; and (4) the collision force is the only force considered. External forces are assumed negligible (for vehicle collisions, this would be tire and aerodynamic forces).

According to the principle of impulse and momentum:

$$P_n = m_1\left(v_{1n,f} - v_{1n,i}\right) = -m_2\left(v_{2n,f} - v_{2n,i}\right) \tag{1.19}$$

$$P_t = m_1\left(v_{1t,f} - v_{1t,i}\right) = -m_2\left(v_{2t,f} - v_{2t,i}\right) \tag{1.20}$$

In these equations,

   P_t is the tangential impulse
   P_n is the normal impulse
   $v_{1n,i}$ is the normal-direction velocity of particle 1 immediately prior to
      the collision
   $v_{1n,f}$ is the normal-direction velocity of particle 1 immediately following
      the collisions

The normal velocities for particle 2 and the tangential velocities for particles 1 and 2 are identified with similar subscripts. Equations (1.19) and (1.20) are statements of *conservation of momentum* along each coordinate axis and they provide two equations for relating the initial and final velocities. Two additional equations are needed.

One equation is provided by the coefficient of restitution (ε), which relates the initial and final relative velocities of the particles along the normal axis and thus controls the energy loss along the normal axis, as follows:

$$\varepsilon = -\frac{v_{2n,f} - v_{1n,f}}{v_{2n,i} - v_{1n,i}} \tag{1.21}$$

The coefficient of restitution will typically fall between 0 and 1, though there are instances in which a negative coefficient of restitution makes physical sense. For instance,

Brach mentions the example of an "errant baseball passing through a window screen." In the context of vehicular crash reconstruction, a similar situation could occur if a corner-to-corner collision occurs between two vehicles and the structures give way before a common velocity can be reached normal to the contact surface. Coefficients of restitution for a given collision type can be determined either experimentally or analytically. Both approaches have been used by crash reconstructionists. Another additional equation is provided by the impulse ratio (μ), which describes the ratio of the tangential to normal impulses generated by this collision and controls the energy loss along the tangential axis, as follows:

$$\mu = \frac{P_t}{P_n} \tag{1.22}$$

In some instances, the impulse ratio can be interpreted as a friction coefficient between the colliding objects, but it is not limited to this interpretation [40, 41, 42, 43, 44]. In addition to the effects of friction, the impulse ratio can also include the effects of forces generated by snagging between the vehicles. The "available friction" can be set at a value that reflects such snagging or furrowing when it occurs. Brach observes that "for an oblique impact when the particles have a nonzero initial relative tangential velocity component, sliding must always occur, at least during initial stages of contact. A question that must be answered is if relative tangential motion continues through separation or ceases prior to separation. Although the laws of Coulomb friction do not apply during all impacts, the concept and mathematical form of a coefficient of friction prove to be very convenient." Brach also notes that "the tangential force and its impulse usually are found to be dissipative, such as from friction or plastic deformation, and cannot add energy to the system. For a particle, the tangential impulse always opposes initial relative tangential motion." This implies that the sign of μ can be either positive or negative and is determined with the following equation:

$$\operatorname{sgn}(\mu) = \operatorname{sgn}\left(\frac{v_{2t,i} - v_{1t,i}}{v_{2n,i} - v_{1n,i}}\right) \tag{1.23}$$

Brach also derived the following expression for the critical impulse ratio, which is the impulse ratio necessary to cause sliding to cease during the collision. The impulse ratio should not be set at a value that exceeds the critical impulse ratio:

$$\mu_c = \frac{1}{1+\varepsilon} \cdot \frac{v_{2t,i} - v_{1t,i}}{v_{2n,i} - v_{1n,i}} \tag{1.24}$$

The relative magnitude of the available friction coefficient to the critical impulse ratio will have physical significance for an impact. The available friction coefficient represents the magnitude of friction force that <u>can</u> be recruited during the impact. The critical impulse ratio represents the magnitude of friction force that <u>must</u> be recruited for relative motion to cease along the contact surface. When the critical impulse ratio is greater than the available friction coefficient, all the available friction will be recruited during the impact, but that friction will be insufficient to cause sliding to cease in the contact region. When the available friction coefficient exceeds the critical impulse ratio, only a portion of the available friction will be recruited and sliding will cease in the contact region. In such cases, the value of the impulse ratio for the impact model should be set at the value of the critical impulse ratio, not the available friction coefficient.

This is because recruitment of the available friction depends on relative velocity being present along the contact surface. Once this relative motion ceases, no additional friction can be recruited.

Brach continues, "in specific applications the appropriate value of μ must be determined experimentally or estimated by means such as analytical modeling of the mechanism of tangential force generation. If Coulomb friction is appropriate, then μ is related to the coefficient of dynamic friction. Otherwise, it can be considered to be an equivalent coefficient of friction." Brach demonstrates that Equations (1.19), (1.20), (1.21), and (1.22) can be solved for the final velocity components, which results in the following set of equations relating the initial velocities to the final velocities:

$$v_{1n,f} = v_{1n,i} + (1+\varepsilon)\frac{m_2}{m_1+m_2}(v_{2n,i} - v_{1n,i}) \tag{1.25}$$

$$v_{2n,f} = v_{2n,i} - (1+\varepsilon)\frac{m_1}{m_1+m_2}(v_{2n,i} - v_{1n,i}) \tag{1.26}$$

$$v_{1t,f} = v_{1t,i} + \mu(1+\varepsilon)\frac{m_2}{m_1+m_2}(v_{2n,i} - v_{1n,i}) \tag{1.27}$$

$$v_{2t,f} = v_{2t,i} - \mu(1+\varepsilon)\frac{m_1}{m_1+m_2}(v_{2n,i} - v_{1n,i}) \tag{1.28}$$

Brach [40, 43] has developed an impulse-momentum impact model applicable to rigid body collisions and incorporating changes in angular velocity. The purpose of this chapter is to give an overview of the physical principles that crash reconstructionists utilize, and so, that full model will not be covered here. The reader is referred to Brach's books for that treatment.

References

1. Toor, A. and Araszewski, M., "Theoretical vs. Empirical Solutions for Vehicle/Pedestrian Collisions," SAE Technical Paper 2003-01-0883, 2003, doi:10.4271/2003-01-0883.

2. Searle, J. and Searle, A., "The Trajectories of Pedestrians, Motorcycles, Motorcyclists, etc., Following a Road Accident," SAE Technical Paper 831622, 1983, doi:10.4271/831622.

3. Searle, J., "The Physics of Throw Distance in Accident Reconstruction," SAE Technical Paper 930659, 1993, doi:10.4271/930659.

4. Aronberg, R., "Airborne Trajectory Analysis Derivation for Use in Accident Reconstruction," SAE Technical Paper 900367, 1990, doi:10.4271/900367.

5. Eubanks, J.J. and Hill, P.F., *Pedestrian Accident Reconstruction*, 2nd ed., (Tucson, AZ: Lawyers & Judges Publishing Company, 1999), ISBN:0-913875-56-2.

6. Han, I. and Brach, R., "Throw Model for Frontal Pedestrian Collisions," SAE Technical Paper 2001-01-0898, 2001, doi:10.4271/2001-01-0898.

7. Happer, A., Araszewski, M., Toor, A., Overgaard, R. et al., "Comprehensive Analysis Method for Vehicle/Pedestrian Collisions," SAE Technical Paper 2000-01-0846, 2000, doi:10.4271/2000-01-0846.

8. Toor, A., Araszewski, M., Johal, R., Overgaard, R. et al., "Revision and Validation of Vehicle/Pedestrian Collision Analysis Method," SAE Technical Paper 2002-01-0550, 2002, doi:10.4271/2002-01-0550.

9. Funk, J. and Luepke, P., "Trajectory Model of Occupants Ejected in Rollover Crashes," SAE Technical Paper 2007-01-0742, 2007, doi:10.4271/2007-01-0742.

10. Funk, J., Beauchamp, G., Rose, N., Fenton, S. et al., "Occupant Ejection Trajectories in Rollover Crashes: Full-Scale Testing and Real-World Cases," *SAE Int. J. Passeng. Cars - Mech. Syst.* 1, no. 1 (2009): 43-54, doi:10.4271/2008-01-0166.

11. Brach, R.M. and Dunn, P.F., *Uncertainty Analysis for Forensic Science*, (Tucson, AZ: Lawyers and Judges Publishing Company, 2004), ISBN:1-930056-20-6.

12. Brach, R., "Uncertainty in Accident Reconstruction Calculations," SAE Technical Paper 940722, 1994, doi:10.4271/940722.

13. Kost, G. and Werner, S., "Use of Monte Carlo Simulation Techniques in Accident Reconstruction," SAE Technical Paper 940719, 1994, doi:10.4271/940719.

14. Wood, D. and O'Riordain, S., "Monte Carlo Simulation Methods Applied to Accident Reconstruction and Avoidance Analysis," SAE Technical Paper 940720, 1994, doi:10.4271/940720.

15. Tubergen, R., "The Technique of Uncertainty Analysis as Applied to the Momentum Equation for Accident Reconstruction," SAE Technical Paper 950135, 1995, doi:10.4271/950135.

16. Rose, N., Fenton, S., and Hughes, C., "Integrating Monte Carlo Simulation, Momentum-Based Impact Modeling, and Restitution Data to Analyze Crash Severity," SAE Technical Paper 2001-01-3347, 2001, doi:10.4271/2001-01-3347.

17. Rose, N., Beauchamp, G., and Bortles, W., "Quantifying the Uncertainty in the Coefficient of Restitution Obtained with Accelerometer Data from a Crash Test," SAE Technical Paper 2007-01-0730, 2007, doi:10.4271/2007-01-0730.

18. Wach, W. and Unarski, J., "Uncertainty Analysis of the Preimpact Phase of a Pedestrian Collision," SAE Technical Paper 2007-01-0715, 2007, doi:10.4271/2007-01-0715.

19. Bartlett, W., Wright, W., Masory, O., Brach, R. et al., "Evaluating the Uncertainty in Various Measurement Tasks Common to Accident Reconstruction," SAE Technical Paper 2002-01-0546, 2002, doi:10.4271/2002-01-0546.

20. Robins, P.J., *Eyewitness Reliability in Motor Vehicle Accident Reconstruction and Litigation*, (Tucson, AZ: Lawyers and Judges Publishing Company, 2001), ISBN:0-913875-92-9.

21. Loftus, E.F., *Eyewitness Testimony*, (Cambridge, MA: Harvard University Press, 1996), ISBN:0-674-28777-0.

22. Loftus, E.F. and Palmer, J.C., "Reconstruction of Automobile Destruction: An Example of the Interaction between Language and Memory," *Journal of Verbal Learning and Verbal Behaviour* 13 (1974): 585-589, doi:10.1016/S0022-5371(74)80011-3.

CHAPTER

23. Fricke, L.B., *Traffic Crash Reconstruction*, 2nd ed., (Evanston, IL: Northwestern University Center for Public Safety, 2010), ISBN:0-912642-03-3.

24. Harris, J.O., "Cause and Contributing Factors," *Accident Reconstruction Journal*, November/December 1990, ISSN: 1057-8153.

25. Beck, R.F., *Bicycle Collision Investigation*, (San Diego, CA: Self-Published by Roman Beck, 2005), ISBN:9780615127941.

26. Association of European Motorcycle Manufacturers (ACEM), "MAIDS: Motorcycle Accidents in Depth Study," Final Report 2.0, April 2009, http://www.maids-study.eu/pdf/MAIDS2.pdf, accessed April 12, 2018.

27. Olson, P.L., *Forensic Aspects of Driver Perception and Response*, 1st ed., (Tucson, AZ: Lawyers and Judges Publishing Company, 1996), ISBN:0-913875-22-8.

28. Robinson, G.H., Erickson, D.J., Thurston, G.L., and Clark, R.L., "Visual Search by Automobile Drivers," *Human Factors*, 14, no. 4 (1972): 315-323.

29. Rahimi, M., "A Task, Behavior, and Environmental Analysis for Automobile Left-Turn Maneuvers," *Proceedings of the Human Factors Society, 33rd Annual Meeting*, Denver, CO, 1989.

30. Van Ness, H.C., *Understanding Thermodynamics*, (New York: Dover Publications Inc., 1969), ISBN:0-486-63277-6.

31. Beer, F.P. and Johnston, E.R., *Vector Mechanics for Engineers: Dynamics*, 5th ed., (McGraw-Hill, 1988), ISBN:0-07-079926-1.

32. Emori, R.I., "Analytical Approach to Automobile Collisions," SAE Technical Paper 680016, 1968, doi:10.4271/680016.

33. Rose, N., Fenton, S., and Ziernicki, R., "An Examination of the CRASH3 Effective Mass Concept," SAE Technical Paper 2004-01-1181, 2004, doi:10.4271/2004-01-1181.

34. Rose, N., Fenton, S., and Ziernicki, R., "Crush and Conservation of Energy Analysis: Toward a Consistent Methodology," SAE Technical Paper 2005-01-1200, 2005, doi:10.4271/2005-01-1200.

35. Kerkhoff, J., Husher, S., Varat, M., Busenga, A. et al., "An Investigation into Vehicle Frontal Impact Stiffness, BEV and Repeated Testing for Reconstruction," SAE Technical Paper 930899, 1993, doi:10.4271/930899.

36. McHenry, "The CRASH Program – A Simplified Collision Reconstruction Program," ZQ-5731-V-1, Calspan, 1975, http://www.mchenrysoftware.com/McHenry%201975%20The%20CRASH%20Program.pdf, accessed April 12, 2018.

37. McHenry, R.R. and McHenry, B.G., "A Revised Damage Analysis Procedure for the CRASH Computer Program," SAE Technical Paper 861894, 1986, doi:10.4271/861894.

38. Woolley, R., "Non-Linear Damage Analysis in Accident Reconstruction," SAE Technical Paper 2001-01-0504, 2001, doi:10.4271/2001-01-0504.

39. Fonda, A., "Principles of Crush Energy Determination," SAE Technical Paper 1999-01-0106, 1999, doi:10.4271/1999-01-0106.

40. Brach, R.M., *Mechanical Impact Dynamics: Rigid Body Collisions*, Revised edition, (South Bend, IN: Brach Engineering, 2007), ISBN:978-1-4028-9462-6.

41. Brach, R.M. and Brach, R.M., "A Review of Impact Models for Vehicle Collision," SAE Technical Paper 870048, 1987, doi:10.4271/870048.

42. Brach, R.M. and Brach, R.M., "Energy Loss in Vehicle Collision," SAE Technical Paper 871993, 1987, doi:10.4271/871993.

43. Brach, R.M. and Brach, R.M., *Vehicle Accident Analysis and Reconstruction Methods*, 2nd ed., (Warrendale: SAE International, 2005), ISBN:978-0-7680-3437-0.

44. Marine, M.C., "On the Concept of Inter-Vehicle Friction and Its Application in Automobile Accident Reconstruction," SAE Technical Paper 2007-01-0744, 2007, doi:10.4271/2007-01-0744.

2

Overview of Motorcycle Crash Analysis

Accident reconstructionists are often tasked with determining the cause, or at least some of the factors that contributed to the cause, of a motorcycle crash. There are many factors that *could* contribute to causing a motorcycle crash. For all categories of motor vehicle crashes, Treat et al. [1] found that human factors contributed to 92.6% of crashes. Environmental factors contributed in 33.8% of crashes and vehicular factors contributed in 12.6% of crashes. Treat noted that "the major human direct causes were improper lookout, excessive speed, inattention, improper evasive action, and internal distraction. Leading environmental causes were view obstructions and slick roads. The major vehicular causes were brake failure, inadequate tread depth, side-to-side brake imbalance, under-inflation, and vehicle-related vision obstructions. Vision (especially poor dynamic visual acuity) and personality (especially poor personal and social adjustment) were found related to accident-involvement."

In relationship to motorcycle crashes, Hurt [2] reported that "the motorcycle is particularly sensitive to environmental problems such as animals in the roadway, oil, water, and gravel contamination of the roadway, grooved freeways, railroad tracks, etc. Also…vehicle mechanical problems have far more serious consequences for the motorcycle than for the contemporary passenger automobile. A puncture flat on the freeway essentially guarantees a disaster for the motorcycle rider while the same occurrence in a passenger car would only cause anxious moments…Of course, in the study of any system of motor vehicle accidents, the problems of inattention, alcohol, risk-taking behavior, etc., will appear and contribute to accident causation." Hurt also noted the following potential factors that are unique to motorcycle crashes: motorcycle conspicuity, rider skill, training, licensing, and protective equipment. In evaluating the degree to which any of these factors may have contributed to a crash, the reconstructionist will need to consider the evidence related to that specific crash.

Motorcycle crashes can be divided into categories based on their attributes. Some are single-vehicle crashes involving the motorcycle, operator, and passengers falling and impacting the ground. Other single-vehicle motorcycle crashes involve the motorcycle exiting the roadway and striking a fixed object, such as a guardrail. Some involve the motorcycle colliding with another vehicle. To reconstruct these various types of motorcycle crashes, the analyst may need to understand the physical evidence each of these crash types creates. They may also need to apply physics-based models and methods to analyze the braking and cornering dynamics of motorcycles and how riders' inputs affect those dynamics. Similarly, the analyst may need to model and explain how motorcycles fall and how different types of falls affect the rider's motion, the way the motorcycle and rider move while sliding and tumbling on the ground, and the physics of an impact between a motorcycle and another vehicle or a roadside barrier. In addition, the analyst may need to develop an understanding of the errors that motorcyclists and the drivers of other vehicles sometimes make and how these play into crash causation. Finally, the they may need to evaluate the visibility of the motorcycle to other drivers or the visibility of other vehicles and objects to the motorcyclist.

Motorcycle accident reconstruction typically proceeds like any other area of accident reconstruction. The crash is separated into phases—the loss-of-control, impact, capsizing, and sliding phases, for a single-vehicle motorcycle crash, for instance. This is analogous to a single-vehicle rollover crash that would be separated into the loss-of-control, trip, and rolling phases. Conceptually, this can be represented with the Equation (2.1), an energy balance equation representing a single-vehicle motorcycle crash. Calculating the initial speed of the motorcycle involves determining the energy dissipated during each phase. The energy loss during each phase of the crash is calculated based on the distance traveled during that phase (d_{loc}, $d_{capsize}$, and d_{slide}) and the corresponding decelerations or drag factors (f_{loc}, $f_{capsize}$, and f_{slide}). Also, m is the vehicle mass, W is the vehicle weight, and v_i is the vehicle's initial velocity. This equation could be amended to include energy loss due to an impact and the initial kinetic energy for a vehicle involved in a collision with the motorcycle. The concept of parsing the crash into phases for analysis would not change, though:

$$\frac{1}{2}m_{mc}v_i^2 = f_{loc}Wd_{loc} + f_{capsize}Wd_{capsize} + f_{slide}Wd_{slide} \tag{2.1}$$

Reconstructing a motorcycle crash will include many, if not all, of the following steps:

- Reviewing investigative reports and photographs from any police investigation that was conducted.

- Reviewing statements and testimony from involved drivers and witnesses.

- Documenting, mapping, and diagraming the geometry of the crash site. This often involves visiting the crash site, but could also rely on aerial imagery [3, 4] and photogrammetric analysis. This may also include documenting changes that have occurred at an accident site to striping, signage, pavement surfaces, or vegetation.

- Documenting, mapping, and diagraming the physical evidence deposited at the scene. Some of this evidence may still be present when the reconstructionist visits the crash site. Other evidence locations may need to be reconstructed based on measurements taken by police or using methods of photogrammetry in conjunction with scene photographs.

- Documenting, mapping, or diagramming the pre-crash geometry of the motorcycle and any other involved vehicle. At times, this may simply involve obtaining manufacturer specifications for the vehicles. At other times, it may involve inspecting or testing an exemplar vehicle or performing calculations related to the inertial properties of the vehicles.

- Documenting and diagramming the physical evidence deposited on the motorcycle and any other involved vehicles. This often involves inspecting the vehicles, but it could also rely on analysis of photographs and photogrammetric analysis.

- Determining the vehicle motion implied by the available physical evidence.

- Applying physical and mathematical models to quantify the vehicle speed at relevant points during the sequence.

- A reconstruction may also include analysis of pre-collision motion of the vehicles and scenarios under which the motorcycle operator or other drivers could have avoided the crash. Rider or driver errors that led to the crash could be analyzed.

- A reconstruction may include analysis of the visibility of a motorcycle to a driver, the visibility of a vehicle or object to the motorcyclists, and the behavior and reactions of the motorcyclist and other drivers.

A reconstruction also typically considers the statements of parties involved in the crash and the statements of witnesses. These statements can often provide valuable information about lane positioning, group riding formation, rider experience, and rider clothing, issues that could be important to a reconstruction. However, as with any area of crash reconstruction, the analyst should be careful about lending too much credence to the accuracy of reported speeds, distances, and time estimates of witnesses and involved parties. As an example, Cummings [5] examined the accuracy of stationary witnesses when estimating the speed of a passing motorcycle. Their study involved 40 participants who each provided estimates of a motorcycle's speed for 20 individual runs (5 runs with each of 4 different motorcycles). This process resulted in 799 useable speed estimates. The results of this study demonstrated "that individual motorcycle speed estimates were often unreliable, even under these ideal experimental conditions." About 27% of the time, the error in the estimates was greater than 10 mph. The maximum errors in speed estimation were an underreporting of the speed by 26 mph and an overreporting of the speed by 41 mph.

This is consistent with what Fricke states in Chapter 12 of *Traffic Crash Reconstruction* [6]: "One caution that should be passed on from experience is that eyewitness accounts of speed in motorcycle collision cases, just as in other vehicle collision cases, tend to be somewhat questionable although they should be taken into account. Eyewitness testimony may suggest that a motorcycle was traveling 'at a high rate of speed.' Such a statement may or may not be true. The eyewitness may be influenced by the lack of experience in observation and knowledge of motorcycles. Eyewitnesses may also be influenced by the existence of a modified motorcycle exhaust system (louder than original equipment). Thus, such information must be judged against the available physical evidence."

2.1 Motorcycle Types

Within the class of motorcycles, NHTSA has included "mopeds, two- or three-wheeled motorcycles, off-road motorcycles, scooters, mini bikes, and pocket bikes" [7]. The Highway Loss Data Institute has defined the following street-legal motorcycle classes: standard, touring, cruiser, chopper, sport, super-sport, unclad sport, dual-purpose, and scooter [8]. They also define the following classes of off-road vehicles: off-road motorcycles, all-terrain vehicles, utility vehicles, and snowmobiles. They observe that "the method used to assign motorcycles to classes includes factors such as riding ergonomics, riding position, body style, features, usability, and driving dynamics." Of the 8.5 million motorcycles registered in the United States, the majority of these are on-road motorcycles. On-road motorcycles are designed for use on public streets and highways and have a huge variety of stylistic designs, sizes, and functions. In addition to the criteria outlined by the Highway Loss Data Institute, the Motorcycle Safety Foundation notes that these styles can be distinguished by their overall size, available features, their engine size, and their performance [9].

Standard motorcycles are the most basic and versatile category of on-road motorcycles. Figure 2.1 depicts a typical standard motorcycle. These motorcycles are also sometimes referred to as "traditional" or "naked" motorcycles. They are characterized by their upright handlebars and intermediate riding position. They are also typically equipped with a gas tank that is too small to go long distances and are usually stripped of advanced features and typically do not have fairings. According to the Highway Loss Data Institute, these motorcycles are generally considered beginner motorcycles with low power-to-weight ratios.

Touring motorcycles are typically the largest of the on-road motorcycles and are designed for comfort and distance. Figure 2.2 depicts a typical touring motorcycle. These motorcycles are large in overall size and engine size and usually accommodate riders with bucket seats and provide cargo carrying areas large enough for long trips.

Cruisers are sized between the touring and standard-size bikes (Figure 2.3). They are styled for looks and performance, without the long-range cargo carrying capabilities. They are characterized by their pulled-back handlebars and a relaxed, feet-forward riding position. The Highway Loss Data Institute states that "cruiser motorcycles mimic the style of earlier American motorcycles from the 1930s to the early 1960s, such as those made by Harley-Davidson and Indian."

Sport motorcycles represent the most powerful class of on-road motorcycles (Figure 2.4). The design of these motorcycles is focused on the motorcycle's capabilities for cornering, maneuverability, braking, and acceleration. Engines sizes have a large range but in general are geared and designed for speed and handling. These motorcycles typically have greater lean angle capabilities than other motorcycle types. Sport motorcycles typically have dropped handle bars, raised foot pegs, and fairings designed for aerodynamic efficiency.

Scooter is a classification of motorbikes above 50cc that are operated differently than a typical motorcycle. For instance, the shifting is typically automatic and does not require clutch operation. Also, both front and rear brakes may be operated by the hands, rather than a foot pedal for the rear brake. Figure 2.5 depicts a typical scooter.

Three-wheeled motorcycles first appeared in the early to mid-1900s. One of the earliest on-road, three-wheeled motorcycles was manufactured by Harley-Davidson from 1932–1975 and was called the Servi-Car. The Servi-Car was designed to transport customer's

FIGURE 2.1 Typical standard motorcycle.

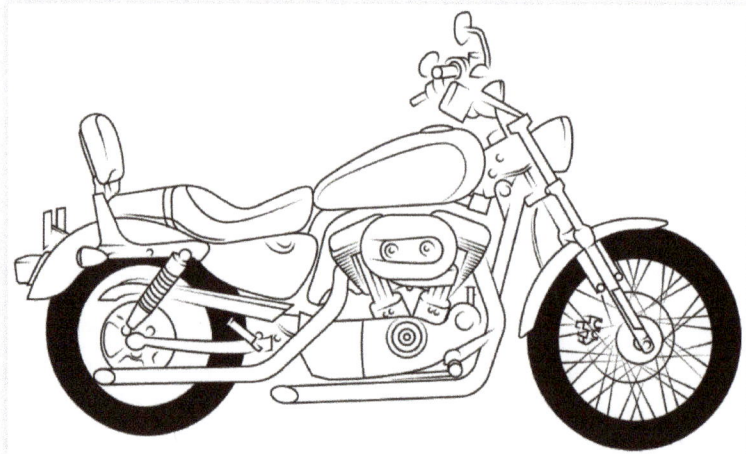

FIGURE 2.2 Typical touring motorcycle.

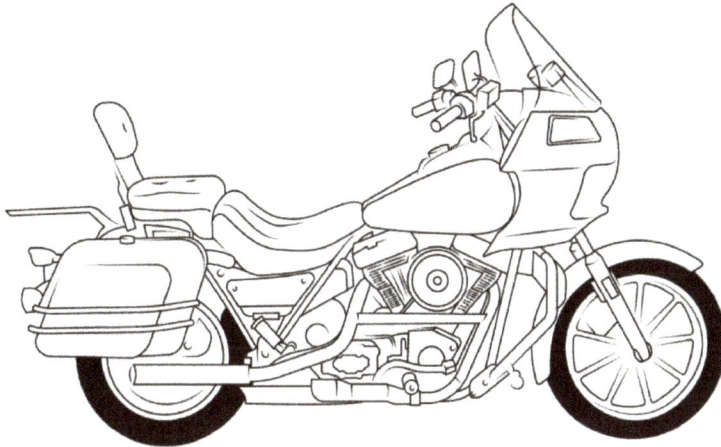

FIGURE 2.3 Typical cruiser motorcycle.

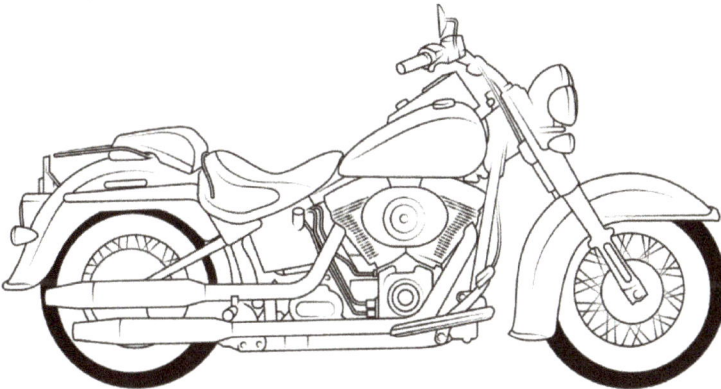

FIGURE 2.4 Typical sport motorcycle.

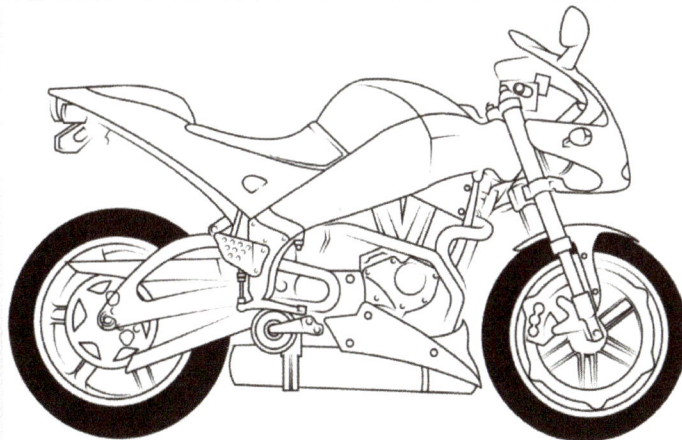

cars from a maintenance garage to the customer's house. Harley-Davidson discontinued the Servi-Car in 1975, and Harley-Davidson did not begin making another three-wheeled motorcycle until the Tri Glide Ultra Classic in 2009. Three-wheeled motorcycles have experienced a surge in popularity recently. These motorcycles perform and handle differently than their two-wheeled counterparts in steering, braking, and acceleration. The analysis of crashes involving these motorcycles may need to account for these differences. Typical three-wheeled motorcycles are shown in Figures 2.6 and 2.7.

Off-road motorcycles are generally referred to as dirt bikes (Figure 2.8). They are designed to handle rough, natural outdoor terrain. Off-road motorcycles, compared to the on-road versions, are typically simpler and lighter, with high clearance for obstacles, ruts, and longer suspension travel. These motorcycles are typically void of fairings and bodywork.

Dual-purpose motorcycles provide the benefits of being roadworthy with the ability to travel off-road as well. As expected from their name, the dual-purpose (or dual-sport) has some of the characteristics of on-road motorcycles, but with a higher ground clearance, greater suspension travel, and knobby tires. A typical dual-purpose motorcycle is depicted in Figure 2.9.

In an accident reconstruction context, there are some instances when the motorcycle type will be relevant to the analysis. The motorcycle characteristics can potentially influence the deceleration rate of the motorcycle under heavy braking or when the motorcycle is sliding on the ground. Different motorcycle types will also generally have different center of gravity heights, which can be relevant to calculations related to the lean angle of the motorcycle for a curve.

2.2 Motorcycle Dimensions and Inertial Properties

Geometric dimensions of the motorcycle will typically need to be obtained when reconstructing a motorcycle crash. These dimensions can be obtained from manufacturer specifications or from inspecting an exemplar motorcycle. Another valuable source of

FIGURE 2.5   Typical scooter.

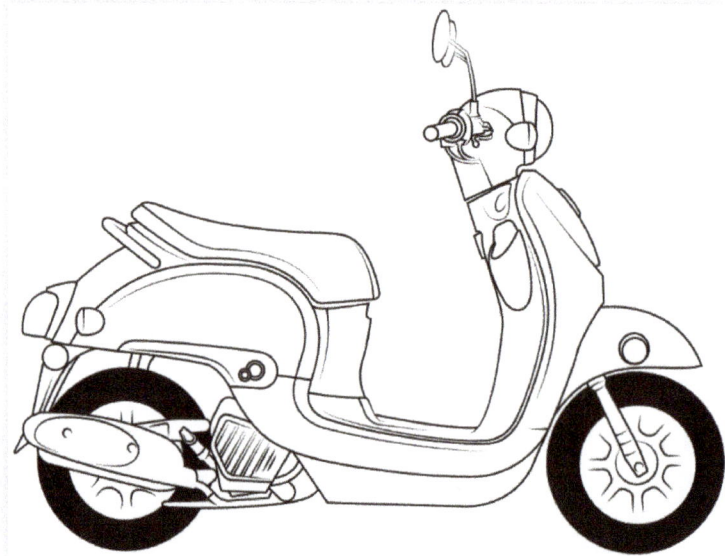

FIGURE 2.6 Typical three-wheeled motorcycle.

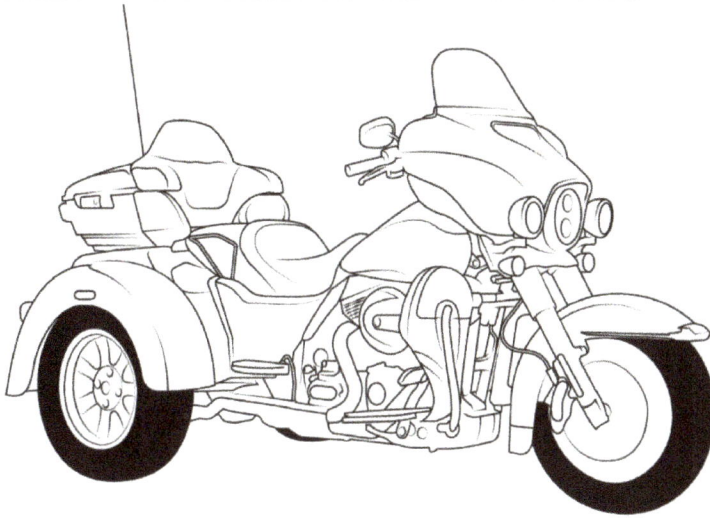

FIGURE 2.7 Another type of three-wheeled motorcycle.

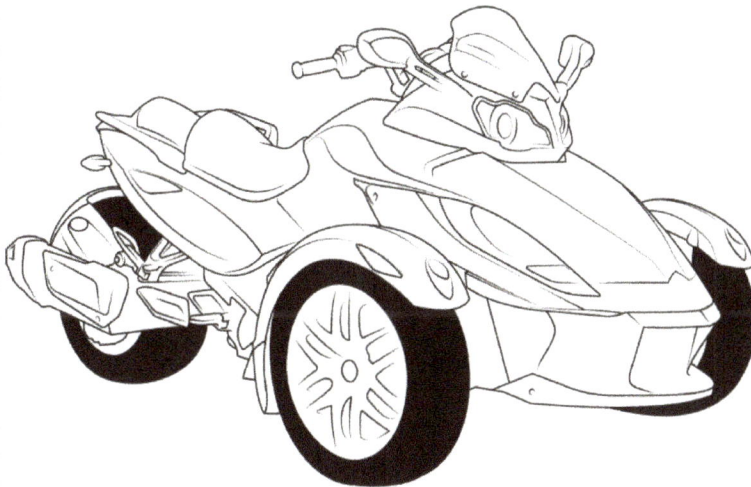

FIGURE 2.8 Typical off-road motorcycle.

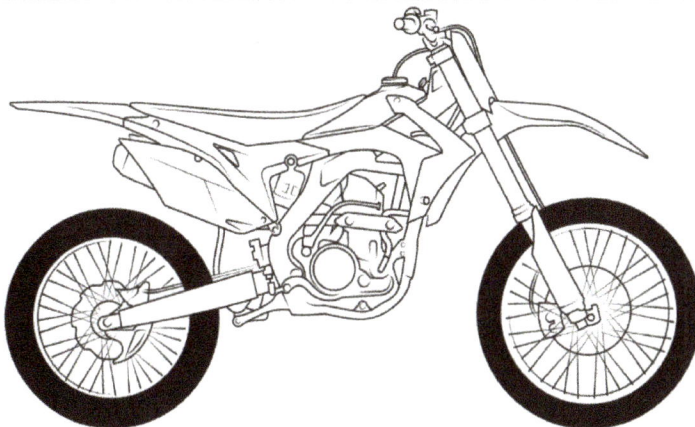

FIGURE 2.9 Typical dual-purpose motorcycle.

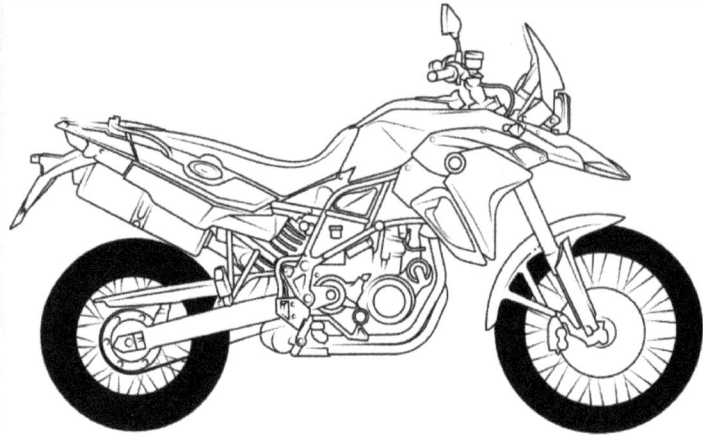

FIGURE 2.9 Typical dual-purpose motorcycle.

motorcycle specifications is Lightpoint Data (http://lightpointdata.com/motorcycle-specs). Depending on the analysis techniques employed, the reconstructionist may also need to determine the weight of the vehicle, its center of gravity location, and its moments of inertia.

Cossalter, Doria, and Mitolo [10] tested two super-sport motorcycles and found that the center of gravity height was equal to approximately 37% of the wheelbase. Foale [11] presented the center of gravity heights for 39 motorcycles. His data is included in Table 2.1, organized by motorcycle type. As this table shows, the center of gravity heights in Foale's data ranged from 11.6 to 24.7 in. (295 to 624 mm). Table 2.1 also includes the wheelbase for each motorcycle, along with the ratio of the center of gravity height to the wheelbase. In Foale's entire dataset, the center of gravity height was, on average, 34.2% of the wheelbase, with a standard deviation of 6.7% of the wheelbase. For the sport motorcycles, the center of gravity height was on average 38.9% of the wheelbase, generally consistent with Cossalter's data. The standard deviation on this was approximately 4.6% of the wheelbase. For cruisers, on the other hand, the center of gravity height was, on average, 27.2% of the wheelbase, with a standard deviation of 4.6% of the wheelbase. The average ratio for the touring motorcycles was 27.1% of the wheelbase, with a standard deviation of 5.8%. For standard motorcycles, the average was 37.2% of the wheelbase, with a standard deviation of 5.2%. Based on these numbers, it appears reasonable to lump cruisers with touring motorcycles and standard with sports motorcycle for developing equations to estimate the center of gravity height of a motorcycle.

DiTallo [12] presented the center of gravity heights for 25 additional motorcycles and his data is included in Table 2.2. In DiTallo's entire dataset, the center of gravity height was, on average, 34.0% of the wheelbase, with a standard deviation of 6.2% of the wheelbase. These numbers are consistent with Foale's dataset. In DiTallo's dataset, the center of gravity height for the sport motorcycles was on average 36.9% of the wheelbase. The standard deviation on this was approximately 5.2% of the wheelbase. For cruisers, on the other hand, the center of gravity height was, on average, 29.0% of the wheelbase, with a standard deviation of 3.5% of the wheelbase. Again, these numbers are consistent with Foale's dataset (and Cossalter's).

To develop equations to predict the center of gravity height of a motorcycle, the Foale and DiTallo datasets were combined. Cruisers and touring motorcycles were lumped together and standard and sports motorcycles were lumped together. These combined datasets were used to calculate an average and standard deviation for each

TABLE 2.1 Center of gravity data from Foale [11]

Motorcycle	Motorcycle type	Motorcycle wheelbase, WB (in.)	Center of gravity height, h (in.)	Ratio (h/WB)
Kawasaki Vulcan 1500 Drifter	Cruiser	65.2	11.6	0.18
Yamaha Road Star	Cruiser	66.5	15.7	0.24
Yamaha V-Star 1100	Cruiser	65.0	16.1	0.25
Yamaha V-Star 1100	Cruiser	65.0	17.4	0.27
Yamaha V-Star 1100 Classic	Cruiser	65.0	17.6	0.27
Harley-Davidson FLHTCUI	Cruiser	62.7	18.2	0.29
Honda Shadow Sabre	Cruiser	65.0	19.5	0.30
Honda Magna	Cruiser	63.8	20.1	0.32
Harley-Davidson FXST Softail STD	Cruiser	66.9	23.2	0.35
BMW R1100GS	Dual-purpose	59.4	22.3	0.38
Kawasaki ZX-6R	Sport	55.1	20.1	0.36
Triumph Daytona	Sport	54.8	20.4	0.37
Suzuki Hayabusa	Sport	58.3	20.6	0.35
Honda CBR600F4i	Sport	55.0	20.8	0.38
Yamaha YZF-R6	Sport	54.3	21.6	0.40
Suzuki GSX-R600	Sport	55.0	21.6	0.39
Kawasaki ZX-6R	Sport	55.1	21.6	0.39
Honda CBR	Sport	54.7	21.6	0.39
Honda CBR1100XX	Sport	58.7	21.7	0.37
Triumph TT600	Sport	54.9	22.1	0.40
Yamaha YZF-R6	Sport	54.3	22.3	0.41
Triumph Sprint	Sport	57.9	22.5	0.39
Suzuki GSX-R600	Sport	55.0	22.7	0.41
Suzuki Bandit 600	Sport	56.0	23.2	0.41
Honda Nighthawk 750	Standard	59.1	18.4	0.31
Suzuki SV650	Standard	56.7	18.7	0.33
BMW F650GS	Standard	62.0	18.7	0.30
Triumph T-Bird Sport	Standard	62.2	20.3	0.33
Suzuki GZ250	Standard	57.1	20.5	0.36
Ducati Monster City	Standard	57.0	21.4	0.38
Buell X1	Standard	55.5	22.4	0.40
Buell Blast	Standard	55.0	22.9	0.42
Triumph Tiger 90	Standard	53.5	23.9	0.45
Buell X1	Standard	55.5	24.7	0.45
Honda Valkyrie Interstate	Touring	66.5	14.1	0.21
Honda GL 1800	Touring	66.6	15.6	0.23
Yamaha Royal Star Venture	Touring	67.1	16.3	0.24
Honda GL 1500 SE	Touring	66.5	19.2	0.29
BMW K1200LT	Touring	62.3	23.4	0.38

population. This resulted in the following equation for *cruisers and touring* motorcycles. In this equation, h is the center of gravity height and WB is the wheelbase of the motorcycle:

$$h = 0.2777 \times WB \pm 0.0454 \times WB \tag{2.2}$$

TABLE 2.2 Center of heights for motorcycles [12]

Motorcycle	Motorcycle type	Motorcycle wheelbase, WB (in.)	Center of gravity height, h (in.)	Ratio (h/WB)
2006 Harley-Davidson XL1200C	Cruiser	64.0	21.8	0.34
2010 Harley-Davidson FXDF	Cruiser	63.7	17.9	0.28
2011 Harley-Davidson FLSTCI	Cruiser	64.6	16.3	0.25
2011 Harley-Davidson FLHRCI	Cruiser	63.5	14.6	0.23
2009 Yamaha XV250	Cruiser	58.8	17.8	0.30
1989 Kawasaki VN1500-A	Cruiser	63.0	19.7	0.31
1996 Kawasaki VN800-A	Cruiser	63.2	17.4	0.28
1998 Honda VT1100C2	Cruiser	65.0	20.9	0.32
1993 Honda XR250L	Dual-purpose	55.6	26.9	0.48
2012 Jmstar YY50QT-6	Scooter	51.0	16.4	0.32
2008 Taizhou Zhongneng GTR150	Scooter	50.5	18.1	0.36
1998 Buell S3 Thunderbolt	Sport	54.6	21.7	0.40
2001 Kawasaki EX500-D	Sport	56.0	14.4	0.26
2001 Honda CBR600	Sport	55.0	21.6	0.39
1997 Kawasaki ZX900-B	Sport	56.0	20.4	0.36
1997 Kawasaki ZX900-B	Sport	57.0	22.4	0.39
1998 Honda CBR900RR	Sport	55.2	26.2	0.47
2000 Yamaha YZF-R6	Sport	54.0	20.3	0.38
2009 Yamaha FZ6R	Sport	56.8	20	0.35
1993 Yamaha FZR600	Sport	56.0	19.9	0.36
1992 Yamaha FZR600	Sport	56.0	17.2	0.31
2005 Suzuki GS500E	Sport	55.0	21.2	0.39
2011 Honda	Standard	55.6	20.2	0.36
2004 Kawasaki EN500C	Standard	62.8	20.8	0.33
2011 Harley-Davidson FLHTCUI	Touring	63.5	16.9	0.27

The following equation resulted for the *standard and sports* motorcycles:

$$h = 0.3759 \times WB \pm 0.0425 \times WB \tag{2.3}$$

The plus/minus on these equations is one standard deviation on each side of the mean. These equations can be used to estimate the center of gravity height for a motorcycle when a measured center of gravity height is not available. The dataset used to generate these equations included 23 cruiser/touring motorcycles and 37 standard/sport motorcycles. This data is plotted in Figure 2.10. Wheelbase is plotted on the horizontal axis and the ratio of center of gravity height to wheelbase is plotted on the vertical axis. From this graph, it is apparent that standard/sport motorcycles generally have shorter wheelbases than cruiser/touring motorcycles and that the center of gravity height for the standard/sport motorcycles is generally a higher percentage of the wheelbase than for the cruiser/touring motorcycles.

Figure 2.11 is a similar graph, but in this graph, the actual center of gravity height is plotted on the vertical axis. From this graph, it is apparent that the standard and sport motorcycles generally have higher centers of gravity than the cruiser and touring motorcycles, though there is overlap of the two datasets.

The moments of inertia characterize a vehicle's resistance to rotation about its principal axes-roll, pitch, and yaw. Cossalter, Doria, and Mitolo [10] reported physical

FIGURE 2.10 Ratio of CG height to wheelbase as a function of wheelbase.

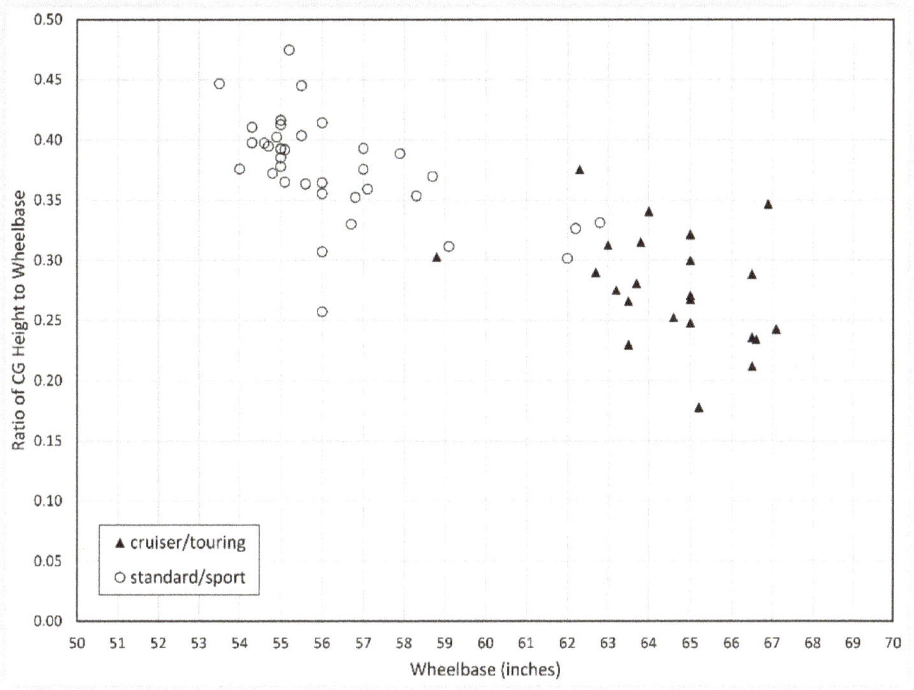

FIGURE 2.11 CG height as a function of wheelbase.

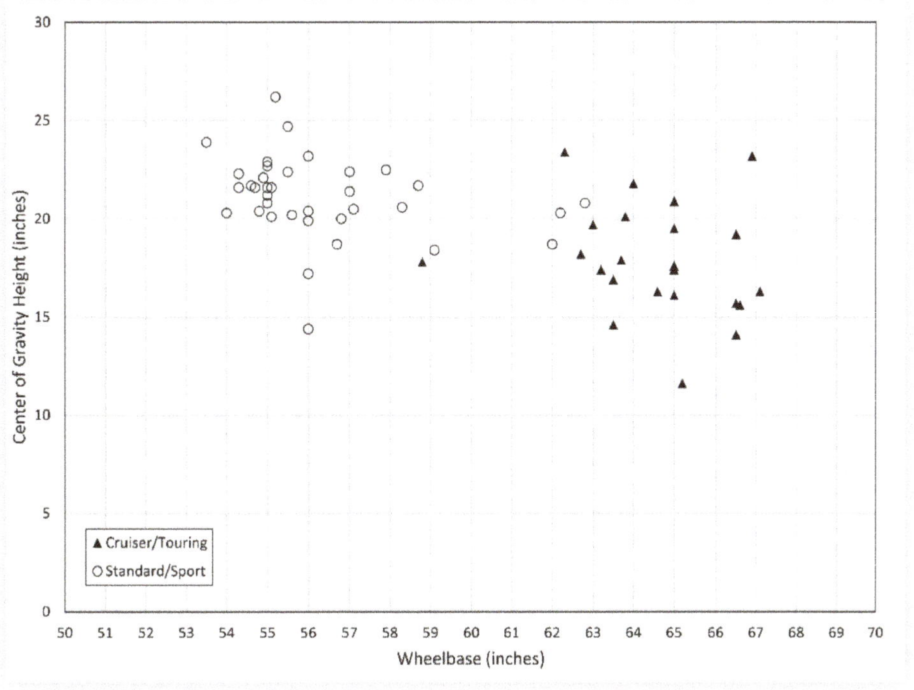

testing of two racing motorcycles to determine their inertial properties. These authors noted that motorcycle moments of inertia would be necessary inputs into a simulation of a motorcycle's dynamic behavior and handling. They also note that "the global center of mass position and moments of inertia around the roll, pitch, and yaw axes gives (sic) simplified but straightforward information about motorcycle handling." In the context of crash reconstruction, there will not be many instances where the analyst needs to evaluate the motorcycle moments of inertia. However, if they are needed, an estimate can be obtained with the prism method (without any testing). The prism method assumes that the vehicle is a solid, homogeneous box. With this assumption, the moments of inertia about the principal axis are given by the following equations:

$$I_{roll} = \frac{1}{2}m \cdot \left(w_{overall}^2 + h_{overall}^2\right) \tag{2.4}$$

$$I_{pitch} = \frac{1}{2}m \cdot \left(l_{overall}^2 + h_{overall}^2\right) \tag{2.5}$$

$$I_{yaw} = \frac{1}{2}m \cdot \left(l_{overall}^2 + w_{overall}^2\right) \tag{2.6}$$

In these equations, I_{roll}, I_{pitch}, and I_{yaw} are the moments of inertia about the roll, pitch, and yaw axes. The vehicle mass is indicated with the letter m, and $l_{overall}$, $w_{overall}$, and $h_{overall}$ are the vehicle length, width, and height, respectively. If precise values are needed, testing could be conducted. Frank [13] reported a measured value for the yaw moment of inertia of a Kawasaki Ninja ZX-10R of 320 in.-lb-s^2.

Geometric and inertial parameters for a *passenger vehicle* involved in a collision with a motorcycle may also be needed for the analysis. For example, if the analyst is using simulation to determine the motorcycle impact speed necessary to cause a documented translation and rotation of a struck vehicle, the yaw moment of inertia will be a necessary input. In these instances, the analyst can reference several studies. MacInnis [14] examined methods for estimating the whole vehicle (as opposed to sprung mass) moments of inertia. He compared each method to actual moments of inertia measured and reported by Garrott of the National Highway Traffic Safety Administration (NHTSA) [15, 16, 17]. In making this comparison, MacInnis divided the vehicles into the following categories: front-wheel-drive passenger cars, rear-wheel-drive passenger cars, sport utility vehicles, pickup trucks, and vans. The article by MacInnis gives a complete listing of the equations he recommended for calculating the center of gravity height and the moments of inertia for each of these vehicle types. Additionally, MacInnis examined the effect of uncertainty in the yaw moment of inertia on the results of planar collision simulation with the crash reconstruction software PC-Crash. He found that varying the yaw moment of inertia by 30% had about a 3% effect on the calculated initial speeds.

The NHTSA published additional moments of inertia data after the MacInnis study [18]. Allen incorporated this additional data and used regression analysis to develop equations for estimating the vehicle center of mass height and moments of inertia [19]. Allen did not partition the data by vehicle type. For each moment of inertia, Allen's equations took the following form:

$$I_i = 10^{k1} \cdot l_{wb}^{k2} \cdot T^{k3} \cdot h_{overall}^{k4} \cdot W^{k5} \tag{2.7}$$

In these equations,

I_i is whichever moment of inertia is under consideration
l_{wb} is the wheelbase (in feet)
T is the average track width (in feet)
$h_{overall}$ is the vehicle height (in feet)
W is the total vehicle weight (in pounds)

The exponents in Equation (2.7) are the regression coefficients. The values of these coefficients for each of the moments of inertia are reported in Table 2.3. With the

TABLE 2.3 Regression coefficients from Allen [19]

	k1	k2	k3	k4	k5
I_{roll}	−2.1363	−0.1596	1.9404	0.3629	0.9421
I_{pitch}	−2.0024	1.5315	0.2526	0.1009	1.0206
I_{yaw}	−1.7797	1.4316	0.3811	0.0188	0.9800

regression coefficients of Table 2.3, Equation (2.7) yields the moments of inertia in units of pounds-feet-s^2.

Allen also reported the following equation for estimating the vehicle center of gravity height (in feet). Allen reported an R^2 value for this equation of 0.8277:

$$h = 0.3891 \cdot h_{overall} + 0.113 \tag{2.8}$$

Garrott tested the effect of adding occupants and cargo on the center of gravity height of several vehicles. In nearly every case, he found that the center of gravity height increased with the addition of occupants [16]. The effect of adding cargo to the vehicle varied depending on how the cargo was placed. Though likely rare given the time and expense, some cases may warrant physical measurement of a vehicle's center of mass location, either in the empty or loaded condition. Should a reconstructionist need to perform such physical measurements, they can refer to the article by Shapiro, who discussed the pros and cons of various methods for making a physical measurement of a vehicle's center of mass height [20].

2.3 Motorcycle Controls

In general, the right side of a motorcycle contains controls for the ignition, braking, and accelerating, while the left side contains controls for shifting gears and signaling. The front and rear brakes are controlled independently on motorcycles with standard braking systems. The front brake is controlled with a lever near the right handgrip and the rear brake is controlled with a foot pedal on the right side (Figure 2.12). The throttle is on the right handgrip, the clutch is actuated using a lever near the left handgrip, and gear changes are commanded using a foot pedal on the left side of the motorcycle. The throttle is increased by rolling the grip towards the rider and decreased by rolling the throttle away from the rider. When released, the throttle will spring back to the idle position. Power from the engine to the wheels is disengaged by squeezing the clutch lever. Power is reengaged by releasing the clutch lever. The shifting pattern for most motorcycles is all the way down to first gear and all the way up for 5th or 6th gear (depending on how many gears there are). This gearing pattern is often referred to as, "one down, five up." Neutral is between 1st and 2nd gears and can be accessed from going up or down in gear. Motorcycle transmissions are sequential, meaning that gears cannot be skipped. However, the gears will only engage if the clutch is released.

2.4 Motorcycle Tires

Motorcycle tires differ from passenger car tires, particularly in terms of their cross-section. Because motorcycle steering and cornering involve the operator leaning the motorcycle, motorcycle tires have a circular or U-shaped profile rather than the flatter profile of a passenger car tire. Because of this, the size and shape of the tire contact patches change as a motorcycle leans. Also, as Obenski [21] notes, "because the consequences of a tire

FIGURE 2.12 Motorcycle controls.

FIGURE 2.12 Motorcycle controls.

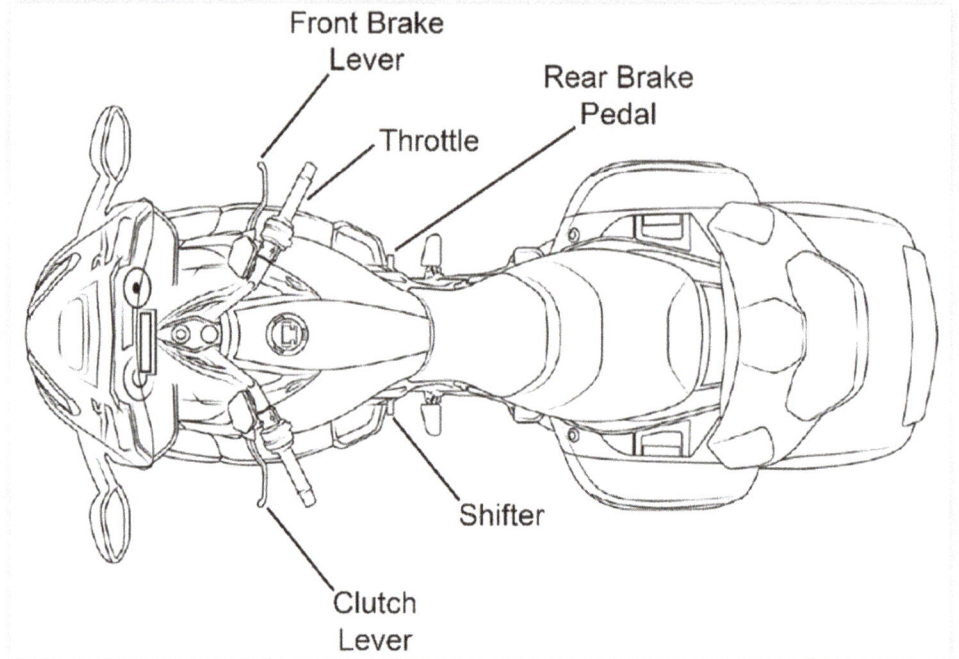

losing its grip can be much more severe to a rider than to other drivers, motorcycle tire construction and rubber compounds are generally optimized for traction at the expense of longevity."

2.4.1 Motorcycle Tire Markings

Figure 2.13 depicts typical markings on the two sides of a motorcycle tire—in this case a Metzeler ME Z2 sport touring radial tire. The markings on this tire include the following:

    Tire Manufacturer—Metzeler

    Tire Model—MEZ2

FIGURE 2.13 Typical markings on a motorcycle tire.

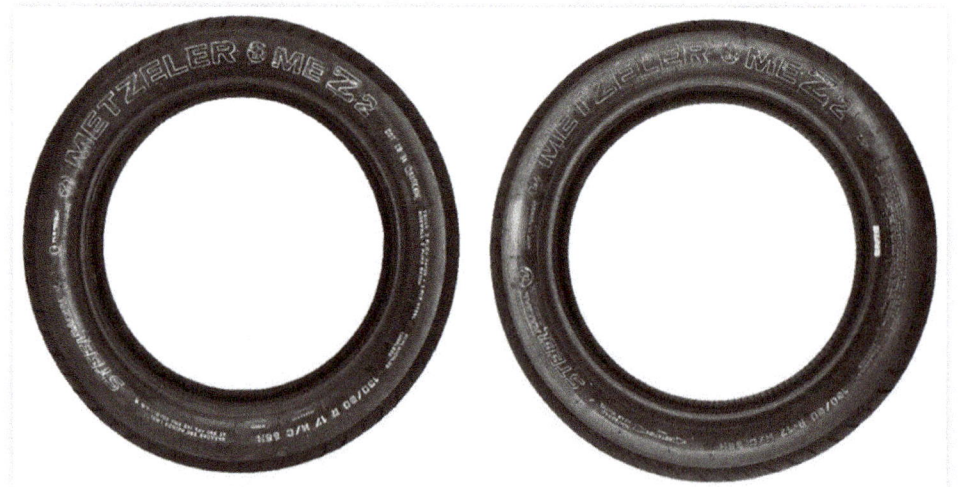

TABLE 2.4 Load indexes for motorcycle tires

Load index	Weight rating (lb)	Load index	Weight rating (lb)	Load index	Weight rating (lb)	Load index	Weight rating (lb)
50	419	56	494	62	584	68	694
51	430	57	507	63	600	69	716
52	441	58	520	64	617	70	739
53	454	59	536	65	639	71	761
54	467	60	551	66	661	72	783
55	481	61	567	67	677	73	805

North American Department of Transportation Compliance Symbol—DOT

DOT is followed by the Tire Serial Number, which ends with a four-digit date code

Tire Construction Details

Size Designation—130/80R17

Nominal Section Width (mm)—130

Aspect Ratio—80

Rim Diameter (inches)—17

Motorcycle Tire Designation—M/C

Load Index (Maximum Capacity at Maximum Pressure)—65

Speed Symbol—H

Maximum Load @ Maximum Pressure—290 kg (639 lb) @ 290 kPa (42 psi)

Tire Construction—Steel Radial

An arrow indicating the correct rotation direction for the tire

The date code, which is the last four digits of the tire serial number, specifies the week and year that the tire was manufactured. For example, the code on the tire in Figure 2.13 is 4116, indicating that the tire was manufactured in the 41st week of 2016. Table 2.4 lists the meaning of several load index numbers for motorcycle tires. Table 2.5 lists the meaning of the speed ratings, given in kilometers per hour. The owner's manual for a motorcycle will specify the tire size, construction, load range, and speed index intended to be installed on both the front and rear of the motorcycle.

As the Motorcycle Industry Council Tire Guide [22] notes, "proper air pressure is critical for tire performance and tire life. Under-inflation or overloading can cause sluggish handling, heavy steering, and internal damage due to over-flexing, and can cause the tire to separate from the rim. Over-inflation can reduce the contact area (and therefore available traction), and can make the motorcycle react harshly to bumps."

2.4.2 Motorcycle Tire Friction Coefficients

Motorcycle tires are softer and stickier than passenger car tires [23]. Lambourn and Wesley [24] used a two-wheeled trailer (designed as a highway friction measuring device) to test three motorcycle tires designed for sports motorcycles to determine their peak and locked-wheel friction coefficients on asphalt

TABLE 2.5 Speed ratings for motorcycle tires

Rating	Speed (kph)
J	100
K	110
L	120
M	130
N	140
P	150
Q	160
R	170
S	180
T	190
U	200
H	210
V or VB	240
Z or ZR	240+
W	270
Y	300

FIGURE 2.14 Pavement friction tester used by Lambourn and Wesley.

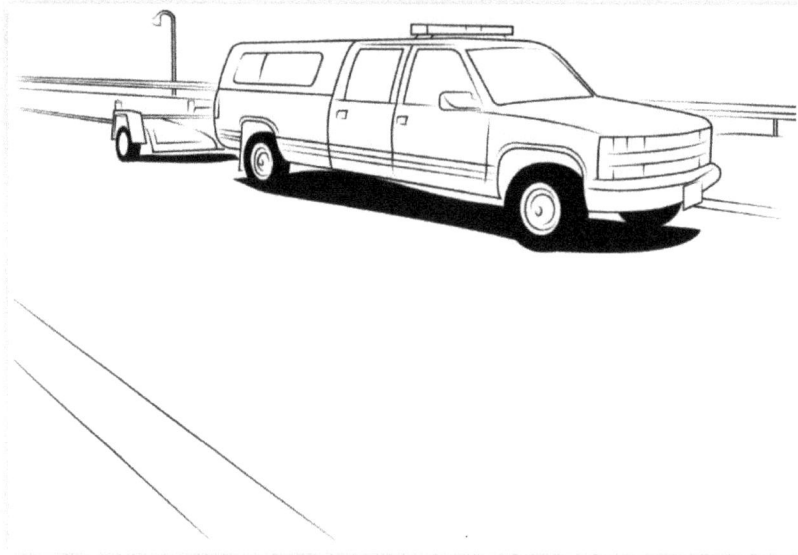

(Figure 2.14). They tested two different asphalt surfaces (hot rolled asphalt and stone mastic asphalt) in both a dry and a wet condition (1 mm water depth). The tires were tested at nominal speeds of approximately 32, 64, and 100 kph (approximately 20, 40, and 60 mph).

On dry, hot rolled asphalt, the motorcycle tires produced average peak friction coefficients between 1.1 and 1.3. These values generally increased with increasing speed. The average locked-wheel coefficients for dry, hot rolled asphalt ranged between 0.7 and 0.9. There was slight speed dependence in these values, with the friction coefficient declining slightly with increasing speed. On the dry stone mastic asphalt, the motorcycle tires produced average peak friction coefficients between 1.1 and 1.25. There was no speed dependence in these values. The locked-wheel coefficients on the dry stone mastic asphalt fell between 0.9 and 0.65. These values exhibited significant speed dependence, with the range at 32 kph (20 mph) falling between 0.8 and 0.9 and the range at 100 kph (60 mph) falling between 0.65 and 0.76.

On wet, hot rolled asphalt, the motorcycle tires produced average peak friction coefficients between 0.99 and 1.36. There was no obvious speed dependence in these values. The average locked-wheel coefficients on the wet, hot rolled asphalt showed significant speed dependence, falling between 0.8 and 0.9 at 32 kph (20 mph) and 0.52 to 0.67 at 100 kph (60 mph). On the wet stone mastic asphalt, the motorcycle tires produced average peak friction coefficients between 1.0 and 1.15. The locked-wheel coefficients exhibited significant speed dependence, falling between 0.68 and 0.76 at 32 kph (20 mph) and between 0.37 and 0.4 at 100 kph (60 mph).

In some situations, the tire temperature could also be an important consideration in assessing the available friction for a motorcycle tire—perhaps, for instance, when determining the friction limits for a motorcycle that has been on a long mountainous ride on a hot day. As Parks observes, "as a tire gets hotter, the rubber becomes more compliant and has a greater ability to interlock with the tarmac, providing greater traction. This increased traction continues until the rubber exceeds its design temperature and begins to degrade...conversely, when tires are cold, the rubber becomes hard and doesn't conform to the peaks and valleys of the road surface as well as when the tires are warm, significantly reducing grip. This is especially true of race compound tires. Pushing too hard on cold tires has caused me and nearly every racer I know to crash. It's also been responsible for a lot of crashes on the street, especially when street bikes are equipped with DOT race tires, which are race-compound tires that have been cut with a tread so that they are approved by the Department of Transportation for street use" [25].

Tests like those reported in Reference [24] can begin to define an upper limit on the performance capabilities of motorcycles. However, these limits will typically be different once the tires are installed on an actual motorcycle. Not only that, in many cases, the performance limits of the motorcycle-rider system will be defined by the rider, not by the tires or the motorcycle. Most riders will not be capable of fully utilizing the peak friction of their tires. In addition to that, the values reported by Lambourn and Wesley are applicable to dry and wet roadway surfaces that are generally free of debris and contaminants. Some motorcycle crashes involve debris or contaminants on the road, placed either intentionally or unintentionally. In such cases, the analyst may need to consider the effect of the debris or contaminants on the friction limits of the motorcycle tires [26, 27].

References

1. Treat, J.R., Tumbas, N.S., McDonald, S.T. et al., "Tri-Level Study of the Causes of Traffic Accidents," DOT HS-034-3-535, May 1979, https://deepblue.lib.umich.edu/handle/2027.42/64993, accessed January 18, 2018.

2. Hurt, H.H., "Human Factors in Motorcycle Accidents," SAE Technical Paper 770103, 1977, doi:10.4271/770103.

3. Wirth, J., Bonugli, E., and Freund, M., "Assessment of the Accuracy of Google Earth Imagery for Use as a Tool in Accident Reconstruction," SAE Technical Paper 2015-01-1435, 2015, doi:10.4271/2015-01-1435.

4. Harrington, S., Teitelman, J., Rummel, E., Morse, B. et al., "Validating Google Earth Pro as a Scientific Utility for Use in Accident Reconstruction," SAE Technical Paper 2017-01-9750, 2017, doi:10.4271/2017-01-9750.

5. Cummings, J.R., Fletcher, H.J., Biller, B.A., Scanlan, S. et al., "Estimates of Motorcycle Speed Made by Eyewitnesses under Ideal Experimental Conditions," *Accident Reconstruction Journal*, January/February 2016, ISSN: 1057-8153.

6. Fricke, L.B., *Traffic Crash Reconstruction*, 2nd ed., (Evanston, IL: Northwestern University Center for Public Safety, 2010), ISBN:0-912642-03-3.

7. NHTSA, "Traffic Safety Facts, 2013 Data, Motorcycles," DOT HS 812 148, May 2015, https://crashstats.nhtsa.dot.gov/Api/Public/ViewPublication/812148, accessed January 18, 2018.

8. Highway Data Loss Institute, "Insurance Motorcycle Comprehensive Report," April 2007, MC-06, accessed online on April 12, 2018.

9. Motorcycle Safety Foundation, *The Motorcycle Safety Foundation's Guide to Motorcycling Excellence*, 2nd ed., (Center Conway, NH: Whitehorse Press, 2005), ISBN:978-1-884313-47-9.

10. Cossalter, V., Doria, A., and Mitolo, L., "Inertial and Modal Properties of Racing Motorcycles," SAE Technical Paper 2002-01-3347, 2002, doi:10.4271/2002-01-3347.

11. Foale, T., *Motorcycle Handling and Chassis Design – The Art and Science*, 2nd ed., (Self-Published by Tony Foale, 2006) and available for purchase at https://tonyfoale.com/book.htm.

12. DiTallo, M. et al., "Motorcycle Center of Gravity Data: Methodology and Reference," *Collision: The International Compendium for Crash Research* 12, no. 1 (September 2017), ISSN: 1934-8681.

13. Frank, T., Smith, J., Fowler, G., Carter, J. et al., "Simulating Moving Motorcycle to Moving Car Crashes," SAE Technical Paper 2012-01-0621, 2012, doi:10.4271/2012-01-0621.

14. MacInnis, D., Cliff, W., and Ising, K., "A Comparison of Moment of Inertia Estimation Techniques for Vehicle Dynamics Simulation," SAE Technical Paper 970951, 1997, doi:10.4271/970951.

15. Garrott, W., Monk, M., and Chrstos, J., "Vehicle Inertial Parameters-Measured Values and Approximations," SAE Technical Paper 881767, 1988, doi:10.4271/881767.

16. Garrott, W., "The Variation of Static Rollover Metrics with Vehicle Loading and between Similar Vehicles," SAE Technical Paper 920583, 1992, doi:10.4271/920583.

17. Garrott, W., "Measured Vehicle Inertial Parameters-NHTSA's Data Through September 1992," SAE Technical Paper 930897, 1993, doi:10.4271/930897.

18. Heydinger, G., Bixel, R., Garrott, W., Pyne, M. et al., "Measured Vehicle Inertial Parameters-NHTSA's Data Through November 1998," SAE Technical Paper 1999-01-1336, 1999, doi:10.4271/1999-01-1336.

19. Allen, R., Klyde, D., Rosenthal, T., and Smith, D., "Estimation of Passenger Vehicle Inertial Properties and Their Effect on Stability and Handling," SAE Technical Paper 2003-01-0966, 2003, doi:10.4271/2003-01-0966.

20. Shapiro, S., Dickerson, C., Arndt, S., Arndt, M. et al., "Error Analysis of Center-of-Gravity Measurement Techniques," SAE Technical Paper 950027, 1995, doi:10.4271/950027.

21. Obenski, K.S., Hill, P.F., Shapiro, E.S., and Debes, J.C., *Motorcycle Accident Reconstruction and Litigation*, 5th ed., (Tucson, AZ: Lawyers and Judges Publishing Company, Inc., 2011), ISBN:978-1-933264-98-1.

22. Motorcycle Industry Council, "Tire Guide: All You Need to Know about Street Motorcycle Tires," https://www.msf-usa.org/downloads/MIC_Tire_Guide_2012V1.pdf, accessed April 6, 2018.

23. Bartlett, W., "Interpretation of Motorcycle Rear-Wheel Skidmarks for Accident Reconstruction," *Proceedings, Fourth International Conference on Accident Investigation, Reconstruction, Interpretation and the Law*, Vancouver, BC, Canada, August 13-16, 2001, ISBN:088865796X.

24. Lambourn, R.F. and Wesley, A., "Motorcycle Tire/Roadway Friction," SAE Technical Paper 2010-01-0054, 2010, doi:10.4271/2010-01-0054.

25. Parks, L., *Total Control: High Performance Street Riding Techniques*, (Minneapolis, MN: MBI Publishing, 2003), ISBN:978-0-7603-1403-6.

26. Hall, G. and Painter, J., "Pavement Friction Reduction Due to Fine-Grained Earth Contaminants," SAE Technical Paper 2007-01-0736, 2007, doi:10.4271/2007-01-0736.

27. Meyers, D. and Austin, T., "Dry Pavement Friction Reductions Due to Sanding Applications," *SAE Int. J. Commer. Veh.* 5, no. 1 (2012): 239-250, doi:10.4271/2012-01-0603.

3

Braking and Acceleration

Motorcycle deceleration during braking is maximized when the rider applies both the front and rear brakes to the maximum extent possible without locking either wheel. During heavy braking, a significant portion of the weight of the motorcycle and rider shift to the front wheel of the motorcycle. This results in the available traction at the front wheel being significantly greater than the available traction at the rear wheel, and thus, the contribution of the front brake to the deceleration is significantly more than the contribution of the rear brake. For a motorcycle without integrated, antilock brakes, a rider's ability to achieve maximum deceleration depends on their skill level. This is because the front and rear brakes are actuated independently and the optimal brake pressure for each brake changes as the weight shifts forward during braking [1].

While expert riders may be able to achieve decelerations approaching or exceeding 1 g on many modern motorcycles, most riders will not be able to achieve this level of deceleration. This is a result of the complex brake actuation required by a rider and the dynamic changing in pressure between the front and rear brakes that needs to occur to maximize braking. The rider needs to roll off the throttle and simultaneously apply both the front and rear brakes. Unless the rider is "covering" the brakes, this requires the rider to move their fingers from the throttle to the front brake lever and their foot from the peg to the rear brake pedal. As they begin to brake, weight shifts to the front of the motorcycle. When this occurs, the rider needs to apply more front brake pressure and less rear brake pressure. The rider needs to modulate the front brake to prevent lockup and to control the rear tire's tendency to lift off the ground. They need to modulate the rear brake to prevent the rear wheel from locking as less weight on the rear tire makes this tire easier to lock. All the while, the rider will be gripping the tank with their knees to maintain body position and keep their butt as far back in the seat as they can to optimize the weight distribution and prevent the rear wheel from lifting. If the rider does lock the front wheel during braking, they will need to react quickly, releasing the brake and starting their brake modulation again. If they lock the rear wheel, the best strategy is typically for the rider to keep it locked until they come to a stop.

3.1 Motorcyclist Braking and Deceleration Capabilities

Tolhurst and McKnight tested and compared five methods of braking in a straight line and three methods of braking in a curve [2]. For all eight methods, the rider applied the front brake to the maximum extent possible without locking the wheel. For the straight-line braking tests, which were run from a nominal speed of 40 mph, the level of rear wheel braking varied as follows: no rear wheel braking, light rear wheel braking, locked rear wheel braking, pumping of the rear brake, and heavy rear wheel braking just below the level necessary to lock the wheel. For the braking in curve tests, which were run from a nominal speed of 30 mph, the level of rear wheel braking varied as follows: no rear wheel braking while keeping the motorcycle leaned, heavy rear wheel braking while keeping the motorcycle leaned, and heavy rear wheel braking while righting the motorcycle.

This study utilized three expert riders operating three different motorcycles—a Yamaha FJ1100 (a sport-touring bike with an approximately 1200 cc engine), a Yamaha 550 Vision (a sport-touring bike with an approximately 500 cc engine), and a Suzuki GS 550. These motorcycles are depicted in Figure 3.1. For the straight-line braking, adding the heavy rear wheel braking to the front wheel braking (below the level necessary to lock the wheel) produced the highest deceleration and the shortest stopping distance. The lowest deceleration and longest stopping distances resulted when only the front brake was applied. This study did not examine rear wheel only braking. For braking in a curve, the highest deceleration and shortest stopping distances were achieved by righting the motorcycle while applying heavy braking to both brakes (without locking the wheels). The lowest deceleration and longest stopping distances were generated by continuing to lean in the curve and not applying any rear brake.

Tolhurst and McKnight noted that there were "highly significant differences among the three [riders]…[these] differences are more easily attributed to differences in the design of motorcycle, particularly the tire 'footprint,' than to the skill of the riders." Unfortunately, they only reported a single average stopping distance for each braking method, and so their article does not enable deeper analysis of motorcycle-to-motorcycle differences.

FIGURE 3.1   Motorcycles used in the testing by Tolhurst and McKnight [2].

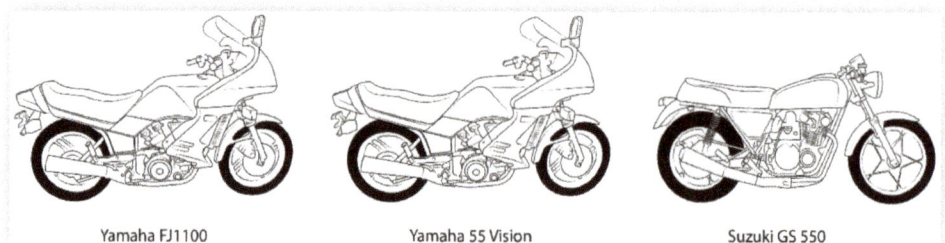

Yamaha FJ1100   Yamaha 55 Vision   Suzuki GS 550

Prem conducted emergency, straight-line braking tests with 59 volunteer riders. He used the Motorcycle Operator Skill Test (MOST) to provide a quantitative assessment of the riders' skill level [3]. The MOST takes the riders through a series of tasks designed to test their steering and braking performance. The braking maneuver from this test required the riders to brake aggressively to a stop from a speed of 32 kph (20 mph). A red signal light was activated to indicate to the riders when they should begin braking. The motorcycles used by the volunteers were instrumented to record the rider's front and rear brake-lever force inputs and motorcycle speed. Prem did not report the make and model of the motorcycle used in this testing.

Prem was interested in determining the differences in braking technique between skilled and less-skilled riders. He found that skilled riders applied higher levels of front brake force than the less-skilled riders. Less-skilled riders preferred the use of the rear brake. The skilled riders also modulated the level of front and rear wheel braking to maintain optimum braking as weight shifted toward the front of the motorcycle during heavy braking. The less-skilled riders maintained a generally constant level of pedal pressure independent of the weight shift. More skilled riders also exhibited shorter braking reaction times.

Fries, Smith, and Cronrath performed testing with five different motorcycles to determine the deceleration of the motorcycles when the rider employed the rear brake only and when the rider employed a combination of front and rear wheel braking [4]. They tested a 1968 Harley-Davidson FLH, a 1978 BMW R90, a 1982 Honda XR500R, a 1972 Honda SL350, and a 1972 Honda SL125S trail bike. These motorcycles are depicted in Figure 3.2. Each motorcycle was tested at nominal speeds of 20, 30, and 40 mph (32.2, 48.3, and 64.4 kph) on worn asphalt. Overall, the deceleration from rear wheel only braking was less than when heavy front wheel braking was also used. The range of deceleration for rear wheel only braking was 0.31 to 0.52 g. The range of deceleration achieved by the riders when they also employed heavy front wheel braking was between 0.54 and 0.88 g.

These authors further stated that "when faced with an emergency stopping situation, or avoidance situation, a motorcycle [rider] has the decision of whether to stop using the rear brake only, front and rear brakes combined, or by laying the motorcycle down. There are several common misconceptions about motorcycles. One is that they will stop faster if they are laid down on their side…. When a motorcycle is stopped by laying it on its side there is a delay in implementing the deceleration…. The test results show that

FIGURE 3.2 Motorcycles used in the testing by Fries, Smith, and Cronrath [4].

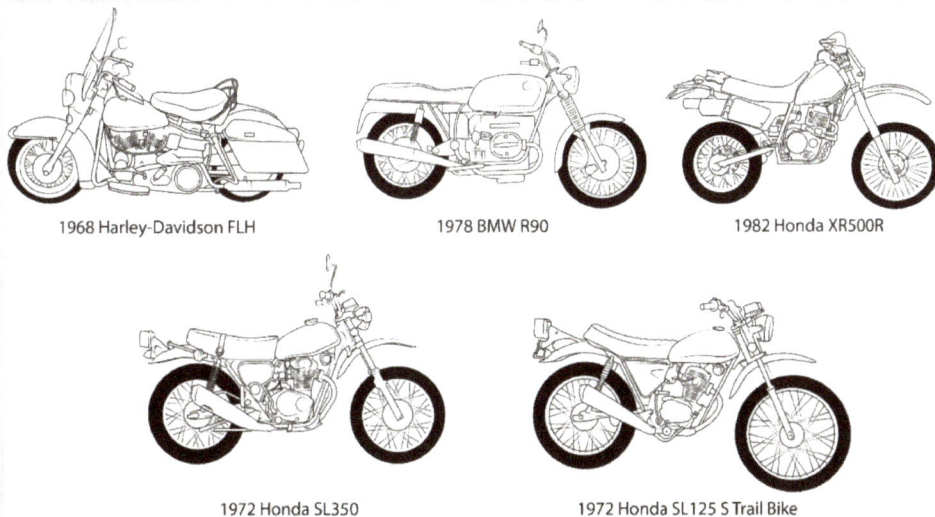

1968 Harley-Davidson FLH   1978 BMW R90   1982 Honda XR500R

1972 Honda SL350   1972 Honda SL125 S Trail Bike

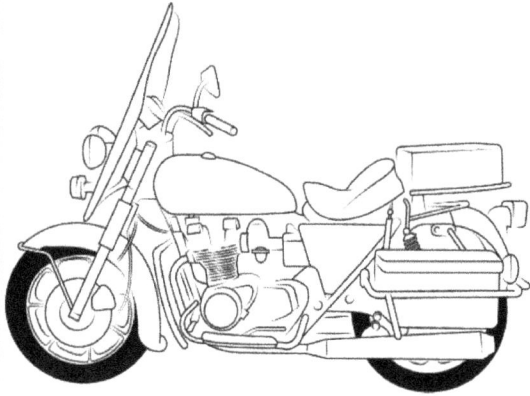

laying a motorcycle over and rear wheel braking have very similar deceleration factors. However, when laying a motorcycle over there is an impact and risk of injury when the motorcycle hits the pavement. Also, all control is lost. If the motorcycle is kept upright, it is possible to reduce braking and steer. Front and rear wheel braking provides the best deceleration factors. Our testing also demonstrates that even during hard braking with front and rear brakes, the experienced driver consistently maintained a straight path without causing the motorcycle to fall…. When a motorcycle rider is presented with an accident situation, proper use of front and rear brakes will produce the most effective stopping…. Laying the bike down results in impact with pavement, total loss of control, and a longer stopping distance."

Hunter reported acceleration and braking tests conducted by the Washington State Patrol on a dry, level roadway with a 1983 and a 1985 Kawasaki 1000 police motorcycle [5]. This motorcycle is depicted in Figure 3.3. For deceleration tests with rear braking only, Hunter reported decelerations between 0.35 and 0.36 g. For deceleration tests with front braking only, Hunter reported decelerations between 0.64 and 0.74 g. For deceleration tests with heavy front and rear braking, Hunter reported decelerations between 0.63 and 0.96 g. For the rapid acceleration tests, Hunter reported accelerations between 0.48 and 0.73 g.

Hugemann and Lange conducted 74 instrumented braking tests with 18 different riders, 15 of whom were riding their own motorcycle [6]. Motorcycle types were not specified. The riders had varying levels of experience (less than 12,500 miles and up to 80,000 miles) and were instructed to brake from 50 kph (31 mph) to a standstill "within the shortest possible distance." Riders characterized as "skilled" exhibited mean decelerations between 0.70 and 0.81 g's. Riders characterized as "novice" exhibited decelerations between 0.44 and 0.52 g's.

Bartlett reported testing with four motorcycles—a Harley-Davidson FXRT, a Yamaha FZ600, a Suzuki Katana 750, and a Kawasaki EX650 [7]. These motorcycles are depicted in Figure 3.4. For tests that utilized only the rear brake, the maximum decelerations between these four motorcycles varied between 0.38 and 0.46 g. For tests that utilized only the front brake, the maximum decelerations varied between 0.88 and 0.89 g. Bartlett reported testing with combined front and rear braking only for the Harley-Davidson. This produced a maximum deceleration of 0.96 g. In this testing, the Yamaha brake pads were deteriorated, resulting in metal-to-metal contact. The maximum deceleration produced with the Yamaha with these deteriorated brake pads was 0.75 g.

Ecker and his colleagues conducted a study comprised of approximately 600 tests performed by more than 300 riders of varying levels of experience (novice to 40+ years) operating an instrumented Honda CB500 [8]. The motorcycle used in this testing is depicted in Figure 3.5. As the riders were operating the Honda around a training facility, the test coordinator would trigger a red light mounted to the instrument cluster, signaling the rider to "make a full stop emergency braking maneuver." The average deceleration for all 600 runs was 0.63 g with a standard deviation of 0.12 g. Assuming a normal distribution, these figures suggest a 68% confidence interval of 0.51 to 0.75 g. Another interesting conclusion of this study was that there was only a minor correlation between braking ability and riding experience, especially for more than 1 year of experience.

Vavryn [9] examined the influence of rider experience level and the effectiveness of antilock braking systems (ABS). He reported the results of 800 tests performed with 181 subjects on two different motorcycles. The riders were asked to "come to a complete stop

FIGURE 3.4 Motorcycles tested by Bartlett [7].

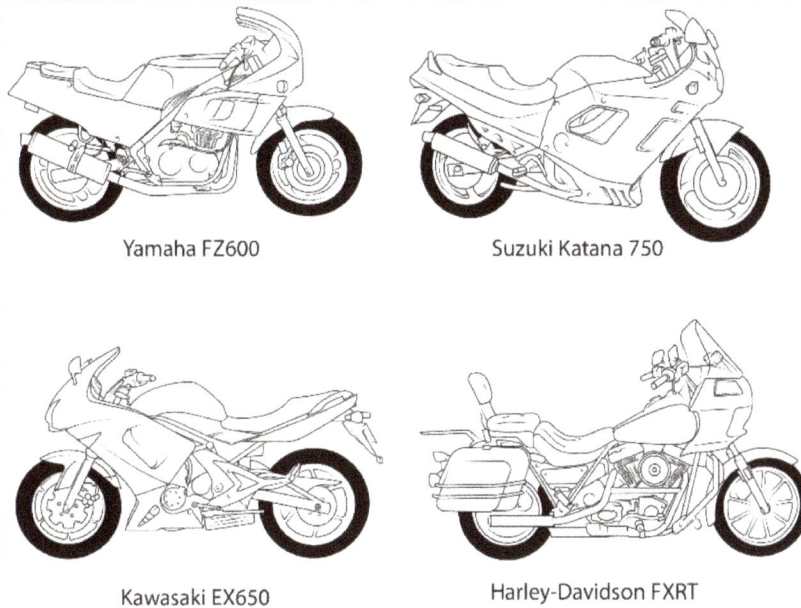

Yamaha FZ600

Suzuki Katana 750

Kawasaki EX650

Harley-Davidson FXRT

as soon as possible without falling off the vehicle." Initial speeds were either 50 or 60 kph (31 or 37 mph), and the subjects performed two tests on their own motorcycle and then two runs on a motorcycle equipped with ABS. One of the ABS-equipped motorcycles was a standard-style BMW, and the other was a scooter equipped with linked ABS. The average deceleration for experienced motorcyclists on their own motorcycle was 0.67 g (SD = 0.14 g). When riding the motorcycles equipped with ABS, that number jumped up to 0.80 g (SD = 0.11 g). Eighty-five percent of the subjects exhibited improved braking with the ABS-equipped motorcycle, and the novice riders achieved almost equal braking decelerations to the experienced riders when operating the ABS-equipped motorcycles. Vavryn also noted that "the deceleration the novice drivers achieved with ABS almost equals the experienced drivers' deceleration. All of the novices improved their deceleration with ABS." Without ABS, the novice riders achieved an average deceleration of 0.57 g.

Bartlett, Baxter, and Robar reported hundreds of brake tests from reconstruction classes conducted at the Institute of Police Technology and Management (IPTM) from between 1987 and 2006 [10]. These tests were conducted at various locations around the country with 112 different motorcycles and riders. They were all conducted on dry asphalt or concrete. Initial speeds in the tests were nominally 20, 30, and 40 mph (32.2, 48.3, and 64.4 kph). The riders in these tests were typically motorcycle unit officers or instructors from a police agency. The data in this study included 275 rear brake only tests, 239 front brake only tests, and 221 tests with combined front and rear braking. This data yielded the conclusion that the decelerations were normally distributed with a mean and standard deviation for the rear only braking of 0.37 g ± 0.06 g, with front only braking of 0.60 g ± 0.16 g, and with combined front and rear wheel braking of 0.74 g ± 0.15 g.

Bartlett and Greer [11] presented brake test data from students in a motorcycle training program

FIGURE 3.5 Honda CB500 used in Ecker's testing [8].

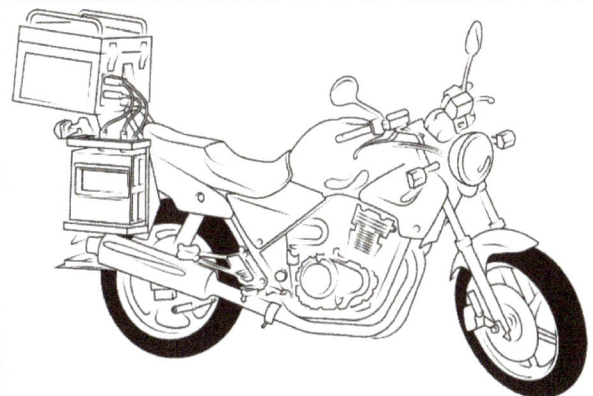

(Skills Training Advantage for Riders from the State of Idaho) with three skill levels—Basic I, Basic II, and Experienced. The authors noted that "the Basic I program is for riders who are new to motorcycling, with virtually no experience, and is conducted on STAR training motorcycles. These bikes are typically 250 cc or smaller, with front disc and rear drum brakes. The Basic II program is for riders who are returning to motorcycling or those who have ridden on dirt, but not on the street, i.e., riders with some experience but not much on street cycles. These riders also use the program's training motorcycles. The Experienced program is for riders who have been riding for more than one year, and is conducted using the riders' own motorcycles."

The culmination of each program was a riding skills test, which included a stopping test. Riders were instructed to approach the stopping area at a steady speed between 15 and 20 mph (24.1 and 32.2 kph). Once in the stopping area, they were to stop the motorcycle as quickly as they could with maximum braking. Bartlett reported the results of 288 tests. The results of these tests "were almost indistinguishable" for the three skill levels. The Basic I group produced decelerations with a mean and standard deviation of 0.60 g ± 0.16 g, the Basic II group produced decelerations of 0.64 g ± 0.14 g, and the Experienced group produced decelerations of 0.61 g ± 0.14 g. The authors note: "The application of this work to reconstruction should not be viewed as a means to interpret speed based on skidmarks. Skidding friction values, to be used when there are marks to measure, have been discussed at length in other articles and publications. Rather, this data should be applied to those circumstances when one is attempting to evaluate how a rider performed or could have performed, given situationally appropriate time and distance limitations based on the scene and circumstances of the event under consideration."

Dunn [12] reported brake test data and tire mark characteristics for the three motorcycles depicted in Figure 3.6—a 1995 BMW R1100RS (sport-touring with antilock brakes), a 2003 Buell XB9R (sport), and a 2005 Harley-Davidson XL 1200 Sportster Custom (cruising/touring). They tested three different braking strategies—best effort front braking only, best effort rear braking only, and best effort front and rear combined braking. Initial speeds for the tests were nominally 25, 45, and 60 mph (40.2, 72.4, and 96.6 kph), and most of the tests were conducted on a flat, dry asphalt surface. One set of tests was conducted on wet asphalt with the BMW, a motorcycle equipped with antilock brakes.

For the BMW, the rear-braking-only strategy produced decelerations between 0.364 and 0.416. The front-braking-only strategy produced decelerations between 0.671 and 0.828. The combined front and rear braking strategy produced decelerations between 0.642 and 0.842. For all three strategies, the decelerations increased with increasing speed. On the wet asphalt surface, the BMW produced decelerations with both brakes between 0.637 and 0.827. For the Buell, the rear-braking-only strategy produced decelerations between 0.345 and 0.380. The front-braking-only strategy produced decelerations between 0.548 and 0.709. The combined front and rear braking strategy produced decelerations between 0.612 and 0.708. Again, for all three strategies, the decelerations increased with increasing speed. For the Harley-Davidson, the

FIGURE 3.6   Motorcycles used in the testing reported by Dunn [12].

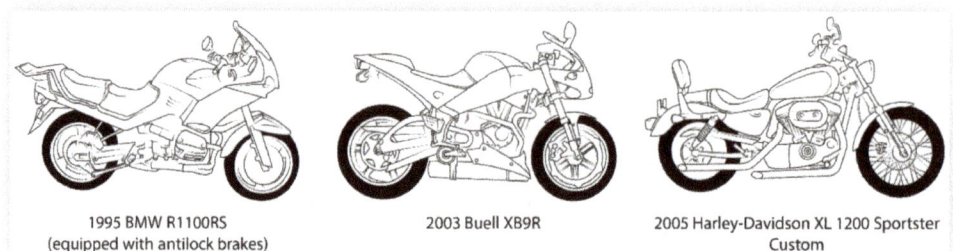

1995 BMW R1100RS
(equipped with antilock brakes)   2003 Buell XB9R   2005 Harley-Davidson XL 1200 Sportster
                                                                  Custom

rear-braking-only strategy produced a deceleration of 0.386 (this strategy was only tested at 45 mph). The front-braking-only strategy produced a deceleration of 0.518 (this strategy was only tested at 45 mph). The combined front and rear braking strategy (tested at 45 and 60 mph) produced decelerations between 0.658 and 0.674.

Dunn found that "at the extreme, the rear tire of the Buell lifted off the ground in some tests." Frank [13] noted that "pitch-over events are common in motorcycle accidents, and can be caused by impact to the front wheel and occasionally by hard brake application.... Provided there is sufficient tire/road friction, at the limit of the braking capacity of the motorcycle the weight on the rear tire is zero. Though not inevitable, this is the point at which the motorcycle can pitch-over." Frank conducted 18 sled tests to evaluate the trajectory and velocity of riders and passengers on motorcycles that pitched over due to braking. This testing used target decelerations of 1.0, 1.15, and 1.3 g, significantly higher decelerations than what could be achieved by most riders. Target speeds for the testing were 20, 30, and 33.5 mph (32.2, 48.3, and 53.9 kph). The lowest braking deceleration that produced a pitch-over in Frank's testing was 1.0 g with a test speed of 30.2 mph (48.6 kph).

Peck, Deyerl, and Rose examined the effect of tire pressure on the deceleration achieved with full application of the rear brake only [14]. This testing utilized a 2003 Suzuki GSF1200 equipped with Michelin Pilot Road radial tires. The tests were run from a nominal speed of 30 mph (48.3 kph)—three tests with the rear tire at 40 psi and three tests with the rear tire at 20 psi. The front tire was inflated to the manufacturer recommended tire pressure of 36 psi for all tests. These authors documented the size of the tire contact patch by using a rear swingarm stand to suspend the rear tire above a piece of brown paper, putting paint on the tire, and then lowering the tire onto the paper. The size of the rear tire contact patch was 46% larger at 20 psi than at 40 psi, and the average deceleration was 5% greater at 20 psi than at 40 psi. For the tests at 40 psi, the three tests yielded the following decelerations (g): 0.324, 0.321, and 0.327 (average = 0.324). For the tests at 20 psi, the three tests yielded the following decelerations (g): 0.341, 0.339, and 0.338 (average = 0.339). These findings related to the influence of tire pressure are consistent with results reported by others for passenger cars [15, 16].

Table 3.1 summarizes the decelerations from the studies reviewed in this section. The decelerations reported in this table can be applied for calculating a motorcycle's speed loss due to maximal braking by the operator.

TABLE 3.1 Summary of braking decelerations from various studies (dry pavement)

Study	Best effort braking decelerations on dry roadway (g)			
	Rear brake only (no ABS)	Front brake only (no ABS)	Front and rear combined (no ABS)	Front and rear with ABS
Tolhurst and McKnight [2]		0.764	0.935	
Fries et al. [4]	0.31 to 0.52		0.54 to 0.88	
Hunter [5]	0.35 to 0.36	0.64 to 0.74	0.63 to 0.96	
Hugemann and Lange [6]				
Bartlett [7]	0.38 to 0.46	0.88 to 0.89	0.96	
Ecker et al. [8]			0.63 ± 0.12	
Vavryn and Winkelbauer [9]			0.67	0.8
Bartlett et al. [10]	0.37 ± 0.06	0.60 ± 0.16	0.74 ± 0.15	
Anderson et al. [21]	0.42	0.65	0.71	0.93
Dunn et al. [12]	0.345 to 0.386	0.518 to 0.709	0.612 to 0.708	0.642 to 0.842
Peck et al. [14]	0.321 to 0.341			
Summary (min to max)	0.31 to 0.52	0.52 to 0.89	0.54 to 0.96	0.64 to 0.842

For many crashes, the braking precedes an impact, and there may be zero, one, or two tire marks deposited by this braking. The following equation can be used to calculate the speed of the motorcycle at the onset of maximal braking or skidding (v_{skid}):

$$v_{skid} = \sqrt{2 f_{skid} g d_{skid} + v_{impact}^2} \qquad (3.1)$$

In this equation,

> f_{skid} is the deceleration of the motorcycle during the skidding or maximal braking in gravitational units
> g is the gravitational acceleration
> d_{skid} is the length of the skid mark(s)
> v_{impact} is the speed of the motorcycle at impact

The impact speed would be determined using methods discussed in a later chapter.

3.1.1 Motorcycles with Integrated, Linked, and Antilock Braking Systems

For an integrated braking system, the lever on the right handlebar actuates the front brake only, and the right-side pedal actuates both the front and the rear brakes. For an independent ABS, the front and rear brakes are controlled independently, but the antilock system prevents either wheel from locking. For an integrated ABS, both brakes are applied regardless of which lever is used, and the antilock system prevents either wheel from locking. For a linked braking system, found only on Honda motorcycles, application of the right-hand lever or pedal will actuate both the front and rear brakes. On this system, the proportioning of the brakes varies with the lever that is used.

Baxter and Robar observed that "the integrated brake system is not very popular with experienced riders. Many operators like to have the option of independent braking on their machines, particularly on surfaces such as gravel and other loose material. Owners unhappy with the integrated systems often replace the integrated parts with parts from sister models that use the standard brake components" [17]. Baxter and Robar noted that, in 1988, BMW became the first manufacturer to offer a motorcycle with an antilock brake system. Yamaha followed in 1991 and Honda in 1996. Baxter and Robar noted that, starting in 2003, Ducati offered an antilock brake system with an on-off switch, giving the operator control over whether the ABS system is active or not. BMW also offered an on-off switch on some of their models. In 2008, Harley-Davidson began offering an optional ABS system with independently controlled front and back brakes.

Mortimer examined the effectiveness of integrated brakes without ABS [18]. His testing utilized a 1979 Yamaha XS-400 with standard brakes as the original equipment and a 1982 Yamaha XS-1100 with integrated brakes as the original equipment. Mortimer modified both motorcycles so that they could be operated in either a standard braking mode or an integrated braking mode. The integrated mode on the XS-400 could only be operated with the right-side rear brake foot pedal. On the XS-1100, the integrated braking would be activated with either the right-side foot pedal or hand lever. Five experienced riders were used in Mortimer's testing. Tests were run from a nominal speed of 25 mph (40.3 kph), and the riders attempted to stop the motorcycle in as short a distance as possible. Each rider performed testing on each motorcycle, and they made five stops in each test condition. The tests were run with the hand brake only, the foot brake only, and then both.

Mortimer noted that "the stopping distances were directly measured at the point where the motorcycle came to a stop in terms of the distance from the cones marking the entrance to the braking course. The stopping distance was translated into the mean deceleration during the stop, assuming an initial speed of 40.3 km/h." This manner of measuring the stopping distance and deceleration is prone to error since there is no way to know, in any given instance, if the riders began braking at the cone or to know that the rider started braking from a speed of precisely 40.3 kph (25 mph). Mortimer found the greatest benefit from integrated brakes for the condition of braking with the foot pedal only. He noted that "use of the foot brake alone of the XS-400 motorcycle produced a 72% greater mean deceleration in the integrated than the separated mode. Similarly, use of the foot brake of the XS-1100 motorcycle in the integrated mode produced a 50% increase in mean deceleration compared with the separated mode.... In addition, when both brakes were used on the larger motorcycle there were significant and consistent increases in deceleration obtained on both the dry and wet pavements in the integrated mode compared with the separated mode, but the increments were not as large as those found for the operation of the foot brake alone."

Vavryn [9] examined the effectiveness of ABS, reporting the results of 800 tests performed with 181 subjects on two different motorcycles. The riders were asked to "come to a complete stop as soon as possible without falling off the vehicle." Initial speeds were either 50 or 60 kph (31 or 37 mph), and the subjects performed two tests on their own motorcycle, and then two runs on a motorcycle equipped with ABS. One of the ABS bikes was a standard BMW, while the other was a scooter equipped with linked ABS. The average braking deceleration for motorcyclists on their own motorcycle was 0.67 g (SD = 0.14 g). However, when riding the motorcycles equipped with ABS, that number jumped up to 0.80 g (SD = 0.11 g). Eighty-five percent of the subjects exhibited improved braking with the ABS-equipped motorcycle, and the novice riders achieved almost equal braking decelerations to the experienced riders when operating the ABS-equipped motorcycles.

Green reported a test program conducted by NHTSA, in cooperation with Transport Canada (TC), "to assess the effectiveness of antilock braking systems (ABS) and combined braking systems (CBS) on motorcycles" [19]. Six motorcycles were tested on both dry and wet asphalt–a 2002 Honda VFR 800 with ABS and CBS, a 2002 BMW F650 with ABS, a 2002 BMW R 1150R with ABS and CBS, a 2002 BMW R 1150R without ABS or CBS, a 2004 Yamaha FJR1300 with ABS, and a 2004 Yamaha FJR1300 without ABS. Green observed that, with ABS, "the stopping distances were very consistent from one run to another." Without ABS, "the stopping distances were less consistent because the rider while modulating the brake force, had to deal with many additional variables at the same time.... Test results from non-ABS were noticeably more sensitive to rider performance variability." On average, ABS reduced the stopping distances by approximately 5%.

Another way to evaluate the effectiveness of motorcycle antilock brakes is to examine its effect on crash rates. Rizzi et al. conducted this kind of study for crashes in Spain, Italy, and Sweden [20]. Rizzi noted that the European Parliament has made ABS mandatory for all new motorcycles over 125 cc, effective in 2016. Using police-reported crashes from 2006 to 2009 in Spain, 2009 in Italy, and 2003 to 2012 in Sweden, Rizzi concluded that "the effectiveness of motorcycle ABS in reducing injury crashes ranged from 24% in Italy to 29% in Spain and 34% in Sweden.... The reduction of severe and fatal crashes was even greater, at 34% and 42% in Spain and Sweden, respectively."

Anderson, Baxter, and Robar [21] reported additional deceleration testing of motorcycles with the following different braking systems: standard brakes (1990 Harley-Davidson Road King FLHTPI), integrated brakes without ABS (1986 Yamaha Venture

TABLE 3.2 Summary of braking decelerations for various systems [21]

	Average deceleration (g)				
	Standard	**Integrated**	**ABS**	**Integrated ABS**	**Linked**
Pedal only	0.42	0.58	0.40	0.98	0.62
Hand lever only	0.65	0.74	0.89	0.92	0.86
Both levers	0.71	0.88	0.93	1.00	0.93

Royale XVZ13), independent ABS brakes (1999 BMW R1100RPT), integrated ABS brakes, and linked brakes (2003 Honda VFR800 Interceptor). The authors tested each of these systems on an asphalt surface (automobile $\mu = 0.83$) with application of the rear pedal only, the front lever only, and with both levers applied. The initial speed for the tests was approximately 56 kph. All the tests utilized the same operator with many years of riding experience. The authors noted that "there was no wheel lockup or skidding during any of the tests runs." Table 3.2 summarizes the results of the testing for each braking system.

Anderson, Baxter, and Robar concluded that "motorcycle braking systems that actuate both front and rear brakes with the application of only one control lever produce more effective braking than independent front and rear brakes on a standard system. When combined with antilock control the benefits of the combined system are increased. Perhaps more importantly, however, is that the motorcycle is also more stable during the braking maneuver. The increased stability along with the simplified brake application combine to reduce the load on the operator during the stressful moment of hard braking to avoid a crash. The operator does not have to concentrate on modulating pressure between two separate controls and simultaneously keep the motorcycle stable and prevent the wheels from locking, as the system performs these functions and permits the operator to focus on avoiding the crash."

Basch, Moore, and Hellinga examined the effectiveness of motorcycle ABS in terms of crash rates [22]. They noted that while prior studies had reported lower crash rates for motorcycles equipped with ABS, these studies had not considered the possibility that "safer" riders are more likely to purchase motorcycles equipped with ABS, and thus, riders with ABS-equipped motorcycles were already less likely to crash. In this study, insurance auto claim frequency was used as a proxy for the crash risk of individual riders. The authors concluded, first, that "there was no evidence that safer riders, as measured by auto claim frequency, were more likely to purchase motorcycles with optional ABS. Rather, riders with higher auto claim frequencies were more likely to ride motorcycles with ABS." Further, they concluded that "after controlling for auto claim frequency, motorcycles equipped with optional ABS were associated with a 21 percent reduction in claim frequency compared with similar motorcycles without ABS."

Dinges and Hoover [23] reported a series of maximal braking tests on a dry, asphalt surface with and without the antilock brakes active on a 2011 BMW S1000RR (a super sport motorcycle). This motorcycle was tested in three modes related to the ABS—sport mode, race mode, and ABS disabled. The BMW was equipped with partially integrated braking when the ABS was active. When the ABS was deactivated, the integral braking was also deactivated. These authors reported a coefficient of friction for the test surface of 0.7, measured using a Ford Expedition with the ABS disabled. Their testing yielded 420 braking runs, with target speeds ranging from 40 to 60 mph. Table 3.3 lists the average decelerations reported by Dinges and Hoover for each mode with three braking conditions—rear brake only, front brake only, and front and rear braking combined.

TABLE 3.3 Average decelerations reported by Dinges and Hoover

	Rear brake only	Front brake only	Front and rear combined
ABS off	0.37	0.79	0.79
Race mode ABS	0.40	0.80	0.80
Sport mode ABS	0.38	0.76	0.72

In addition to these decelerations, Dinges and Hoover reported hydraulic pressure build times, noting that "the average time it takes to build pressure in the front brake system is between 0.2 and 0.3 seconds.... The rear brake system is similar, but a range of 0.2 to 0.4 seconds is shown from the data."

3.1.2 What Deceleration Can Motorcyclists Be Expected to Achieve?

Crash reconstructionists are frequently asked to determine how a crash could have been avoided. In conducting this analysis, there will be instances in which an assumption will be made about the level of deceleration a motorcyclist should have been able to achieve. Based on the data summarized in Table 3.1, motorcyclists would be able to achieve a deceleration of 0.5 g and above by utilizing only their front brakes. By utilizing both brakes, most motorcyclists will typically be able to achieve a deceleration of 0.6 g and above. That said, the level of deceleration that can be achieved during a specific emergency must consider conditions present that may have affected a rider's ability to achieve these expected levels. External factors such as roadway conditions, other traffic, the presence of cargo or passengers, or what the specific avoidance decision a rider makes may need to be considered when assigning an expected braking level to a specific crash scenario.

Another way to look at this question is to examine what braking skill level is required by the states to issue an endorsement to operate a motorcycle. In other words, when a motorcyclist takes a state licensing exam, what level of deceleration is required to successfully complete the braking portion of the test? Consider the Quick Stop, one of several skills tests that are evaluated and scored when a student attempts to obtain a license. The student accelerates from a stop up to a speed between 12 and 18 mph, in second gear. The student then maintains that speed until the front wheel of the motorcycle reaches the cue cones. When the front wheel reaches the cue cones, the student applies both the front and rear brakes, downshifts to first gear, and stops as quickly and safely as possible. If a student does not stop within the standard distance for their speed, points are added for each additional foot of travel. Only so many points can be accrued during the licensing skills test before the student reaches a failing score. The standard distance equates to them achieving a deceleration of approximately 0.51 to 0.61g. Additional points can be added for other errors such as failing to use both brakes, failing to downshift to first gear, going too slow, or anticipating the cue cones by braking early.

3.2 Motorcycle and Rider Acceleration Capabilities

Bartlett [24] studied motorcycle accelerations and reported that "maximum motorcycle acceleration rates are highly nonlinear.... In a perfect world, the investigator will have access to the accident motorcycle or an identical unit for testing with reliable and accurate

TABLE 3.4 Bartlett's motorcycle acceleration equations

Parameter	Equation	R^2
Quarter mile time (lb/hp < 30)	$t = 6.5729 \cdot x^{0.278}$	0.97
Quarter mile speed (lb/hp < 30)	$S = 239.90 \cdot x^{-0.351}$	0.97
Quarter mile time (lb/hp > 30)	$t = 5.9504 \cdot x^{0.322}$	0.90
Quarter mile speed (lb/hp > 30)	$S = 172.78 \cdot x^{-0.267}$	0.70
0–30 mph	$t = 0.0023x^2 - 0.01x + 1.23$	0.78
0–60 mph	$t = 0.0067x^2 - 0.1x + 2.13$	0.97
0–90 mph	$t = 0.0342x^2 - 0.1x + 3.47$	0.89
0–100 mph	$t = 0.0312x^2 - 0.45x + 2.55$	0.92

measurement equipment. In the real world, though, this is often not the case. This leaves the investigator to review published data on their motorcycle capabilities." Bartlett discussed two techniques reconstructionists could use to estimate accelerations for a motorcycle. However, these techniques only provide a maximum rate.

The first technique is applicable to instances when the reconstructionists has access to some time/speed data, typically from an enthusiast magazine. In this instance, Bartlett proposed that the analyst should (1) plot the data points available as speed versus time, (2) determine the best-fit curve for the speed versus time data, (3) calculate the predicted speed for every 0.1 s using the equation for the best-fit curve, (4) calculate the distance covered in each 0.1 s, and (5) calculate the cumulative distance across the data.

The second technique is applicable to instances when no time/speed data is available. In this instance, Bartlett suggests that the analyst should determine the combined weight of the motorcycle (wet) and rider and the motorcycle's horsepower. Bartlett noted that "the horsepower measured at the rear wheel using the most common type of dynamometer is commonly expected to be about 85% of that reported at the crankshaft due to losses in the driveline. In the current analysis, comparing 30 such pairs of claimed/measured data from published sources reveals the average loss from the claimed value to be approximately 13%, which matches the expectation quite well. If only published 'crankshaft' or 'claimed' horsepower values are available, they should be degraded by 15% to approximate rear wheel horsepower." Bartlett reported the following table of equations (Table 3.4). In these equations x is the weight-to-horsepower ratio. These equations yield points for use with the first technique.

These equations can be used to place an upper limit on the speed a motorcycle could have been traveling in scenarios where a crash was preceded by the motorcycle accelerating. However, in most situations, motorcyclists will not choose or be able to utilize the full acceleration capabilities of their motorcycles.

3.3 Determining Speed Based on Gear

In certain instances, on-scene investigators will document the gear the motorcycle was in at the time of the crash. If not, this determination can sometimes be made during a later inspection of the motorcycle. If the reconstructionist can determine the gear the motorcycle was in at the time of a collision or loss of control, this information can be used to place an upper limit on the speed of the motorcycle [25]. To make this determination, the analyst will need to determine the rolling radius of the rear tire of the motorcycle (r_{rear}), the maximum engine speed in rotations per minute ($S_{rpm,max}$), the primary reduction ratio (r_{pr}), the final reduction ratio (r_{fr}), and the gear ratio for the gear of interest (r_i). The primary reduction ratio is the reduction that occurs from the engine to the transmission. The final reduction ratio is the ratio of the crank sprocket to the wheel sprocket. Assuming the rolling radius of the rear tire of the motorcycle has been obtained in units of inches, Equation (3.2) will yield the distance this tire rolls for each revolution, in units of feet (c_{rear}). Then, Equation (3.3) will yield the maximum road speed ($S_{road,max}$) for the gear of interest, in units of mph.

$$c_{rear} = \frac{2\pi \cdot r_{rear}}{12} \tag{3.2}$$

$$S_{road,max} = \frac{S_{rpm,max}}{r_{pr} \cdot r_{fr} \cdot r_i} \cdot c_{rear} \cdot \frac{60}{5,280} \tag{3.3}$$

In applying the results of these calculations, the reconstructionist should keep in mind that a motorcyclist may downshift during pre-collision braking.

3.3.1 Case Study: Determining Speed Based on Gear

To test the accuracy of Equation (3.3), physical testing was conducted to determine the maximum speed of a 2008 Lifan 200GY-5 dual-sport motorcycle (Figure 3.7) in each of its five gears. This motorcycle had a 15 horsepower, 200 cc single cylinder gasoline engine, a five-speed manual transmission, and original equipment tires. The engine on this motorcycle reaches the redline at 10,500 rpms. Manufacturer specifications were obtained to determine the gearing parameters for this motorcycle. The manufacturer specifications also reported that this motorcycle had a maximum speed of 100 kph (62 mph). The maximum engine speed was controlled by an ignition limiter.

Additional parameters used in the gear train calculations are included in Table 3.5. Static testing was conducted, and it was determined that the rear tire would compress approximately 0.7 in. with a rider sitting on the motorcycle. In the calculations, this value was reduced slightly—to 0.5 in.—in recognition of tire recovery that would occur

FIGURE 3.7 Lifan motorcycle utilized for physical testing.

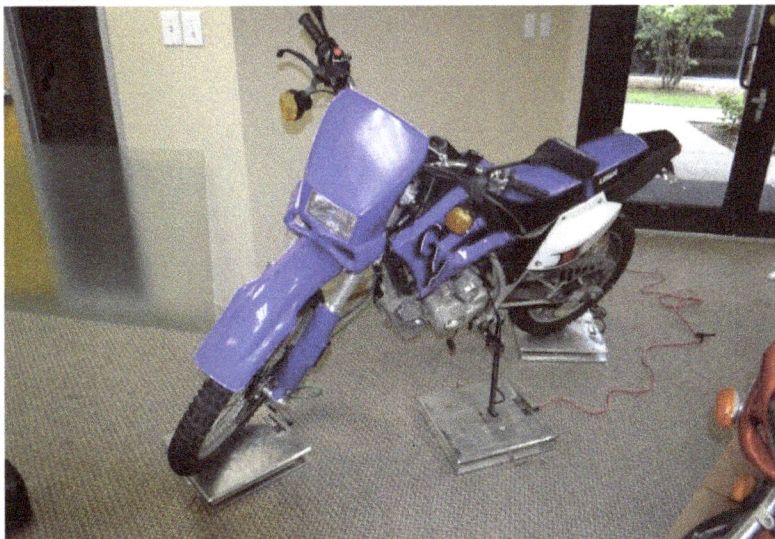

TABLE 3.5 Gearing parameters for the Lifan motorcycle

Theoretical rear tire diameter (in.)	24.9
Rear tire compression (in.)	0.5
Rear tire diameter (ft)	2.03
Tire rolling distance/rev (ft)	6.39
Engine idle speed (rpm)	1500
Maximum engine speed (rpm)	10500
Maximum road speed (km/h)	100.0
Maximum road speed (mph)	62.1
Primary reduction ratio	3.333
Final reduction ratio	2.706
Gear ratio, first gear	2.769
Gear ratio, second gear	1.882
Gear ratio, third gear	1.400
Gear ratio, fourth gear	1.130
Gear ratio, fifth gear	0.960

at speed. The calculations based on Equation (3.3) are included below in Table 3.6. These calculations provided the road speed for each gear and rpm combination over the range of 7500 to 10,500 rpm (in 250 rpm increments). These calculations predicted that the motorcycle would reach a maximum speed of approximately 29.9 mph in first gear, 44.0 mph in second gear, 59.1 mph in third gear, 62 mph in fourth gear, and 62 mph in fifth gear.

Prior to testing, the Lifan motorcycle was warmed to operating temperature, and the tires were checked to verify they were inflated to manufacturer specifications. Testing was performed on a nearly flat roadway at Front Range Airport in Watkins, CO, on August 1, 2017. Each test run consisted of accelerating the motorcycle up to its maximum speed for a given gear with the operator attempting to achieve the greatest acceleration possible. Each gear was tested in both directions on the roadway, since the road had a slight grade. This allowed for any roadway grade effects on the speed test results to be eliminated. A VBOX Sport data acquisition system was attached to the motorcycle to document vehicle speed during each run. The motorcycle operator also wore a chest-mounted Go-Pro camera to document the engine speed as reported by an aftermarket digital tachometer. Five separate tests were completed by the operator—one for each gear.

The data from each of the five test runs is depicted in Figure 3.8. Time is plotted on the horizontal axis and speed on the vertical axis. In first gear, the motorcycle achieved an average maximum speed of approximately 30.3, 0.3 mph greater than what Equation (3.3) predicted. In second gear, the motorcycle achieved an average maximum speed of approximately 43.6 mph, 0.4 mph lower than what Equation (3.3) predicted. In third gear, the motorcycle achieved an average maximum speed of 54.4 mph, approximately 4.7 mph lower than what Equation (3.3) would predict for a redline engine speed of 10,500 rpm. However, in third gear, the video revealed that the maximum engine speed was limited to approximately 9800 rpm. At this engine speed, Equation (3.3) predicted a speed of 55.2 mph, 0.8 mph greater than what was achieved. In fourth gear, the motorcycle achieved an average maximum speed of 58.4 mph. In fourth gear, the video revealed that the maximum engine speed was limited to approximately 8300 rpm. At this engine speed, Equation (3.3) predicts a road speed of 57.9 mph, 0.5 mph less than what was achieved.

In fifth gear, the motorcycle achieved an average maximum speed of 59.9 mph. This was the run with the greatest discrepancy between the downhill and uphill directions. In the downhill direction, the motorcycle achieved a speed of 62.4 mph and, in the uphill direction, a speed of 57.4 mph. In fifth gear, the video revealed that the maximum engine

TABLE 3.6 Gear train calculations for the Lifan motorcycle

	Engine speed (rpm)												
Gear	7500	7750	8000	8250	8500	8750	9000	9250	9500	9750	10,000	10,250	10,500
1	21.35	22.06	22.78	23.49	24.20	24.91	25.62	26.34	27.05	27.76	28.47	29.18	29.89
2	31.42	32.46	33.51	34.56	35.61	36.65	37.70	38.75	39.79	40.84	41.89	42.94	43.98
3	42.23	43.64	45.05	46.46	47.86	49.27	50.68	52.09	53.50	54.90	56.31	57.72	59.13
4	52.32	54.07	55.81	57.56	59.30	61.05	62.79	64.53	66.28	68.02	69.77	71.51	73.25
5	61.59	63.64	65.70	67.75	69.80	71.86	73.91	75.96	78.01	80.07	82.12	84.17	86.23

FIGURE 3.8 Curves for testing of top speed in each gear.

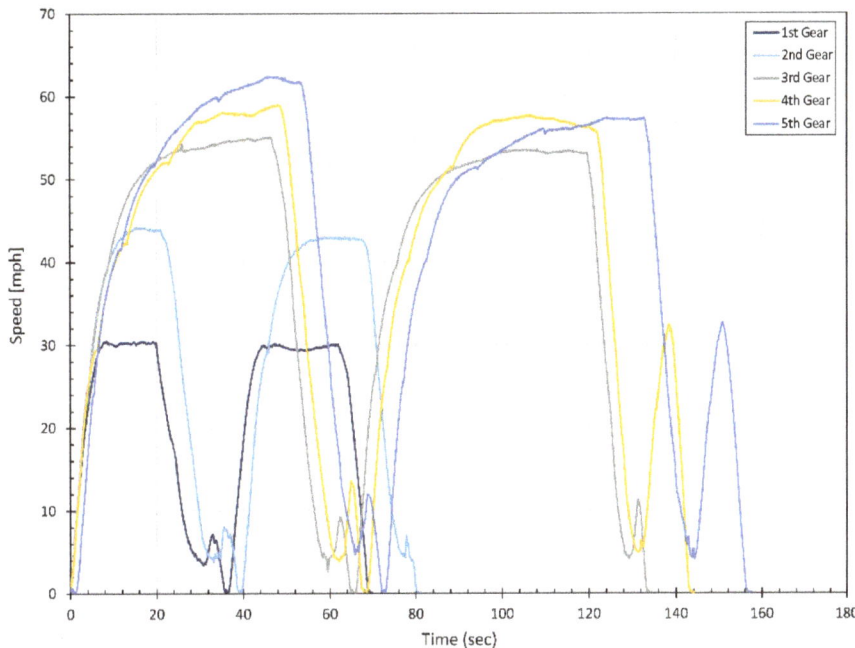

TABLE 3.7 Summary of the results from testing of the Lifan motorcycle

Gear	Calculated maximum speed (mph)	As tested maximum speed (mph)	Difference, calculated versus actual (mph)	Percent difference
1	29.9	30.3	−0.4	−1.3%
2	44.0	43.6	+0.4	+0.9%
3	55.2	54.4	+0.8	+1.5%
4	57.9	58.4	−0.5	−0.9%
5	62	59.9	+2.1	+3.4%

speed was limited to approximately 7600 rpm. At this engine speed, Equation (3.3) predicts a road speed should be able to reach the maximum of 62 mph, 2.1 mph greater than the average of what was achieved, but in line with the downhill maximum. Thus, Equation (3.3) provided a reasonable estimate of the maximum speed achievable in each gear, as long as the analyst recognized the rpm limits in each gear. Unfortunately, in this instance, this required testing of the motorcycle, which would eliminate the need for Equation (3.3). This likely would not be an issue for a more powerful motorcycle because the rpm limits would be higher. The maximum error was the 2.1 mph in fifth gear. This is a 3.4% overestimate. These results are summarized in Table 3.7.

References

1. Cossalter, V., Lot, R., and Maggio, F., "On the Braking Behavior of Motorcycles," SAE Technical Paper Number 2004-32-0018, 2004, doi:10.4271/2004-32-0018.

2. Tolhurst, N. and McKnight, A., "Motorcycle Braking Methods," SAE Technical Paper 860020, 1986, doi:10.4271/860020.

3. Prem, H., "The Emergency Straight-Path Braking Behaviour of Skilled versus Less-Skilled Motorcycle Riders," SAE Technical Paper 871228, 1987, doi:10.4271/871228.

4. Fries, T.R., Smith, J.R., and Cronrath, K.M., "Stopping Characteristics for Motorcycles in Accident Situations," SAE Technical Paper 890734, 1989, doi:10.4271/890734.

5. Hunter, J.E., "The Application of the G-Analyst to Motorcycle Acceleration and Deceleration," SAE Technical Paper 901525, 1990, doi:10.4271/901525.

6. Hugemann, W. and Lange, F., "Braking Performance of Motorcyclists," 1993, http://www.calculamus.de/pdf/vuf_1993_motorcycle_englisch.pdf.

7. Bartlett, W., "Motorcycle Braking and Skidmarks," Mechanical Forensics Engineering Services, LLC, 2000, unpublished article available at https://www.mfes.com/motorcyclebraking.html, accessed June 1, 2017.

8. Ecker, H., Wasserman, J., Hauer, G. et al., "Braking Deceleration of Motorcycle Riders," *International Motorcycle Safety Conference*, Orlando, FL, March 1-4, 2001.

9. Vavryn, K. and Winkelbauer, M., "Braking Performance of Experienced and Novice Motorcycle Riders – Results of a Field Study," *International Conference on Traffic & Transport Psychology*, Nottingham, England, 2004.

10. Bartlett, W., Baxter, A., and Robar, N., "Motorcycle Braking Tests: IPTM Data through 2006," *Accident Reconstruction Journal*, July/August 2007, ISSN: 1057-8153.

11. Bartlett, W. and Greer, C., "Braking Rates for Students in a Motorcycle Training Program," *Accident Reconstruction Journal* 20, no. 6 (November/December 2010), ISSN: 1057-8153.

12. Dunn, A.L. et al., "Analysis of Motorcycle Braking Performance and Associated Braking Marks," SAE Technical Paper 2012-01-0610, 2012, doi:10.4271/2012-01-0610.

13. Frank, T., Smith, J., Hansen, D., and Werner, S., "Motorcycle Rider Trajectory in Pitch-Over Brake Applications and Impacts," *SAE Int. J. Passeng. Cars - Mech. Syst.* 1, no. 1 (2009): 31-42, doi:10.4271/2008-01-0164.

14. Peck, L., Deyerl, E., and Rose, N., "The Effect of Tire Pressure on the Deceleration Rate of a Motorcycle Under Application of the Rear Brake Only," *Accident Reconstruction Journal*, July/August 2017, ISSN: 1057-8153.

15. Baumann, F.W., Schreier, H., and Simmermacher, D., "Tire Mark Analysis of a Modern Passenger Vehicle with Respect to Tire Variation, Tire Pressure and Chassis Control Systems," SAE Technical Paper 2009-01-0100, 2009, doi:10.4271/2009-01-0100.

16. Rievaj, V., Vrabel, J., and Hudak, A., "Tire Inflation Pressure Influence on a Vehicle Stopping Distances," *International Journal of Traffic and Transportation Engineering* 2, no. 2 (2013): 9-13, doi:10.5923/j.ijtte.20130202.01.

17. Baxter, A. and Robar, N., "An Examination of the Performance of Motorcycle Brake Systems," *Accident Investigation Quarterly*, no. 47 (2007): 28-31, ISSN: 1082-6521.

18. Mortimer, R., "Braking Performance of Motorcyclists with Integrated Brake Systems," SAE Technical Paper 861384, 1986, doi:10.4271/861384.

19. Green, D., "A Comparison of Stopping Distance Performance for Motorcycles Equipped with ABS, CBS and Conventional Hydraulic Brake Systems," *USDOT, NHTSA, International Motorcycle Safety Conference*, Long Beach, CA, March 2006.

20. Rizzi, M., Strandroth, J., and Tingball, C., "The Effectiveness of Antilock Brake Systems on Motorcycles in Reducing Real-Life Crashes and Injuries," *Traffic Injury Prevention* 10 (2009): 479-487, doi:10.1080/15389580903149292.

21. Anderson, B., Baxter, A., and Robar, N., "Comparison of Motorcycle Braking System Effectiveness," SAE Technical Paper 2010-01-0072, 2010, doi:10.4271/2010-01-0072.

22. Basch, N., Moore, M., and Hellinga, L., "Evaluation of Motorcycle Antilock Braking Systems," *The 24th Enhanced Safety of Vehicles Conference*, Paper Number 15-0256, Gothenburg, Sweden, June 2015.

23. Dinges, J. and Hoover, T., "A Comparison of Motorcycle Braking Performance with and without Anti-Lock Braking on Dry Surfaces," SAE Technical Paper 2018-01-0520, 2018, doi:10.4271/2018-01-0520.

24. Bartlett, W., "Estimating Maximum Motorcycle Acceleration Rates," *Collision* 6, no. 1 (2011), ISSN: 1934-8681.

25. Baxter, A.T., *Motorcycle Crash Investigation*, (Jacksonville, FL: Institute of Police Technology and Management, 2017), ISBN:978-1-934807-18-7.

4

Cornering and Swerving

A curve, a reconstructionist may need to calculate the lean angle that a motorcyclist would have achieved to traverse their chosen path at a given speed. In some instances, calculating this lean angle can reveal the degree to which a rider was operating at the limits of the motorcycle's capabilities or at their own psychological (or willingness) limits. This analysis may reveal factors that contributed to a crash. Similarly, in evaluating a motorcyclist's ability to avoid a crash, a reconstructionist may need to analyze the distance that would be required for a motorcyclist to swerve laterally or make a lane change. This chapter introduces equations that can be used to analyze cornering, swerving, and lane change maneuvers.

4.1 Analysis of a Motorcycle Traversing a Curve

The lean angle required for a motorcycle traversing a curved path is the angle that brings the overturning moment generated by the tire frictional forces into balance with the opposing moment generated by the tire forces perpendicular to the road surface. The required lean angle increases with increasing speed and decreasing path radius.

Fricke [1] and Cossalter [2] report that the lean angle of a motorcycle for a given path and speed can be calculated with the following equation:

$$\theta = \tan^{-1}\left(\frac{v_{mc}^2}{g \cdot r}\right) \tag{4.1}$$

In this equation:

θ is the lean angle of the motorcycle
v_{mc} is the forward velocity of the motorcycle
g is the gravitational acceleration
r is the path radius

This equation assumes that the motorcycle is traveling a steady speed high enough that the rider is using countersteering to initiate the lean, that the rider is leaning at the same angle as the motorcycle, and that the part of the tire contacting the road does not change as the motorcycle leans. For a real motorcycle tire, as the motorcycle leans, the portion of the tire contacting the road will change.

4.1.1 Incorporating Roadway Superelevation

Rose, Carter, and Pentecost derived a form of Equation (4.1) that included the roadway superelevation and yielded the lean angle relative to the road surface [3]. In deriving this equation, they used the nomenclature identified in Figure 4.1, which is a diagram of a motorcyclist traversing a leftward curve with a superelevation. The superelevation angle has been given the symbol ϕ, and θ designates the lean angle of the motorcycle relative to the road surface. Thus, the lean angle of the motorcycle and rider relative to the vertical direction is $\phi + \theta$. In this derivation, counterclockwise rotations are positive, and therefore, the superelevation and lean angles for a leftward curve are positive. Figure 4.1 also depicts the forces applied to the cornering motorcycle—the combined weight of the motorcycle and rider applied at their effective center of mass (W), the lateral friction force ($F_{friction}$) applied at the tire contact patch, and the normal force (F_{normal}) also applied at the tire contact patch.

To remain in equilibrium as it traverses the curve, the resultant of the normal and friction forces must act along the line connecting the tire contact patch to the center of mass of the motorcycle and rider. For this to be the case, the friction and normal forces will be related to the lean angle as defined by the following equation:

$$F_{friction} = F_{normal} \cdot \tan \theta \tag{4.2}$$

Newton's second law dictates that the sum of the forces in the lateral direction is equal to the mass multiplied by the lateral acceleration:

$$\sum F_{lat} = m \cdot a_{lat} \tag{4.3}$$

By examination of Figure 4.1, it can be seen that:

$$\sum F_{lat} = F_{lat} \cdot \sin \phi + F_{friction} \cdot \cos \phi \tag{4.4}$$

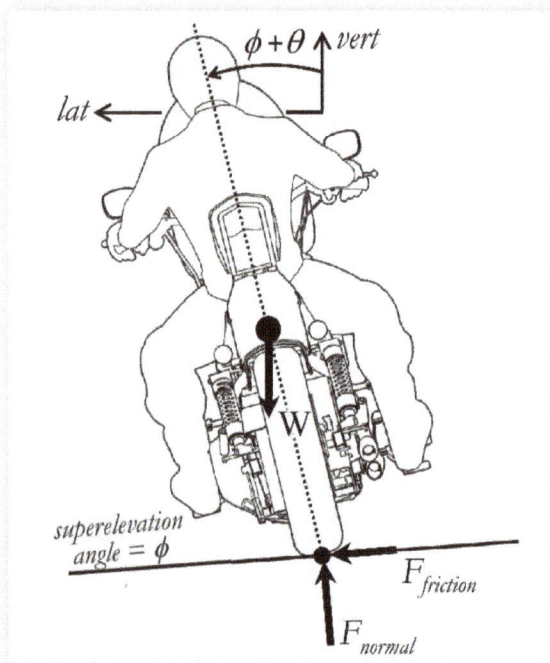

FIGURE 4.1 Forces applied to a cornering motorcycle.

Further, for a motorcycle traversing a curved path:

$$a_{lat} = \frac{v_{mc}^2}{r} \tag{4.5}$$

Therefore, Equation (4.3) can be rewritten as follows:

$$F_{normal} \cdot \sin\phi + F_{friction} \cdot \cos\phi = \frac{W}{g} \cdot \frac{v_{mc}^2}{r} \tag{4.6}$$

Substituting Equation (4.2) into Equation (4.6) yields:

$$F_{normal} \cdot (\sin\phi + \tan\theta\cos\phi) = \frac{W}{g} \cdot \frac{v_{mc}^2}{r} \tag{4.7}$$

As it traverses the curve, the motorcycle depicted in Figure 4.1 is in static equilibrium in the vertical direction. Therefore, the sum of the forces in the vertical direction is equal to zero. This can be written as follows:

$$-W + F_{normal}\cos\phi - F_{friction}\sin\phi = 0 \tag{4.8}$$

Substituting Equation (4.2) into Equation (4.7) and solving for F_{normal} yields:

$$F_{normal} = \frac{W}{\cos\phi - \tan\theta\sin\phi} \tag{4.9}$$

Substituting Equation (4.9) into (4.7) yields the following equation:

$$\frac{1}{g} \cdot \frac{v_{mc}^2}{r} = \frac{\sin\phi + \tan\theta\cos\phi}{\cos\phi - \tan\theta\sin\phi} \tag{4.10}$$

Roadway superelevation typically does not exceed 6° or 7° [4]. Given this, we can employ small-angle assumptions to simplify Equation (4.1). Specifically:

$$\cos\phi \approx 1 \tag{4.11}$$

$$\sin\phi \approx \tan\phi \tag{4.12}$$

Substituting Equations (4.11) and (4.12) into (4.10) yields the following equation:

$$\frac{1}{g} \cdot \frac{v_{mc}^2}{r} = \frac{\tan\phi + \tan\theta}{1 - \tan\phi\tan\theta} \tag{4.13}$$

Using trigonometric identities, it can be show that:

$$\frac{\tan\phi + \tan\theta}{1 - \tan\phi\tan\theta} = \tan(\phi + \theta) \tag{4.14}$$

Therefore:

$$\theta = \tan^{-1}\left(\frac{v_{mc}^2}{g \cdot r}\right) - \phi \tag{4.15}$$

Equation (4.15) shows that the superelevation angle simply reduces the required lean angle relative to the road surface by one degree for each degree of superelevation.

From Equations (4.1) and (4.15), the following relationships can be observed: (1) as a motorcyclist's speed around a curve increases, their lean angle will also increase to maintain the same path of travel; (2) superelevation in a curve reduces the magnitude of lean relative to the roadway; (3) the larger the radius of a curve, the less lean angle required for a motorcyclist to traverse that curve.

4.1.2 Example Lean Angle Calculation

As an example, consider a motorcycle following a curve with a radius of 300 feet and a superelevation of 5° at a speed of 55 mph. Equation (4.15) would be applied as follows. Within the equation, the 55 mph speed is multiplied by 1.4667 to convert it to units of feet per second. The calculated lean angle relative to a line normal to the road surface is 29°. The lean angle relative to vertical would be 34°.

$$\theta = \tan^{-1}\left(\frac{(55 \cdot 1.4667)^2}{32.2 \cdot 300}\right) - 5 = 29°$$

4.1.3 Assumptions

Equations (4.1) and (4.15) were developed with several assumptions. First, these equations assume the motorcycle is traveling a constant velocity of great enough magnitude that the rider is initiating lean through countersteering. Second, they assume that the motorcycle and its rider have the same lean angle. This is often an accurate assumption, but clearly a rider has the option of leaning either more than or less than the motorcycle, and reconstructionists should be attentive to situations where it might not apply. As Cossalter has noted [2]:

> The motorcycle roll angle on a turn is influenced, in a significant way, by the rider's driving style. By leaning with respect to the vehicle, the rider changes the position of his center of gravity with respect to the motorcycle…if the rider remains immobile with respect to the chassis, the center of gravity of the motorcycle-rider system remains in the motorcycle plane…if the rider leans towards the exterior of the turn, the center of gravity is also moved to the exterior of the turn with respect to the motorcycle. As a result, he needs to incline the motorcycle further so that the tires, being more inclined than necessary, operate under less favorable conditions…If the rider leans his torso towards the interior of the turn and at the same time rotates his leg so as to nearly touch the ground with his knee, he manages to reduce the roll angle of the motorcycle plane. When racing, the riders move their entire bodies to the interior of the turn, both to reduce the roll angle of the motorcycle and to better control the vehicle on the turn.

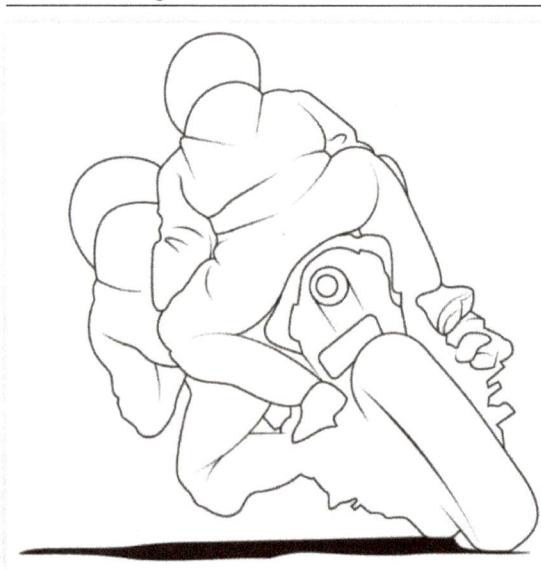

FIGURE 4.2 Motorcycle, operator, and passenger with different lean angles while cornering.

Along these same lines, when there is a passenger on the motorcycle, the passenger may lean more than or less than the operator, and this influences the trajectory of the motorcycle (see Figure 4.2). As Baxter [5] has noted, "a passenger who is unfamiliar with a motorcycle and will not lean with the operator, or leans in the opposite direction during a turn, makes steering and handling much more difficult. If the passenger leans in the wrong direction, it has a negative effect on the operator's lean and steering inputs, canceling them out, so that the motorcycle continues in a straight line." In instances where there is a passenger on the motorcycle in addition to the operator, this is a factor worth considering when analyzing a motorcycle crash involving a curve.

Finally, Equations (4.1) and (4.15) assume that the motorcycle tires have no width, such that the part of the tire contacting the roadway does not change as the motorcycle leans. In reality, as the motorcycle leans, the portion of the tire contacting the road changes, and the contact patch moves in the direction of the lean. This reduces the effective lean angle of the motorcycle. Thus, due to this assumption, the actual lean angle required for a curved path will be higher than that predicted by Equation (4.1) or (4.15).

4.1.4 Case Study: Application of the Lean Angle Equations at the Apex of a Curve

To test the accuracy of Equations (4.1) and (4.15), physical testing was conducted with two motorcycles—a 2012 Suzuki DR650SE Enduro and a 2007 Kawasaki VN900-D [6]. The photographs of Figure 4.3 show these motorcycles. The photographs of Figure 4.4 show cross-sectional views of the rear tires of these motorcycles. Figure 4.5 is an aerial photograph showing the area where the testing was conducted. Because this lot was used for teaching the Motorcycle Safety Foundation's (MSF) Basic Rider's Course and Advanced Rider's Course, this range was pre-marked for the various exercises in those courses. This testing utilized the two semi-circle paths that form a large oval marked with blue paint, visible near the center of Figure 4.5.

FIGURE 4.3 Motorcycles used for testing.

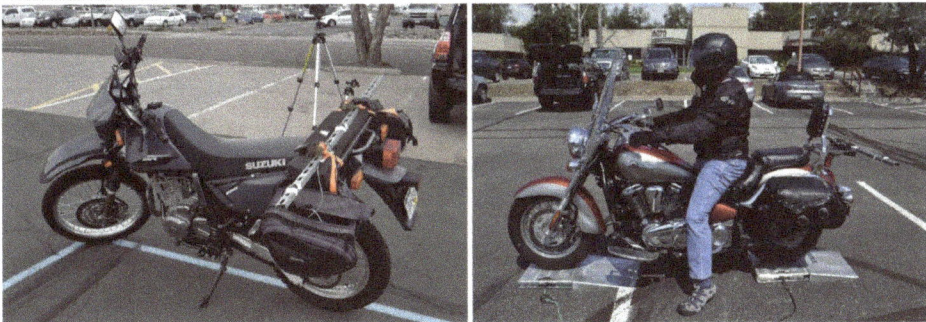

FIGURE 4.4 Contact between the Suzuki's tire and the test surface.

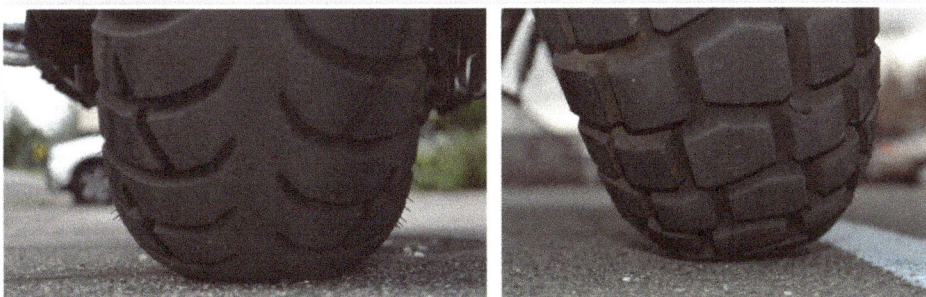

FIGURE 4.5 Parking lot and range used for testing.

FIGURE 4.5 Parking lot and range used for testing.

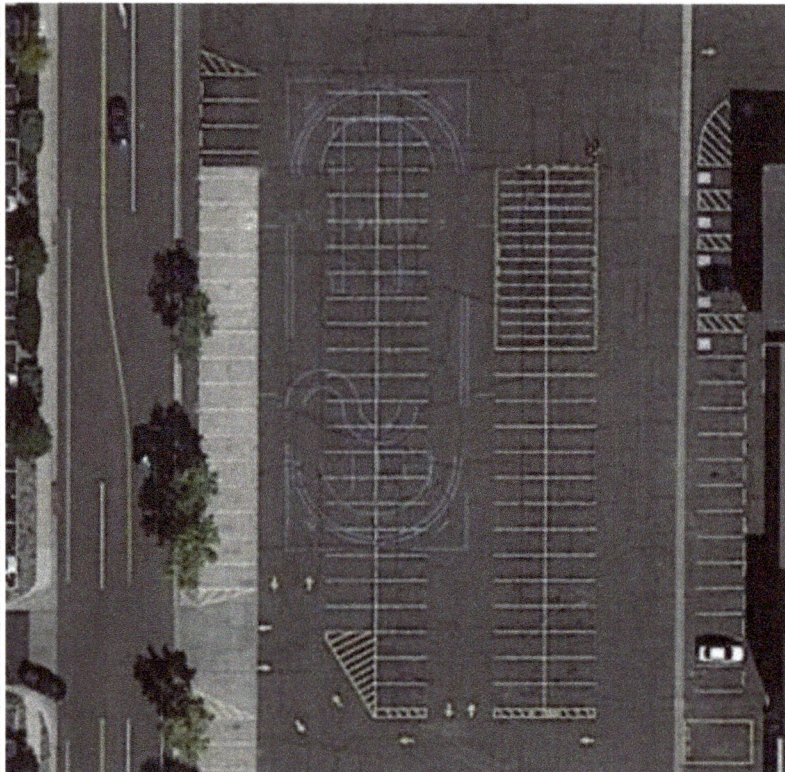

Map data © 2018 Google

Three riders were utilized for this testing—one a novice and two expert riders (these are self-characterizations). The riders were instructed to make turns at different speeds while trying to maintain a constant velocity during the turns. The riders also attempted to lean their body to the same degree that the motorcycle leaned during each turn. Each rider rode the motorcycle around the oval path numerous times, varying their speed and direction of travel. The path, speed, and lean angle of the motorcycle were continuously documented using a Racelogic VBOX that measured speed, position, and roll angle at 20 Hz. The VBOX system utilized two GPS antennae. A metal crossbar was strapped to the rear of the motorcycle, and the GPS sensors were magnetically attached to this crossbar (Figures 4.3 and 4.6).

One sensor was attached at the motorcycle centerline and another near the left extent of the crossbar. The metal crossbar was damped with a piece of Styrofoam placed between the crossbar and the rack on the back of the bike. The VBOX data logger was placed in the left saddlebag of the motorcycle. This testing was also captured with two video cameras recording at a rate of 30 fps. Testing was conducted on two separate days. On both days, the range was clear and dry, and the wind was below a level that would have required the riders to make any adjustment to their riding.

The VBOX data from each cornering maneuver was analyzed to determine the motorcycle's path radius, speed, and lean angle relative to gravity (rather

FIGURE 4.6 Motorcycle and rider at apex of curve during one test.

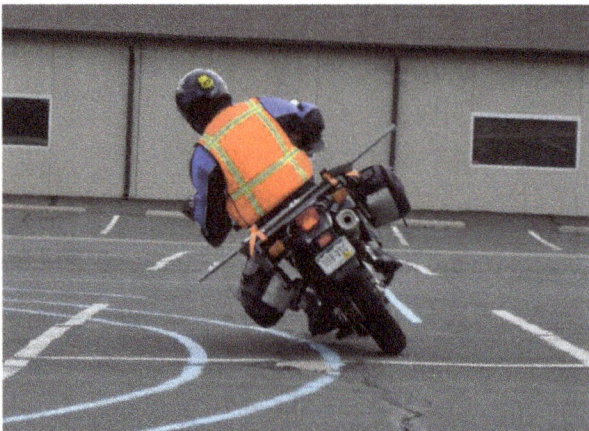

than relative to the road surface). These values were tabulated for the time during each cornering maneuver when the lean angle reached a maximum. The path radius was determined by fitting a curve to the VBOX positional data for each curve. To normalize the results from the testing and plot them all on one graph, the path radius and speed were used to calculate a lateral acceleration for each maneuver.

Figure 4.7 is a graph that depicts the lateral acceleration, and resulting lean angle from each cornering maneuver from our testing compared to the lean angle Equation (4.1) would predict. Lateral acceleration in g's is plotted on the horizontal axis, and the lean angle in degrees is plotted on the vertical axis. This is the lean angle of the motor-cycle itself since the instrumentation was attached to the motorcycle. Points plotted in gray are for the Suzuki motorcycle, and points plotted in purple are for the Kawasaki motorcycle. Points plotted with an "x" are for the novice rider, and points plotted with a circle are for the expert riders.

Several trends emerge in Figure 4.7. First, while Equations (4.1) and (4.15) prescribe a particular lean angle for a given lateral acceleration, the test data we gathered shows scatter in the actual lean angle for any particular lateral acceleration level. Second, the actual lean angle is nearly always greater than the lean angle predicted by Equations (4.1) or (4.15). To some degree, this trend is expected since Equations (4.1) and (4.15) neglect the effects of the motorcycle tires having width.

Cossalter [2] showed that the additional lean angle required due to the tire width could be calculated using Equations (4.16) and (4.17). In these equations, t is the tire width, and h is the combined motorcycle and rider center of gravity height;

$$\theta = \theta_{Equation(1)} + \Delta\theta_{tire\ width} \tag{4.16}$$

$$\Delta\theta_{tire\ width} = \sin^{-1}\left(\frac{\frac{t}{2} \times \sin\left(\theta_{Equation(1)}\right)}{h - \frac{t}{2}}\right) \tag{4.17}$$

FIGURE 4.7 Test results compared to lean angle equation.

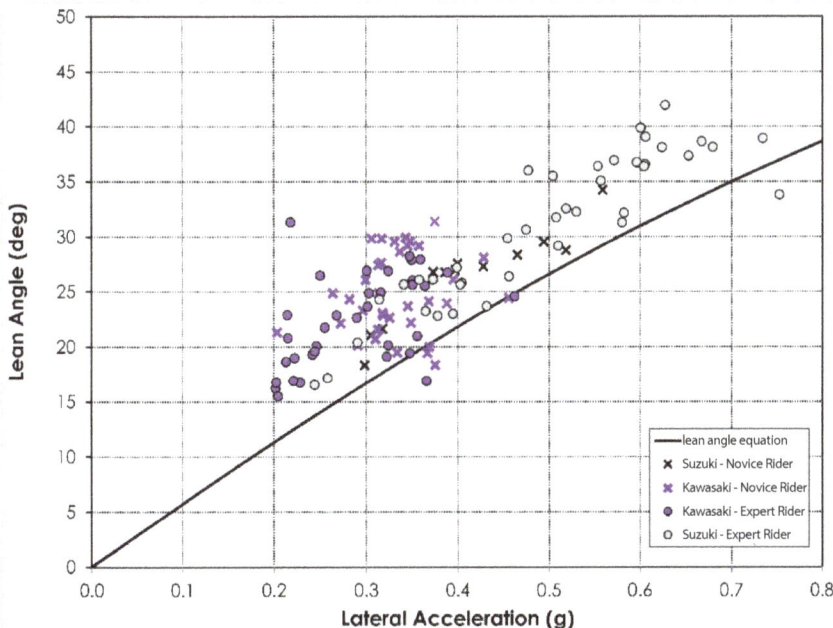

Figures 4.8 and 4.9 are similar to Figure 4.7. Figure 4.8 only plots the test points for the Suzuki motorcycle, and Figure 4.9 only plots the points for the Kawasaki motorcycle. These figures also plot Equation (4.16) for each motorcycle with a dashed line. For purposes of calculating the curve for Equation (4.16), the average of the front and rear tire widths of each motorcycle was used. The center of gravity height of the Suzuki was estimated with Equation (2.3) and with Equation (2.2) for the Kawasaki. Each rider's seated center of gravity height was estimated to be at their navel. Each motorcycle and

FIGURE 4.8   Test results for Suzuki compared to lean angle equation with tire width.

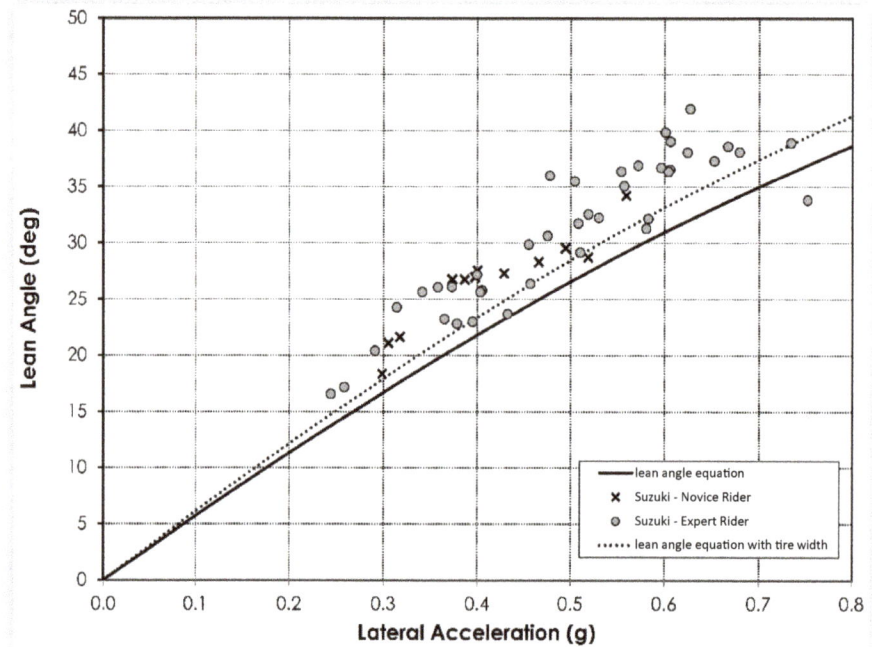

FIGURE 4.9   Test results for Kawasaki compared to lean angle equation with tire width.

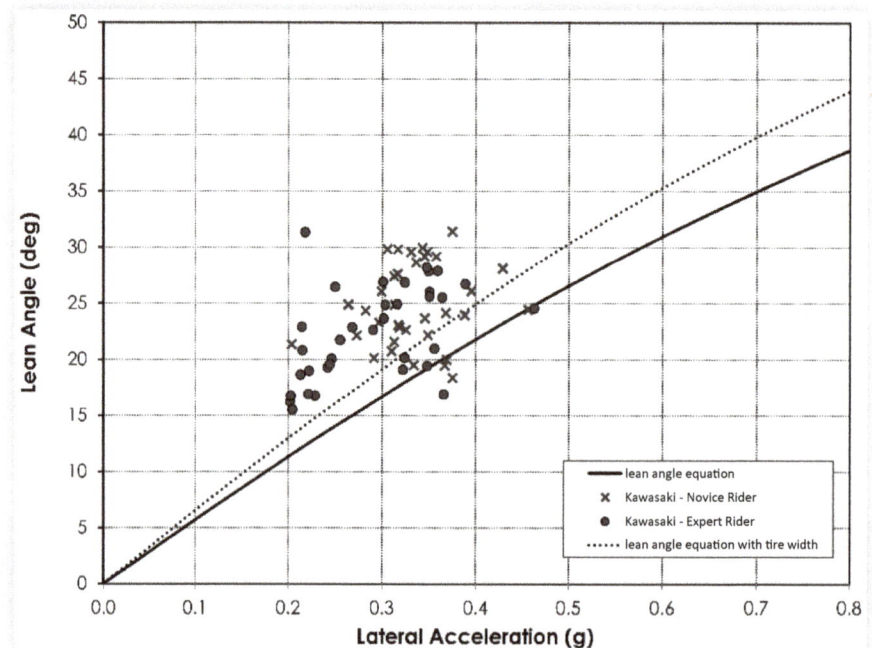

rider were then weighed, and a combined center of gravity height for the motorcycle and rider was calculated using the formula of Equation (4.18):

$$CG_{combined} = \frac{CG_{mc} \times W_{mc} + CG_r \times W_r}{W_{total}} \qquad (4.18)$$

The results displayed on these graphs demonstrate that incorporating the tire width into the calculation of lean angle reduces the average error in the calculation. However, it did not fully explain the error. There are other factors that likely explain the difference between the theoretical and actual lean angles. This research did not measure or quantify the _rider_ lean angle during the cornering maneuvers. A discrepancy between the motorcycle and rider lean angles could further explain why the motorcycle lean angle was consistently under-predicted by Equations (4.1) and (4.15). If this was the case, it would imply that both the novice and expert riders consistently leaned less than they leaned their motorcycles. Review of the testing video revealed that the novice rider did tend to lean less than the motorcycle and had a tendency when riding the Kawasaki to turn the front wheel during low-speed cornering, which reduces the motorcycle lean angle required for a given maneuver. The expert riders had similar tendencies, but to a lesser degree. The next section will examine motorcycle cornering at significantly higher speeds where the rider would use counter-steering to initiate lean and there would not be a contribution from significant handlebar steer.

Two additional areas deserve comment. First, the Kawasaki motorcycle had a geometric limit of around 30° of lean. Based on Equation (4.16), this geometric limit should have allowed the riders to reach a lateral acceleration level of 0.5 g. While the expert rider achieved a lateral acceleration of 0.46 g on this motorcycle and the novice rider achieved 0.45 g, the bulk of the data points for this motorcycle fell below 0.4 g. Both riders reported repeatedly scraping components of this motorcycle during the testing. The Suzuki, on the other hand, had a geometric limit exceeding 40° of lean. Neither rider reported scraping components of the motorcycle during the testing with this motorcycle. The expert rider achieved a lateral acceleration level of 0.75 g with this motorcycle, whereas the novice only achieved 0.56 g. In the test results with the Kawasaki, it is difficult to discern any difference in the lean angle behavior of the novice and expert riders. With the Suzuki, the novice rider, for the most part, kept the lean angle below 30°. The expert rider achieved lean angles with this motorcycle that approached and exceeded 40°. These results indicate that the observed limits for lean angle on the Kawasaki are being driven by the geometric limit defined by component of this motorcycle contacting the road surface. Initially, it was thought that a willingness limit could be driving the results for the Suzuki. However, in discussing the Suzuki tests with the expert rider, he indicated that the limiting factor for his lean angles was due to the geometry of the motorcycle, not to a willingness limit.

4.1.5 Case Study: Application of the Lean Angle Equations in the Time Domain

To test the accuracy of Equations (4.1) and (4.15) in the time domain, physical testing was conducted using a 2007 Suzuki GSX-R750 motorcycle (Figure 4.10) [7]. This testing utilized a single experienced rider who was a certified safety instructor through the MSF. The rider traversed the route with the goal of maintaining safety and varying his speed in accordance with the characteristics of the roadway. No special instructions were given to the rider in terms of how he should lean his body relative to the motorcycle. The risks of this ride were discussed with the rider, and he was aware of and consented to these risks.

FIGURE 4.10 Suzuki motorcycle used for testing.

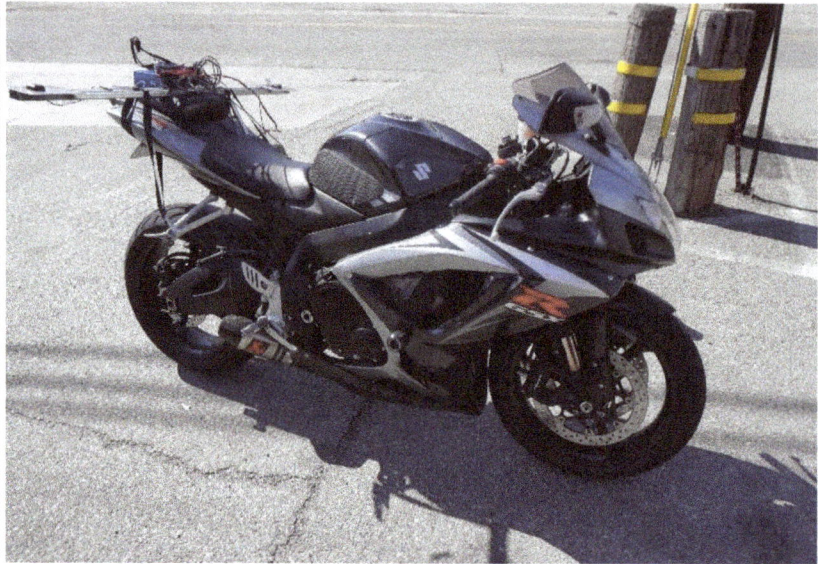

This testing involved the rider driving the motorcycle westbound along County Road 95 between Frazier Park, California, and State Highway 33. Seven curves were identified for analysis on this section of roadway. The rider also drove southbound along Highway 33, and three additional curves were identified for analysis on this section. Three of the ten curves were digitally mapped with a Faro laser scanner. One of these three was also mapped with a total station. The remaining seven were mapped with aerial imagery. The images below depict the geometry of the curve that was mapped with both a total station and a Faro scanner. Figure 4.11 is an aerial photograph showing this curve. This photograph is oriented such that north is up on the page. Riders traveling southbound through this curve would first traverse from the top left to the top right of this photograph and then exit the curve traveling from right to left across the image. Figure 4.12 is a photograph showing the overall geometry of the curve from a ground

FIGURE 4.11 Aerial photograph showing one of the curves.

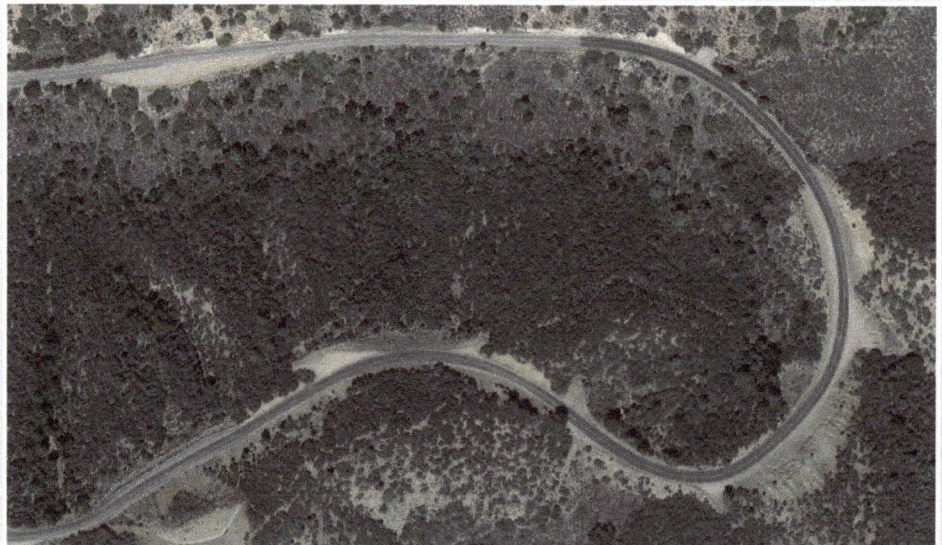

Map data © 2018 Google

FIGURE 4.12 Photograph showing the same curve.

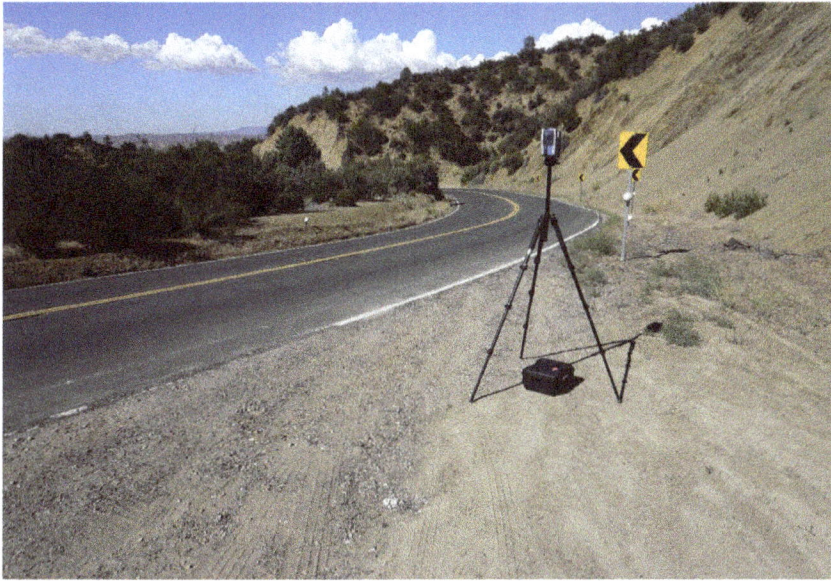

level perspective. Riders traveling southbound through this curve would travel toward the viewer of this image. Figure 4.13 shows the 45,784,170 scan data points that were captured around this curve.

Throughout the entire route, the path, speed, and lean angle of the motorcycle were continuously recorded using a Racelogic VBOX that measured speed, position, and roll angle at 20 Hz (a similar setup to that used in the previous section). The VBOX system utilized two GPS antenna. A metal crossbar was strapped to the rear of the motorcycle, and the GPS sensors were magnetically attached to this crossbar, near its outer extents (Figure 4.14). The motorcycle was scanned with a Faro laser scanner both before and after the ride, so that any displacement of this bar that might occur over the course of the ride could be quantified. The VBOX data logger was carried in the rider's backpack. This testing was also captured with a video camera and a GoPro camera attached to a chase vehicle and with two GoPro cameras attached to the rider (helmet and chest). These cameras were recording at a rate of 30 fps. At the time of the testing, the road surface was dry.

FIGURE 4.13 Scan data capturing the geometry of the curve.

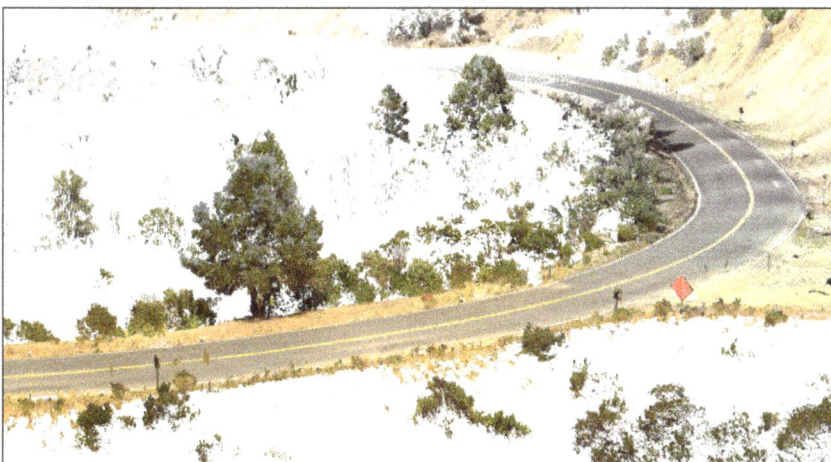

FIGURE 4.14 VBOX sensors attached to motorcycle.

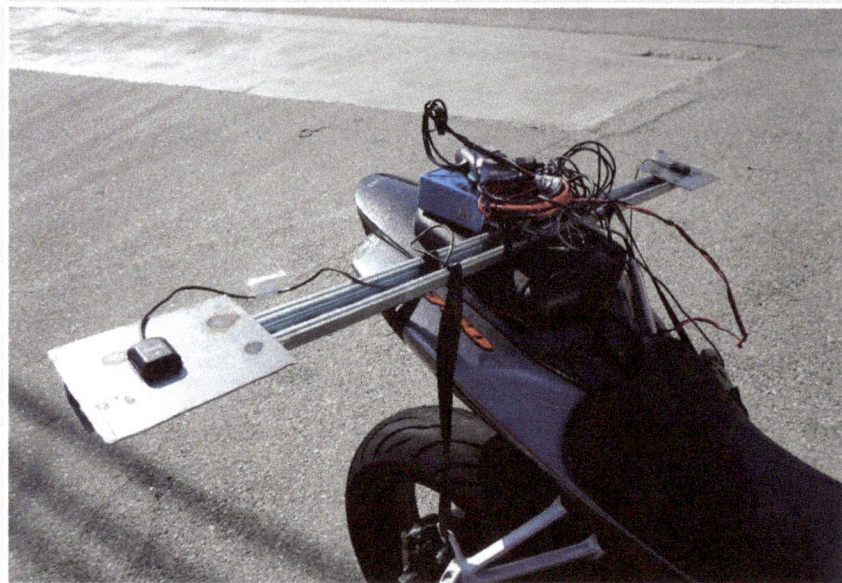

The VBOX data from each of the 10 curves was analyzed to determine the motorcycle's actual path radius, speed, and lean angle relative to gravity (rather than relative to the road surface). These values were tabulated for the motorcycle's entire traversal of each curve. The path radius was calculated using positional data from the VBOX. When the motorcycle was instrumented, the authors attempted to position the antenna bracket perpendicular to the vertical axis of the motorcycle. The motorcycle was then scanned with a Faro laser scanner in its instrumented state. The scan data was examined, and it was found that the bar had a 2.2° angle relative to the roll axis of the motorcycle. The measured lean angles were adjusted to reflect this offset. Adjustments were also made to the radius to compensate for the primary antenna placement relative to the center of gravity of the motorcycle. The positional data from the VBOX was analyzed to determine the instantaneous radius of the path of the motorcycle at each point along each curve. To eliminate excessive noise due to the sensitivity of the radius calculation to small changes in positional data, points selected for this calculation were selected ½ s apart. Thus, the "instantaneous" radius was calculated over 1 s intervals.

Figure 4.15 is a graph that compares the VBOX measured lean angles (dashed black) to the lean angles calculated with Equation (4.1) (green) and with Equation (4.16) (red) for turn 4. Positive values for lean angle indicate a leftward lean, while negative values indicate a rightward lean. Examination of this graph reveals that Equation (4.1) tends to underestimate the fully developed lean for each curve. Equation (4.16), on the other hand, closely predicts the lean angle throughout the course of this curve.

The results depicted here were typical for the curves tested. Table 4.1 lists the average differences between the measured lean angle and the lean angle calculated with Equation (4.16). This difference was calculated in two ways. First, it was calculated simply as the average of the point-to-point differences, with consideration for the positive and negative signs associated with left and right turns. Second, it was calculated as the average of the absolute value of the difference. The average difference between the predicted lean angle of Equation (4.16) and the actual lean angle for all the data was −0.10°. Thus, the average error was near zero, and the differences that existed were sometimes smaller and sometimes larger than the actual lean angle. The average of the absolute differences between the predicted and actual lean angles for all the data was 0.94°. Equation (4.16) typically predicted

FIGURE 4.15 Comparison of measured and calculated lean angles for turn 4.

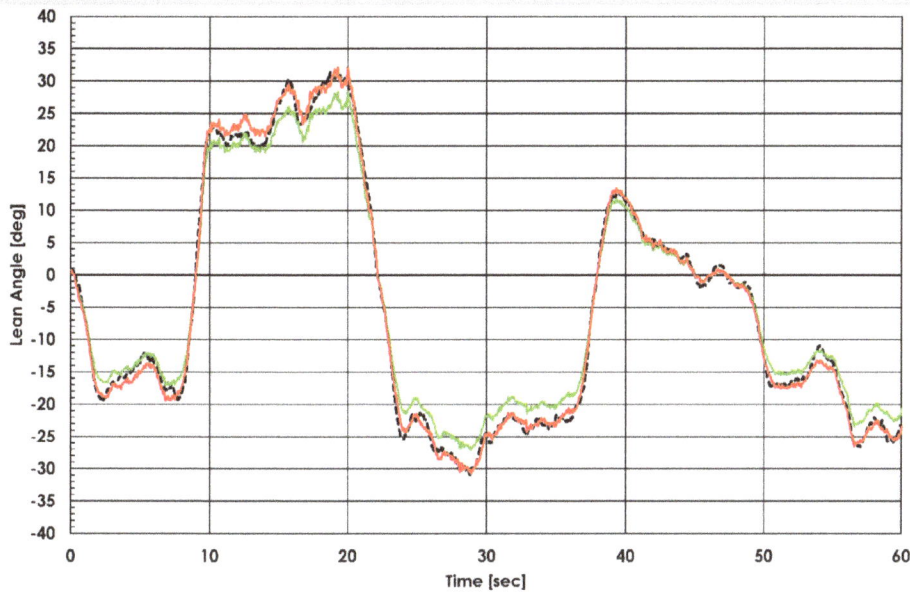

---- VBOX Measured Lean Angle ——— Calculated Lean Angle ——— Calculated Lean Angle with Tire Width Adjustment

the actual lean angle within 3° (sometimes underestimating and sometimes overestimating). The difference between calculated and actual was seldom greater than 5°. This equation also reasonably models the buildup of lean angle through the progression of a curve (in the time domain). Thus, it could be used to compare the rate at which a motorcyclist would need to lean when traversing a curve at various speeds.

4.1.6 Friction-Limited Speed

Three factors limit the speed at which a motorcycle can traverse a curve. The first of these is the limit of the available friction between the motorcycle tires and the roadway. The second is a geometric limit that is defined by the lean angle at which the motorcycle's foot peg—or some other component—contacts the roadway. The third is the limit imposed by the rider's willingness limits—their willingness to approach either the geometric or friction limits of their motorcycle.

On a curve with no superelevation, the friction limit is reached when the lateral acceleration (in gravitational units) of the motorcycle/rider combination is equal to the coefficient of friction between the roadway and the motorcycle tires. Equation (4.19) expresses this limit:

$$v_{mc,max} = \sqrt{\mu g r} \qquad (4.19)$$

Roadway superelevation decreases both the necessary friction force and the angle a motorcyclist needs to lean relative to the road to traverse a curve. In determining the limits for a motorcycle or rider on a curve, the superelevation needs to be considered,

TABLE 4.1 Average differences between measured lean angle and calculated lean angle for each curve

Turn number	Average difference (°)	Average of absolute value of difference (°)
1	−0.25	0.84
2	−0.05	1.56
3	−0.58	0.90
4	0.05	0.73
5	0.10	0.89
6	0.10	0.89
7	−0.02	0.82
8	−0.28	1.18
9	0.32	0.77
10	−0.42	1.14
All data	−0.10	0.94

since most curves are banked in a way that reduces the lean angle the motorcycle and rider will achieve relative to the roadway. To develop a comparable equation for a curve with superelevation, the lateral forces depicted in Figure 4.1 can again be equated to the lateral inertial force, as written in Equation (4.6). When the motorcycle reaches its friction limits:

$$F_{friction} = \mu F_{normal} \tag{4.20}$$

Substituting Equation (4.20) into (4.6) yields the following equation:

$$F_{normal}\left(\sin\phi + \mu\cos\phi\right) = \frac{W}{g}\cdot\frac{v_{mc}^2}{r} \tag{4.21}$$

Returning now to the sum of forces in the vertical direction, Equation (4.8), and substituting Equation (4.20) into this equation yields:

$$F_{normal} = \frac{W}{\cos\phi - \mu\sin\phi} \tag{4.22}$$

Substituting Equation (4.22) into (4.21) yields the following equation:

$$\frac{\sin\phi + \mu\cos\phi}{\cos\phi - \mu\sin\phi} = \frac{1}{g}\cdot\frac{v_{mc}^2}{r} \tag{4.23}$$

Again, employing small-angle assumptions and then solving for the maximum, friction-limited speed in Equation (4.23) results in the following equation:

$$v_{mc,max} = \sqrt{\frac{\mu + \tan\phi}{1 - \mu\tan\phi}gr} \tag{4.24}$$

Lambourn [8] examined friction coefficients between motorcycle tires and dry asphalt roadways and found peak friction coefficients of 1.2. With this level of friction, a motorcycle traversing a flat, 250 ft radius curve would have a friction-limited speed of 67 mph. On a flat, 500 ft radius curve, the same motorcycle would have a friction-limited speed of 95 mph. If superelevation is present, these speeds would increase. As the next section discusses, many motorcycles do not have the geometric clearances necessary for the lean angle that these speeds would require. Thus, a motorcycle's physical limits are likely to be determined by its maximum lean angle, not the friction limits of its tires.

4.1.7 Geometric Limit on Speed

The second factor that limits the speed of a motorcycle around a curve is the geometric limit that is defined by the lean angle at which motorcycle components other than the tires—a foot peg or crash bar, for instance—contact the roadway. This limit is defined by the geometry of each motorcycle but is generally in the range of 25° to 50° [9]. On a flat, 250 ft curve, a motorcycle that can lean 25° can achieve a speed of 42 mph before components begin to contact the roadway. A motorcycle that can lean 50° can achieve the friction-limited speed of 67 mph.

Suspension loading and compression have a small effect on the geometric limit for a motorcycle on a curve. As the load on the suspension increases, the springs compress more, and the ground clearance of components on the motorcycle decreases. To account for this in evaluating the geometry-limited speed of a motorcycle around a curve, an equation can be developed to calculate the suspension load for a rider operating a motorcycle through a curve at a given speed. Developing this equation begins by parsing the weight of the motorcycle/rider combination into individual components as follows:

$$W = W_{rider} + W_{mc-sprung} + W_{mc-unsprung} \tag{4.25}$$

In this equation, the weight of the motorcycle has been divided into sprung and unsprung components. The sprung weight of the motorcycle is the portion of the motorcycle weight that is supported by the suspension, and the unsprung weight is the weight of the motorcycle components that support the suspension. The unsprung portion of the motorcycle weight does not contribute to compressing the suspension springs. Thus, when the motorcycle is upright, the force compressing the suspension is as follows:

$$F_{suspension} = W_{rider} + W_{mc-sprung} \tag{4.26}$$

The force compressing the suspension increases during cornering. To quantify this increase, the lateral component of the force on the suspension can be equated to the inertial force of the rider and sprung weight of the motorcycle, as follows:

$$F_{suspension} \sin(\theta + \phi) = \frac{W_{rider} + W_{mc-sprung}}{g} \cdot \frac{v_{mc}^2}{r} \tag{4.27}$$

Substitution into Equation (4.15) and solving for $F_{suspension}$ yields the following equation:

$$F_{suspension} = \left(W_{rider} + W_{mc-sprung}\right) \frac{1}{\cos(\theta + \phi)} \tag{4.28}$$

Equation (4.28) demonstrates that the force on a motorcycle's suspension depends on the superelevation of the roadway and the motorcycle lean angle. Since the lean angle depends on the motorcycle speed and the radius of the curve being traversed, so does the force on the suspension and thus, the compression of the suspension. This means that the maximum lean angle of a motorcycle depends, to some degree, on the speed and curve radius.

To explore and illustrate the significance of these suspension effects, the suspension on a 2003 Harley-Davidson FXD motorcycle was tested, and the motorcycle's ground clearance under various loading conditions was documented (Figure 4.16). For each loading

FIGURE 4.16 2003 Harley-Davidson FXD.

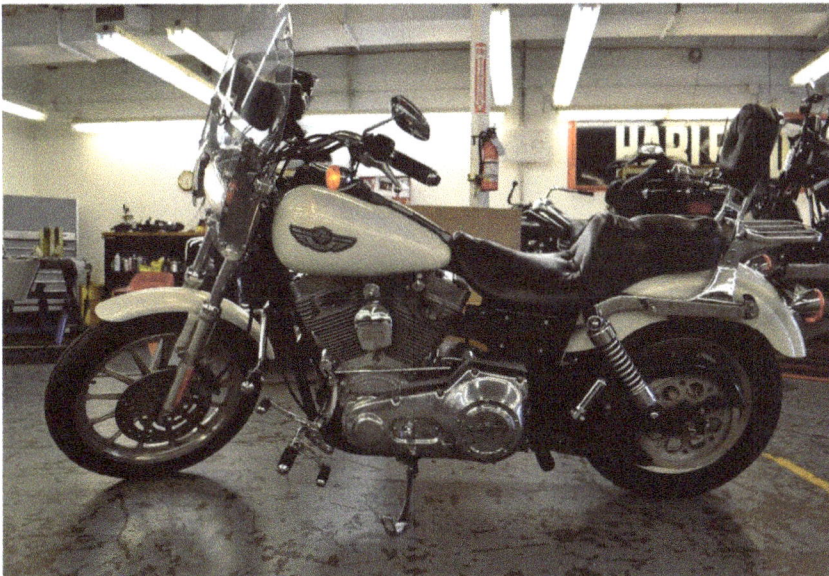

FIGURE 4.17 2003 Harley-Davidson FXD with rider.

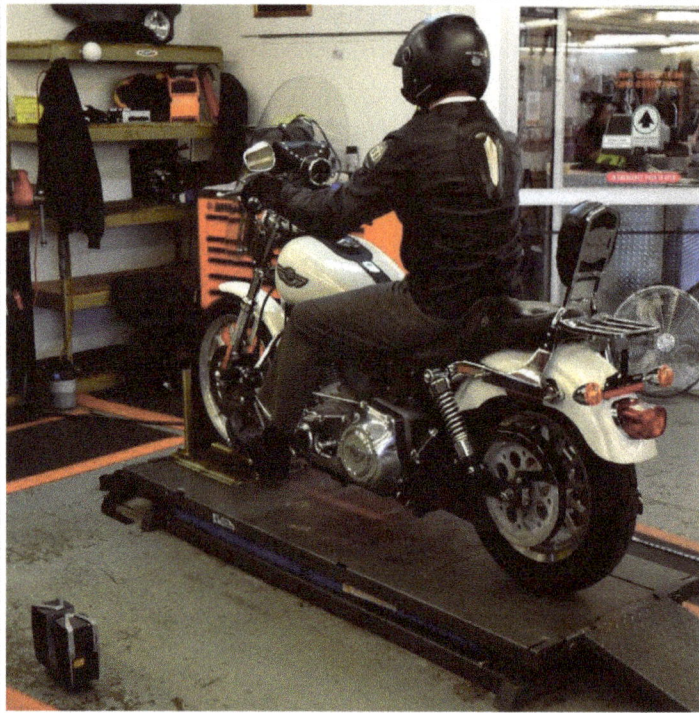

configuration, a Faro Laser Scanner Focus³ᴰ was used to document the position of the motorcycle undercarriage relative to the test platform and to measure the ground clearance. With the fuel tank approximately five eighths full, this motorcycle weighed 671 lb. Without a rider, the motorcycle had 5.34 in. of ground clearance, as measured at the kickstand stop.

The following four additional configurations were tested: (1) the motorcycle with a 201 pound rider, including his gear (Figure 4.17), (2) the motorcycle with a 201 pound rider and 51 lb of ballast placed on the fuel tank in front of the rider, (3) the motorcycle with a 201 pound rider and 105 lb of ballast placed on the fuel tank in front of the rider, and (4) the motorcycle with a 201 pound rider and 155 lb of ballast placed on the fuel tank in front of the rider.

Table 4.2 lists the ground clearance for the motorcycle undercarriage for the various loading conditions. With the ground clearance that resulted from loading the suspension of this motorcycle with a rider, this motorcycle would have a maximum lean angle of 33°. With the ground clearance that resulted from loading the suspension of this motorcycle with a rider and 155 lb of ballast, this motorcycle would have a maximum lean angle of 32°. These values show that the suspension load has an effect, though relatively minor, on the maximum lean angle.

The maximum lean angle for a motorcycle can often be reasonably estimated from what is reported in manufacturer specifications, without the need for any physical testing. The maximum lean angle reported in these specifications will typically have been determined according to the procedure described in Society of Automotive Engineers (SAE) Recommended Practice J1168 [10]. This recommended practice specifies that the front and rear suspension systems on the motorcycle be compressed to 75% of their maximum travel. The motorcycle is then leaned until a component contacts the test

TABLE 4.2 Harley-Davidson FXD ground clearance under various loading conditions

Loading condition	Ground clearance (in.)
No rider	5.34
Rider (201 lb)	4.90
Rider + 51 lb	4.77
Rider + 105 lb	4.67
Rider + 155 lb	4.48

surface and the lean angle is measured. Because this procedure specifies the motorcycle suspension being compressed, the resulting value will be a reasonable approximately of the geometric limit in most cases.

4.1.8 Willingness to Lean

The amount of lean required by a rider as they traverse a curve is determined by their speed in the curve. Many riders reach a limit on their willingness to continue to lean their motorcycle before they reach the maximum lean angle of their motorcycle. Watanabe and Yoshida found that the maximum lean angles utilized by novice riders were typically in the range of 15° to 25° and those used by experienced riders were in the range of 34° to 40° [11]. These results imply that the experienced riders in the study by Watanabe and Yoshida would approach the lean angle limits of many motorcycles, whereas novice riders stopped well short of the motorcycle limits. Using the middle values of these ranges, these results further imply that on a flat, 250 ft curve, an experienced rider would be willing to lean far enough to traverse the curve at a speed of 53 mph, whereas a novice rider would only be willing to lean far enough to traverse the curve at a speed of 37 mph.

Thus, speed can contribute to causing a motorcycle crash in a curve even if the motorcyclist's speed has not reached either the friction-limited or geometric limited speeds. If a motorcyclist enters a curve at a speed that requires them to lean beyond the angle they are willing to achieve, then the motorcycle will drift toward the outside of the curve (assuming no other action is taken by the rider) and may cross out of its lane and off the shoulder or into oncoming traffic, depending on whether the subject curve is toward the left or right.

4.2 Lane Change, Swerve, and Turn-Away

In some situations, a motorcyclist will need to complete a lane change, swerve, or turn-away to avoid a hazard. Hurt and DuPont [12] noted that if a hazard appears in the roadway which requires that the motorcycle turn to the left for collision avoidance, the first control input must be steering to the right. This initial steering to the right is necessary to allow the wheels to track to the right and lean the motorcycle to the left, eventually causing the motorcycle to turn to the left.

For the discussion here, a *lane change* is defined as a complete lateral move by a vehicle from one lane to another. For a motorcyclist completing a lane change to the left, this would involve an initial rightward countersteer and lean (at least of the motorcycle) to the left, followed by a subsequent return to an upright position, and then a leftward countersteer and lean to the right, followed by a return to an upright position. The term *swerve* refers to a maneuver that is like a lane change in the sense that it involves a complete lateral movement, but it is not referenced to any marking on the roadway and will typically be smaller laterally and quicker than a lane change. The term *turn-away* is defined as half of a swerve.

Rice [13] examined the effect of skill level on the technique used by motorcyclists making lane changes. He studied the degree to which riders of various skill level used countersteering and body lean to initiate and execute these maneuvers. The lane change tests involved a 12 ft lateral move to the left for which the riders were afforded 60 ft in which to complete the maneuver. All the tests utilized a 1974 Honda CB 360G. Four riders of varying skill level were utilized, and they were instructed to continue increasing their speed through the course until they could no longer successfully complete the required lane change. Rice observed that "the rider has great flexibility in selecting a combination of leaning motions and steer torque applications [countersteering] for successfully performing a simple lane change maneuver. This result alone points strongly to the need for considering motorcycle performance in terms of the rider-vehicle combination – the handling qualities problem – rather than on vehicle dynamics alone (given, of course, reasonable response characteristics in the machine)." Rice noted that the most experienced rider used a large initial countersteer to initiate the lane change. For the least experienced rider, Rice found significant variability from run-to-run in the degree to which the rider utilized countersteering and body lean. One moderately experienced rider tended to emphasize control of the motorcycle through lean of his body rather than through the large countersteers utilized by the most experienced rider.

In his discussion of motorcycle avoidance maneuvers, Limpert suggested a maximum lateral acceleration of 0.65 g for motorcyclists [14, 15]. However, this is contrary to the lean angles that actual riders were willing to utilize, according to Watanabe and Yoshida. Their finding that novice riders utilized maximum lean angles in the range of 15° to 25° would imply a maximum lateral acceleration for those riders in the range of 0.268 to 0.466 g. Their finding that experienced riders utilized maximum lean angles in the range of 34° to 40° would imply a maximum lateral acceleration for those riders in the range of 0.675 to 1.0 g. This means that, in evaluating a motorcyclist's ability to avoid a crash by swerving, the rider's experience and skill level may need to be considered.

Daily, Shigemura, and Daily [16] presented the following equation for calculating the turn-away distance. In this equation, S is the vehicle speed in mph, L is the lateral turn-away distance in feet, f_y is the average lateral acceleration in gravitational units, and $d_{turn-away}$ is the longitudinal distance required for the maneuver. For a complete lane change or swerve, Daily, Shigemura, and Daily recommended doubling the coefficient in this equation to 0.732. It is important to note when applying the Daily approach for a complete lane change or swerve, the lateral distance entered into the equation is half of the total lateral distance traversed.

$$d_{turn-away} = 0.366 \cdot S \sqrt{\frac{L}{f_y}} \qquad (4.29)$$

Bartlett and Meyers reported [17] testing conducted with four experienced and skilled motorcyclists on four motorcycles, swerving 2 m (6.5 ft) to their left after passing through a gate at speeds of 40 to 88 kph (25 to 55 mph). The riders were instructed to swerve as rapidly as safely possible "to cross a line 2 m (6.5 ft) away from the left edge of the approach chute…A group of observers on the sidelines marked the point where the motorcycle's front tire crossed the line." The following motorcycles were tested: a 2010 Kawasaki Ninja 250, a 2005 Yamaha R6, a 2009 Harley-Davidson FLHTPI, and a 1990 Harley-Davidson FXRT. The testing was conducted on a dry roadway with a coefficient of friction, measured with a Ford Crown Victoria police cruiser, of 0.75. Bartlett and Meyers reported the speed, distance, and time for each swerve maneuver. Unfortunately, they did not measure or calculate the lean angles (of the motorcycles or the riders) or the actual lateral accelerations utilized by the riders. They simply assumed a lateral acceleration of 0.65 g—the maximum value suggested by Limpert—and used that to refine the empirical coefficient for Equation (4.29) and other equations taking similar form. It is unlikely that every rider would swerve with a lateral acceleration of 0.65 g, so the assumption made by Bartlett and Meyers is not likely to be valid. The data reported by Bartlett and Meyers was reanalyzed here using Equation (4.29). Instead of assuming the same lateral acceleration for each maneuver, Equation (4.29) was used to calculate an apparent lateral acceleration for each test. The resulting lateral accelerations are reported in Table 4.3. These are not measured lateral accelerations but rather calculated lateral accelerations assuming the validity of Equation (4.29). That being the case, they should be applied in conjunction with that equation. Based on the average acceleration reported in this table for each rider, there does appear to be dependence on the rider in this data.

Figure 4.18 is a graph that plots the lateral acceleration from these tests against the maneuver speed. Each motorcyclist's runs are depicted with a different point style (open circles, open squares, x's, and filled triangles). No relationship is apparent between speed and lateral acceleration, but rider-to-rider differences are apparent. The rider on motorcycle D (filled triangles), for instance, generated apparent lateral accelerations between 0.46 and 0.72, whereas the rider on motorcycle C (open circles) generated apparent lateral accelerations between 0.22 and 0.40. Since the riders were instructed to "swerve left as rapidly as possible," these differences likely reflect something about these riders' willingness limits on these motorcycles (which could reflect their familiarity with the motorcycle, the geometry of the motorcycle, their personality, and other factors).

Shuman and Husher [18] reported a series of swerve tests on a level, dry asphalt roadway with a single rider on his own 2004 Honda RC51 sport motorcycle. They conducted

TABLE 4.3 Lateral acceleration for the Bartlett and Meyers testing calculated with Equation (3.31)

	MC ID and test #	Speed (mph)	Longitudinal turn-away distance (ft)	Lateral acceleration (g)	Average (g)
Police cruiser	A1	29	45.5	0.35	0.38
	A2	31	44.3	0.43	
	A3	40	65.8	0.32	
	A4	39	61.0	0.36	
	A5	51	78.0	0.37	
	A6	50	67.5	0.48	
Sport motorcycle	B1	32	45.5	0.43	0.49
	B2	28	41.5	0.40	
	B3	41	57.3	0.45	
	B4	50	70.3	0.44	
	B5	49	54.7	0.70	
	B6	55	69.2	0.55	
Sport motorcycle	C1	30	50.2	0.31	0.31
	C2	32	52.7	0.32	
	C3	40	64.6	0.33	
	C4	38	56.0	0.40	
	C5	44	77.6	0.28	
	C6	43	85.7	0.22	
Cruiser	D1	29	39.7	0.46	0.59
	D2	28	34.4	0.58	
	D3	38	41.8	0.72	
	D4	35	42.4	0.59	
	D5	43	56.6	0.50	
	D6	46	52.1	0.68	
	D7	54	72.1	0.49	
	D9	53	60.6	0.67	

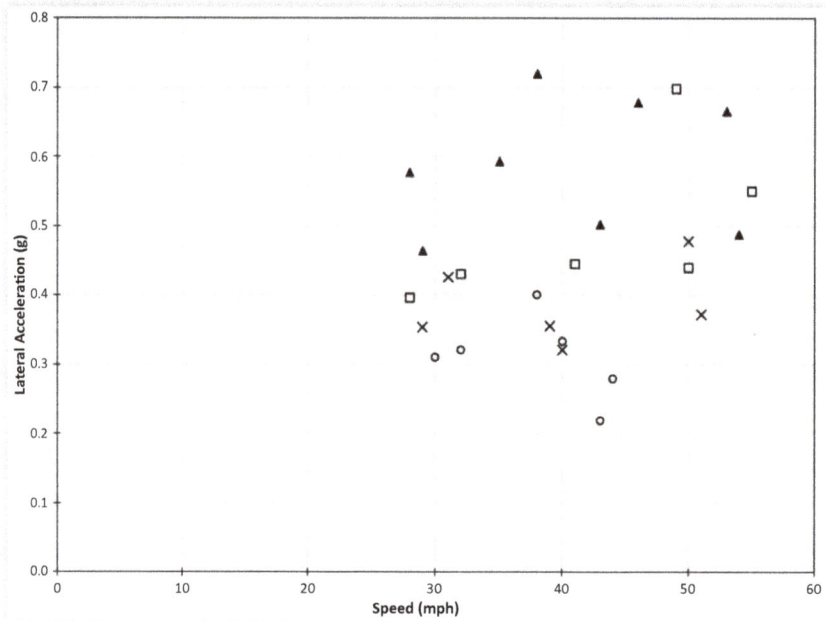

FIGURE 4.18 Lateral acceleration versus speed graph for the Bartlett and Meyers turn-away testing

tests with lateral offsets of 6.5 and 13 ft (2 and 4 m) at speeds between 25 and 40 mph (40 and 64 kph). They stated that "the swerve type maneuver is investigated using active, purposeful countersteering with minimal rider body lean." This statement is contradicted, however, by the images in their report, which show the rider leaning his body. These tests were captured with video and documented with a Racelogic VBOX III 100 Hz data acquisition system. Shuman and Husher observed that "the beginning and end points of the swerve have the motorcycle upright and proceeding down the roadway at laterally offset road positions. The total swerve distance involves multiple steering inputs by the rider and a sequence of responses by the motorcycle. This total swerve distance is contrasted with the shorter distance whereby the front and rear tires have successfully moved laterally the desired distance. This wheel clearance distance may be sufficient to clear short roadway hazards even if the total swerve is not yet complete. Since obstacle size varies in the real world, it is helpful to consider both the total distance for the swerve as well as the time for the wheels to clear the desired lateral offset…it takes less time and distance to avoid an object near ground level than to avoid larger obstacles."

Table 4.4 lists data reported by Shuman and Husher. The lateral accelerations listed were not reported in the paper. The lateral accelerations for the turn-aways were calculated

TABLE 4.4 Turn-away and swerve data from Shuman and Husher [18]

	Speed (mph)	Lateral movement (ft)	Longitudinal turn-away distance (ft)	Lateral acceleration (g)	Average (g)	Longitudinal swerve distance (ft)	Lateral acceleration (g)	Average (g)
Sport motorcycle	30	6.5	47	0.35	0.42	69	0.33	0.40
	30	13	56	0.50		78	0.52	
	35	6.5	50	0.43		73	0.40	
	35	13	65	0.50		100	0.43	
	40	6.5	60	0.39		95	0.31	
	40	13	86	0.38		115	0.42	

with Equation (4.29). The lateral accelerations for the full swerves were calculated with this same equation, with the exception that a coefficient of 0.732 was used and only half of the full lateral distance was input (consistent with how the formula is derived in Daily's text).

4.3 Crashes Involving Passengers

The addition of a passenger to the motorcycle adds mass that the operator will have to account for, and this additional mass can influence the path of the motorcycle and affect the operator's ability to brake or swerve. Not only will the passenger increase the total stopping distance, due to the added weight and changed weight distribution, but the ability for an operator to lean the bike, and hence traverse a curve or swerve to avoid a hazard, can be overwhelmed by the passenger leaning the opposite direction of the operator.

When braking with a passenger, the distance required to come to a stop may increase because the passenger adds weight to the system and, being unrestrained, the passenger adds pressure and potentially discomfort to the operator. As the operator applies the brakes and the motorcycle begins to decelerate, the passenger moves forward into the back of the operator. The willingness of the operator to maximize braking may be reduced as the operator negotiates balancing the motorcycle and the passenger who are moving independently while also maintaining control the bike. The uncertainty in exactly how braking is going to affect the balance and control of the passenger and the motorcycle will limit to comfort the operator has in maximizing it. The combination of the operator's discomfort in supporting the load of the rear passenger, balancing and controlling the motorcycle, and the additional loading to the front brakes results in additional stopping distance.

4.4 Additional Data Acquisition Techniques

4.4.1 Harry's Lap Timer

In the case studies related to calculating the motorcycle lean angle, this chapter covered a data acquisition setup that could be used for tracking a motorcycle's speed, path, and lean angle. Other data acquisition setups could also be used, particularly if the lean angle is not needed. For example, McDonough, Danaher, and Neale [19] tested the use of the smart phone application Harry's Lap Timer in conjunction with an external Sky Pro GPS antenna to track the speed and path of vehicles. In their testing, they compared the data from Harry's Lap Timer to data collected with a 20 Hz VBOX SL3 paired with a RLVB IMU 03 3-axis accelerometer. The VBOX was chosen as the control for this testing due to its wide use in the automotive industry and in accident reconstruction and the fact that it is specifically designed to monitor and record vehicle movement. Other data acquisition systems can sample at higher data rates, and these may be required for events where data needs to be sampled greater than 20 cycles per second, such as an impact crash test. Additionally, if the location where the test is taking place does not have good satellite coverage, then the use of different systems, or combination of systems, may be needed.

Harry's Lap Timer has four different versions: the Rookie Edition, the Petrolhead Edition, the ToGo Edition, and the Grand Prix Edition. For the examples described here, the Grand Prix Edition was used. This edition allows for pairing with an external GPS sensor that can record up to 20 Hz. It also allows for pairing with multiple cameras and can produce a video reference lap. Harry's Lap Timer is one of several that are designed to record a vehicle's speed, position, distance, and acceleration. Other examples are Track Attack, Track Master, Dynolicious, and Track Addict. These applications vary in their features, costs, and phone operating system, as well as in what data they collect. Harry's Lap Timer is available on both iOS and Android platforms, can record video, uses the phone's internal accelerometer, and uses Doppler shift to determine the vehicle's speed. Harry's Lap Timer can also overlay the speed, position, and acceleration data onto video. The video overlay feature allows the speed and acceleration data to be synchronized with the video as a real-time feedback. The video can be recorded separately, as its own video file or as a video file with the data imprinted in the lower left corner.

Two configurations of Harry's Lap Timer were tested. One configuration limited the reported data to 1 Hz and utilized the phones' internal GPS and accelerometer. The second configuration added the external Sky Pro GPS sensor, a small, lightweight Bluetooth-enabled GPS antenna that has a maximum sample rate of 10 Hz. Harry's Lap Timer will access the highest available sample rate through the external GPS, up to 20 Hz. If it was paired with an antenna that had a sample rate of 20 Hz, Harry's Lap Timer would track speed and position at 20 Hz. Figure 4.19 shows a smart phone with the Harry's Lap Timer home screen and the Sky Pro GPS accessory antenna.

The smart phones used in this testing were the iPhone 6 Plus and the Motorola Droid Turbo 2. These phones are equipped with an internal magnetometer, three-axis gyroscope, and three-axis accelerometer which can track the motion and acceleration of the phone. Harry's Lap Timer accesses the phone's accelerometer to measure the acceleration of the device directly. The accelerometers in the smart phones have a higher sample rate than the GPS system utilized in our testing. The accelerometer sensor in the iPhone 6 Plus, for instance, is a InvenSense MP67B (MPU-6500) which samples at 200 Hz. The accelerometer has a user-programmable full-scale range of ±2 g, ±4 g, ±8 g, or ±16 g. The gyroscope has a programmable full-scale range of ±250, ±500, ±1000, or ±2000 degrees/s. The accelerometer in the Droid has tri-axis Kionix KXTF9 with a programmable range of ±2 g, ±4 g, or ±8 g. The sample rate for the accelerometer is 25 to 800 Hz,

FIGURE 4.19   Harry's Lap Timer home screen and Sky Pro GPS XGPS160.

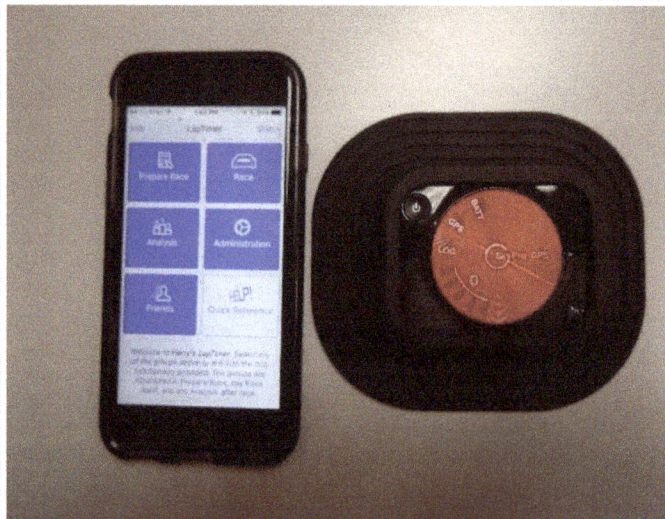

FIGURE 4.20 Exterior of test vehicle.

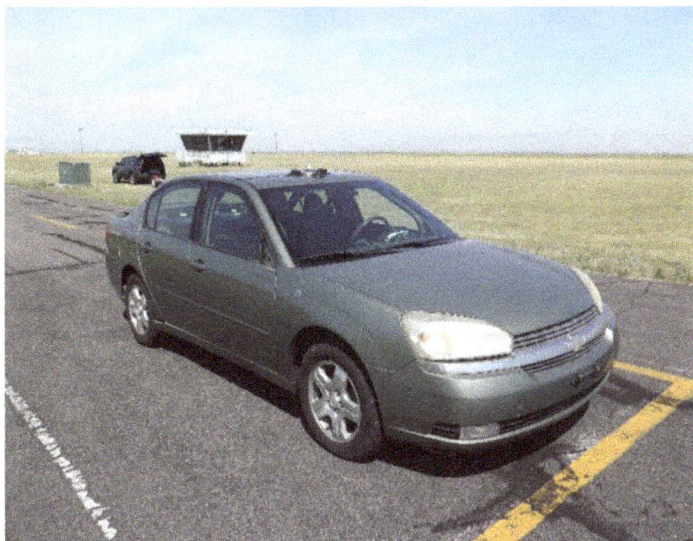

with a typical output of 50 Hz. When Harry's Lap Timer accesses the acceleration data, it samples the data to match the sample rate of the GPS.

Testing was performed with a 2004 Chevrolet Malibu. Both the iPhone (iOS 9.3.4) and the Droid (Android 6.0) were mounted on the inside of the windshield. The Bluetooth Sky Pro GPS antenna connected to the Droid was placed on the roof of the test vehicle above the vehicle's previously measured center of gravity and as close to the VBOX GPS receiver as possible. The VBOX accelerometer was mounted to a rigid plate directly above the vehicle's airbag control module. The test vehicle is shown in Figure 4.20, and the interior is shown in Figure 4.21.

In Harry's Lap Timer, there is a help section that shows how to setup the phone to record data, and there are also multiple guides and instructional videos on the application's web site. However, the process is relatively straightforward and requires minimal setup, such as connecting the phone via Bluetooth to the GPS antenna. Once the phones were paired with the sensors, both phones were then positioned onto independent mounts and rotated to have a level landscape orientation with a view through the windshield. Leveling the phones in the vehicle prior to testing insures that the longitudinal and lateral accelerations are zero. This can be accomplished by using the acceleration circle on the bottom left of the video display as shown in Figure 4.22.

The phones were located laterally as close to the center line of the vehicle as possible and mounted to the windshield though a suction style mount. Once the VBOX system and the phones were ready to collect data, they were initialized, and the car was held stationary for approximately 5 s. This established a zero state for the entire system before testing which created a baseline for data comparison. The following four groups of tests were performed on a closed course: (1) long distance, (2) slalom maneuvers, (3) left and right turns, and (4) hard acceleration and braking. An aerial view of the testing course outlining the location of each test is shown in Figure 4.23.

FIGURE 4.21 Interior of test vehicle.

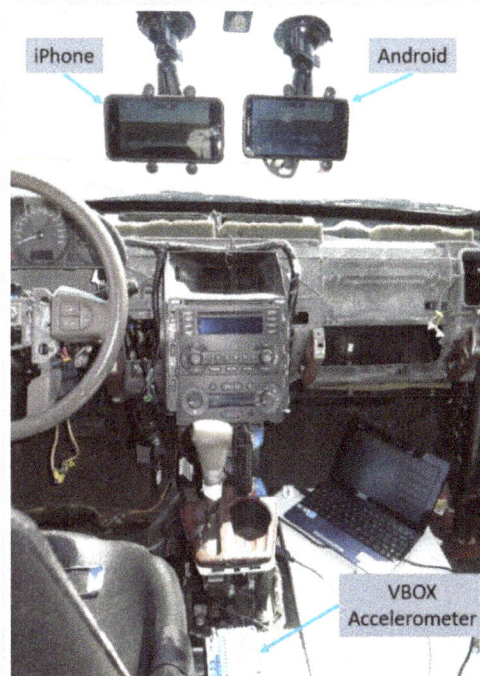

FIGURE 4.22   Acceleration circle shown in Harry's Lap Timer.

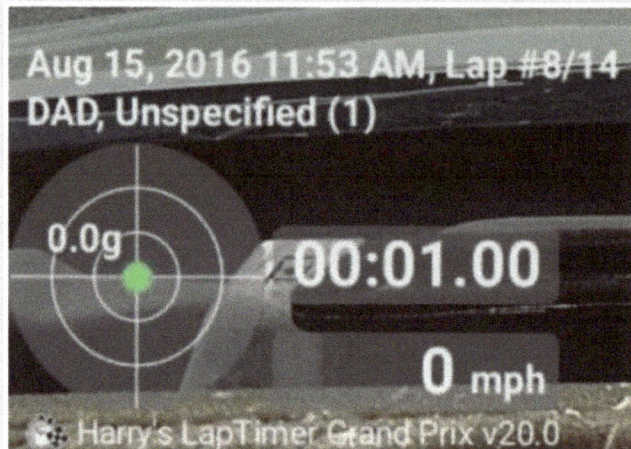

FIGURE 4.23   Aerial view of testing area.

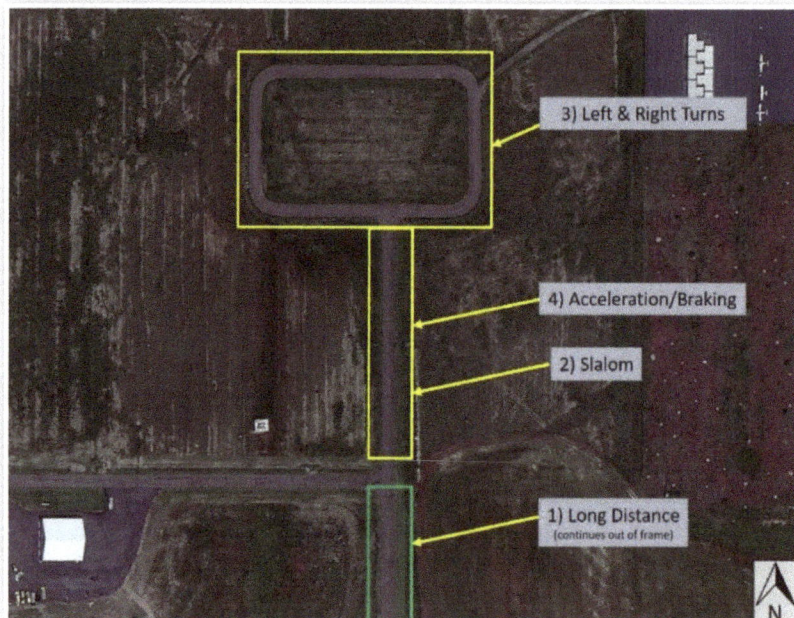

The right turns were performed traveling clockwise around the loop, and the left turns were performed driving counterclockwise. The slalom, braking, acceleration, and distance testing were performed on the straight section of road south of the loop. A sample of the GPS mapping for one of the left turn tests is shown in Figure 4.24. The three colors are visualizations of the paths of the three different devices (Droid, iPhone, and VBOX) during the run. The VBOX path is shown in red, the Droid (sampling at 10 Hz) in yellow, and the iPhone (sampling at 1 Hz) in green. The vehicle began each run traveling north (up) on the straight portion of the track, heading toward the loop. At the loop, the vehicle was driven either counterclockwise (left turn) or clockwise (right turn) for two full laps then returned to the initial position.

Review of the GPS positional data between the phones and the VBOX shows that there are certainly positional errors in the data (consistent with the manufacturer-stated 3 m positional accuracy). The data would be accurate enough for determination of the

FIGURE 4.24 GPS tracking of left turn Run 1.

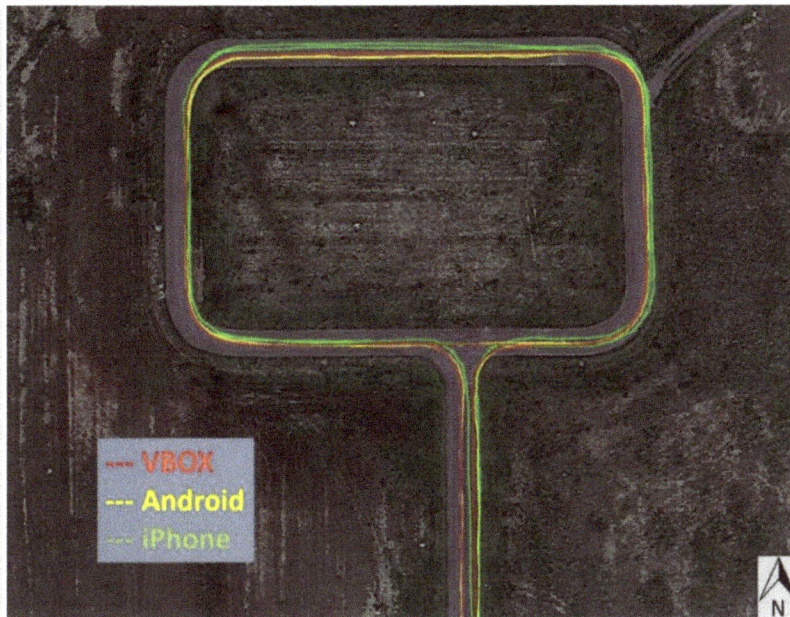

route the vehicle took, but not accurate enough to determine the lane position of the vehicle at any instant in time. If this setup was being used to document the motion of a motorcycle through a curve, the setup would need to be supplemented with video footage (perhaps aerial footage from an unmanned aerial vehicle) that would yield the path through the curve.

A total of 13 tests were performed, including 4 long distance runs, 3 slalom runs, 2 left turn runs, 2 right turn runs, and 2 straight-line acceleration and braking runs. The acceleration data from the VBOX accelerometer was filtered using a Butterworth 4-channel low-pass filter with a cutoff frequency of 3.3 Hz. The acceleration from Harry's Lap Timer is smoothed automatically by the software using a three-point moving average. This feature cannot be turned off. Speed and distance data collected by Harry's Lap Timer was not filtered, nor was the speed and distance data from the VBOX.

At the onset of each test, the VBOX and both phones began recording data at slightly different times. The VBOX was started first, then one phone, and then the other phone. With the difference in start times and the different rates that which each device recorded data, a time offset to synchronize the data needed to be determined. Harry's Lap Timer records video, but the VBOX used in the testing did not; therefore video synchronization was not an option. Instead, the data was synchronized first by using the initial steady-state condition created when the vehicle sat at rest for the 5 seconds prior to testing. The Harry's Lap Timer data was shifted to match the initial resting period with the data collected by the VBOX. The syncing was refined by calculating the total error using the sum of the square root of the differences squared from each data point. The total error was divided by the number of data points to get the average error. The solver function in Excel was then used to adjust the initial time offset to minimize the error in the data set.

Distance testing was performed on both phones, one at 1 Hz (iPhone) and the other at 10 Hz (Droid). Review of the distance data reported by each device showed a larger difference than expected (around 3% over approximately 3500 ft). It was determined that the difference was due to differences in the way the distances were calculated by

VBOX and Harry's Lap Timer. Distance reported by the VBOX is calculated based on speed and time. However, Harry's Lap Timer determines the distance by using a Haversine approximation between discrete GPS points. With the associated error inherent with any GPS system, the Haversine method used by Harry's Lap Timer can produce errors exceeding 3% to 5%, even over a small distance (under 350 ft). We achieved significantly better agreement with the VBOX data by calculating our own distance based on the Harry's Lap Time speed and time data. This reduced the error to about 0.4% over 3500 ft. Therefore, it is recommended that a distance be calculated from the speed and time reported by Harry's Lap Timer rather than relying on the distance directly reported by Harry's Lap Timer.

Figure 4.25 shows the vehicle speed data from the VBOX and Harry's Lap Timer (1 Hz) for one of the test runs (Run 1—left turn). The VBOX data is shown in black and Harry's Lap Timer data in green. Figure 4.26 is a close-up view of the speed comparison shown in the square on Figure 4.25. The speed data from Harry's Lap Timer shows good

FIGURE 4.25 Comparison of the HLT speed data at 1 Hz to the VBOX data from Run 1 (left turn).

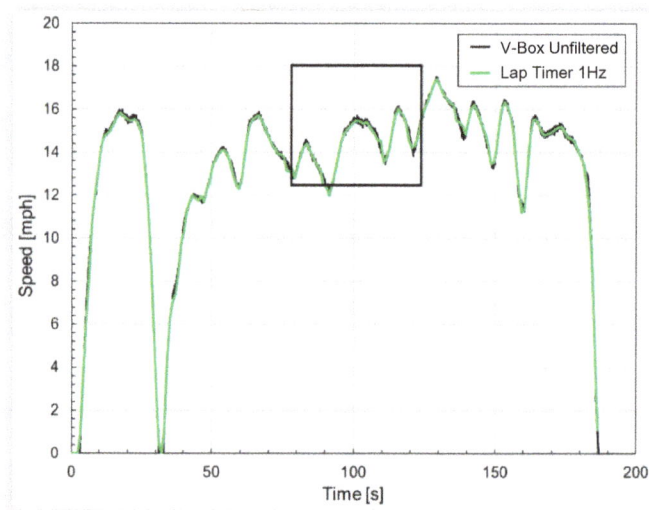

FIGURE 4.26 Close-up view comparison of the speed data from Run 1 (left turn).

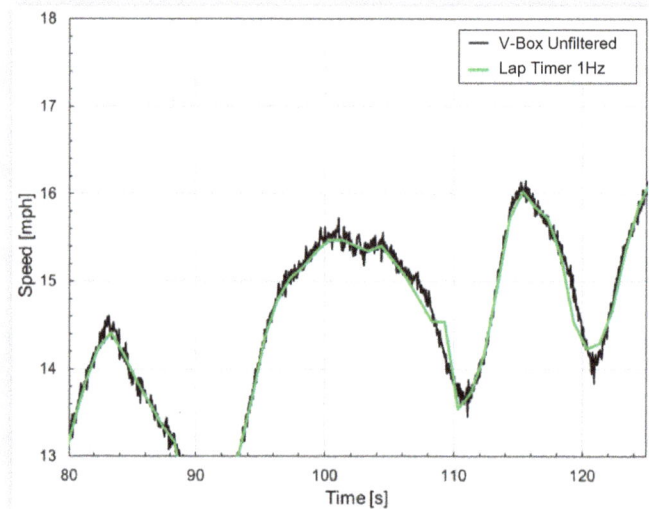

FIGURE 4.27 Comparison of the 10 Hz HLT speed data to the VBOX data for Run 1 (left turn).

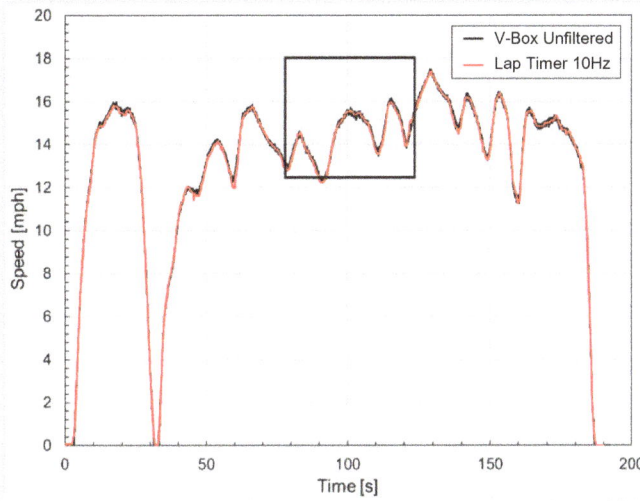

agreement with the VBOX data. The average difference between Harry's Lap Timer and the VBOX data was 0.09 mph.

When Harry's Lap Timer accessed the external antenna, the sample rate increased to 10 Hz. Figure 4.27 shows the comparison of the 10 Hz test data for Run 1 and the VBOX data. Figure 4.28 shows a close-up view of the data outlined by the square box in Figure 4.27. The VBOX data is in black and Harry's Lap Timer data is shown in red. The average difference between Harry's Lap Timer and the VBOX was ±0.07 mph. Similar results were obtained for the other test runs.

Lateral and longitudinal accelerations from Harry's Lap Timer were also compared to the VBOX acceleration data. Generally, a sampling frequency of 1 Hz would be inadequate for measuring acceleration during testing for accident reconstruction purposes, so the 10 Hz data is discussed here. Figure 4.29 is a comparison of the Harry's Lap Timer and VBOX data for the first left turn test. The filtered VBOX data is shown

FIGURE 4.28 Close-up of the comparison of the 10 Hz HLT speed data to the VBOX data for Run 1 (left turn).

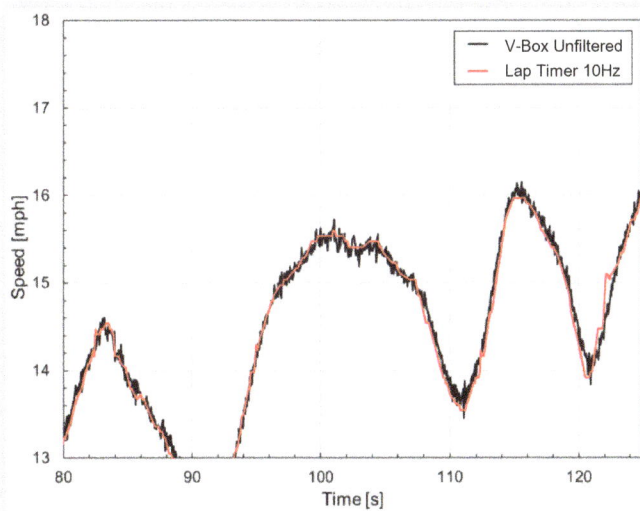

FIGURE 4.29 Comparison of lateral accelerations from Run 1 (left turn).

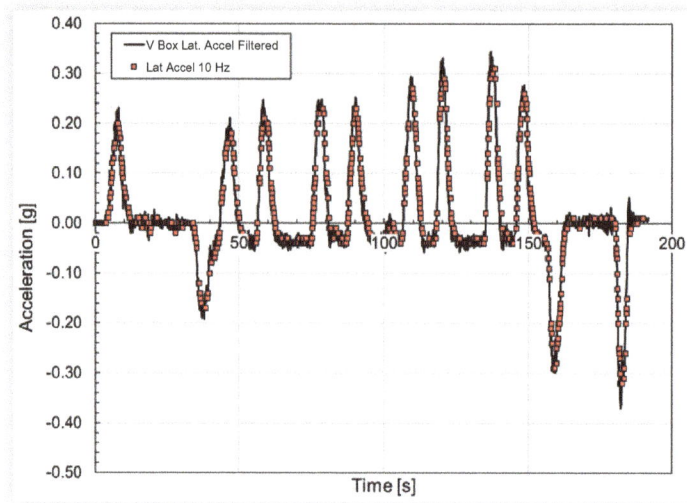

in black, and Harry's Lap Timer data is shown with red squares. The average difference between the Harry's Lap Timer data and the VBOX data was ±0.01 g.

Figure 4.30 is a similar comparison for the first slalom run. This test was run at a nominal speed of 35 mph with cone spacing of 100 ft. The filtered VBOX data is shown in black and Harry's Lap Timer data is shown with red squares. In this case, that lateral acceleration peaks are underreported by approximately 0.1 g. The average difference between the Harry's Lap Timer data and the VBOX data was ±0.04 g.

Harry's Lap Timer acceleration data (10 Hz) is compared to VBOX data for hard acceleration and braking in Figures 4.31 and 4.32. The hard acceleration data shows that the initial acceleration from 4.1 to 5.1 s does not track well. From 7 to 10 s, the acceleration reaches a steady-state condition resulting in an average acceleration of 0.33 g from both Harry's Lap Timer and the VBOX. The average difference between the acceleration from Harry's Lap Timer and the VBOX was 0.05 g. For the hard braking, the average difference between the Harry's Lap Timer data and the VBOX data was 0.05 g.

Analysis of the hard acceleration and braking data showed that the location of the phones during the testing compared to the location of the VBOX accelerometer was a

FIGURE 4.30 Comparison of lateral accelerations from Run 1 (slalom).

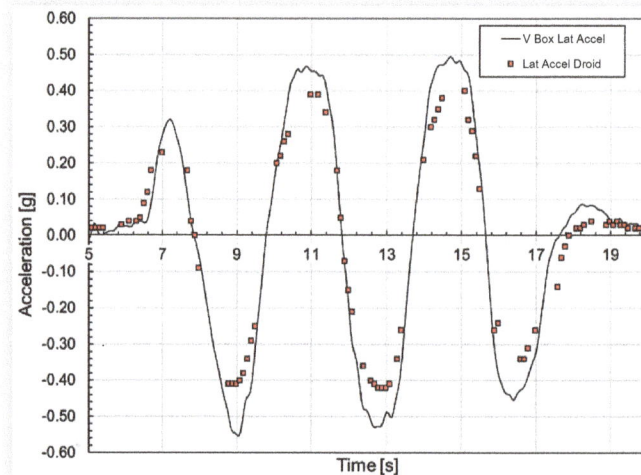

FIGURE 4.31 Comparison of longitudinal accelerations at 10 Hz, hard acceleration Run 1.

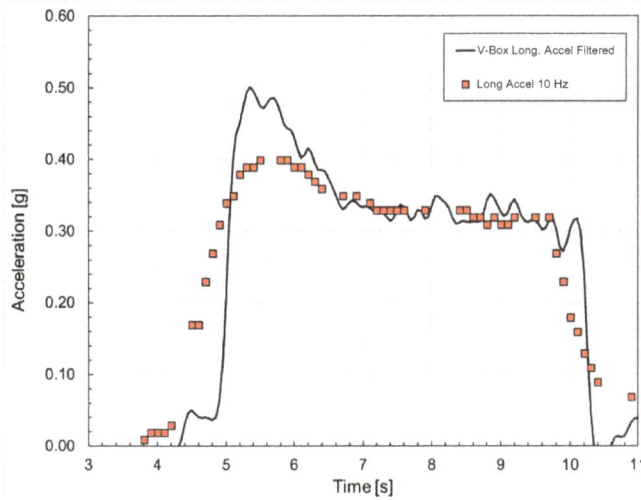

FIGURE 4.32 Comparison of longitudinal decelerations at 10 Hz, hard braking Run 1.

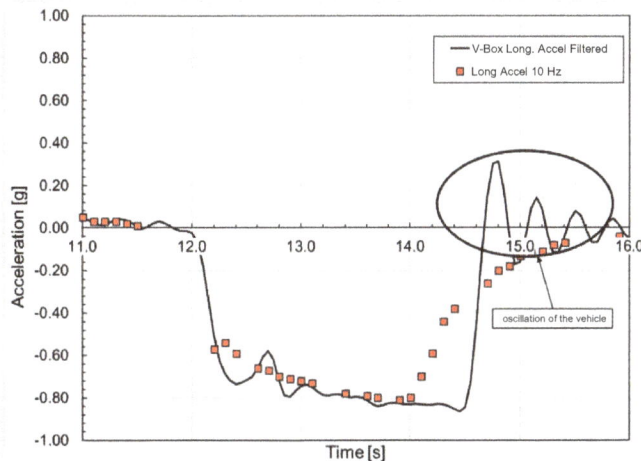

contributing factor in the data fit, along with the smoothing done by Harry's Lap Timer. The phones were mounted on the windshield, while the VBOX accelerometer was mounted on the floorboard of the vehicle. During events where the accelerations are moderate, such as 0.3 to 0.4 g, the body of the vehicle stays relatively flat. However, during heavy acceleration and braking where the vehicle saw accelerations over 0.5 g, the body pitch became much more pronounced. The location of the phones on the windshield created a moment arm away from the location of the VBOX accelerometer when the vehicle squats during acceleration or dives during braking. Therefore, the data does not track well with the VBOX data during hard acceleration and braking.

As part of the data collection, the phones were mounted to the windshield and oriented, so the camera was facing forward. This setup allowed the use of Harry's Lap Timer's video feature. Figure 4.33

FIGURE 4.33 Phones mounted to the windshield.

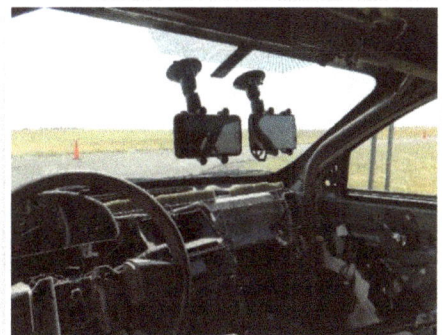

FIGURE 4.34   Video image from Harry's Lap Timer overlaid with data.

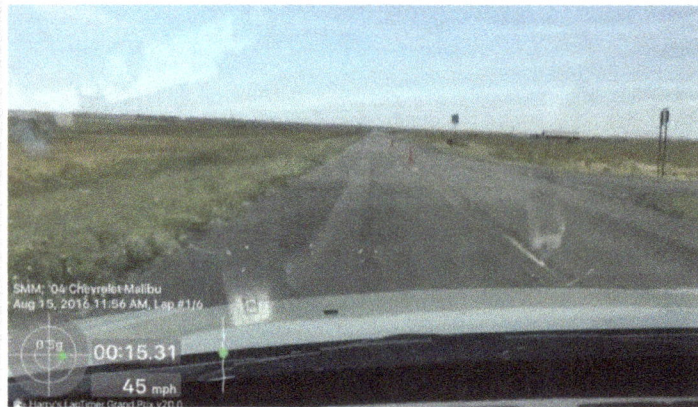

shows the two phones used in the testing mounted to the windshield, side by side. The mounts oriented the phones' level and plumb to provide a baseline for the accelerometer, and they also allowed the phones' cameras a level view from the interior of the vehicle. As the vehicle performs the maneuver, the data is visually overlaid onto the video by Harry's Lap Timer, providing real-time feedback. Figure 4.34 shows an example frame of video from Harry's Lap Timer. After the testing, the video can be downloaded with or without the data overlay. Harry's Lap Timer can also synchronize with other Bluetooth or Wi-Fi capable video devices such as GoPro to allow a wider range of options.

Similar testing was conducted using a 2007 Bonneville Triumph motorcycle. Again, Harry's Lap Timer was compared to the VBOX data. Harry's Lap Timer was operated using a Pixel 2 phone with Android 8.1.0. This phone has an internal accelerometer. Harry's Lap Timer was connected via Bluetooth to the Sky Pro GPS XGPS160. Both the phone and the Sky Pro GPS were mounted to the front of the motorcycle, and data was recorded at 10 Hz. The VBOX was attached at the rear. Figure 4.35 shows this setup

FIGURE 4.35   Data acquisition setup on the Triumph Bonneville.

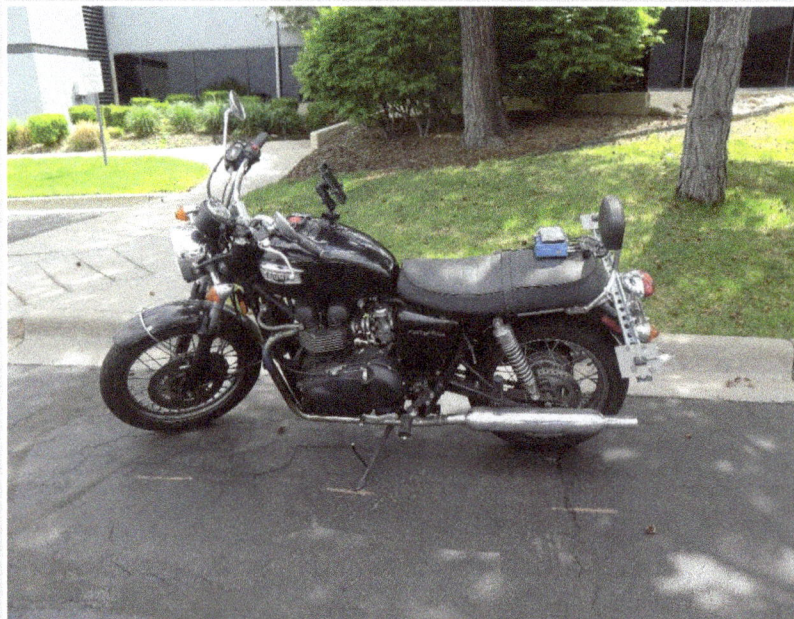

FIGURE 4.36 Motorcycle test route.

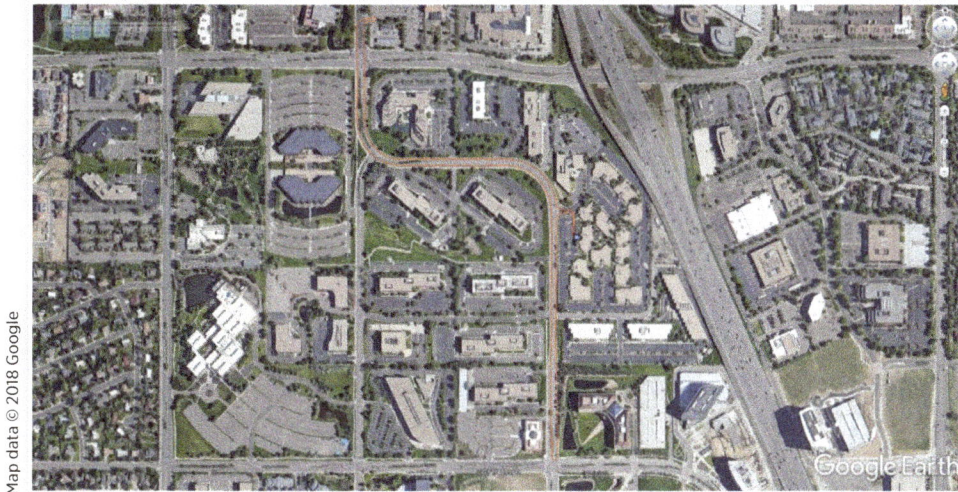

Map data © 2018 Google

on the motorcycle. The motorcycle was ridden through a 1.7 mile loop, shown in Figure 4.36. This route included a U-turn, left and right turns, and stop signals, and it lasted approximately 400 s. Figure 4.37 shows a comparison of the speed data from Harry's Lap Timer and the VBOX. Figure 4.38 shows a close-up of one section of the data. Again, Harry's Lap Timer collected speed data that compared well to the VBOX speed data. The average difference between the speed readings from the two devices was ±0.12 mph. In this test, Harry's Lap Timer did not report acceleration.

FIGURE 4.37 Comparison of the HLT speed data to the VBOX data for motorcycle test.

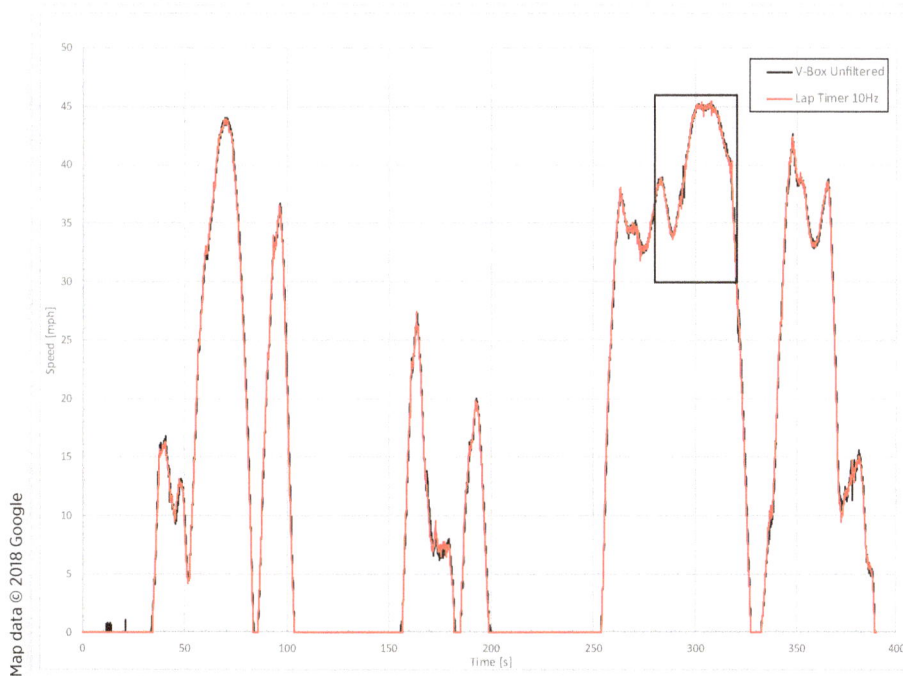

Map data © 2018 Google

FIGURE 4.38 Close-up comparison of the HLT speed data to the VBOX data for motorcycle test.

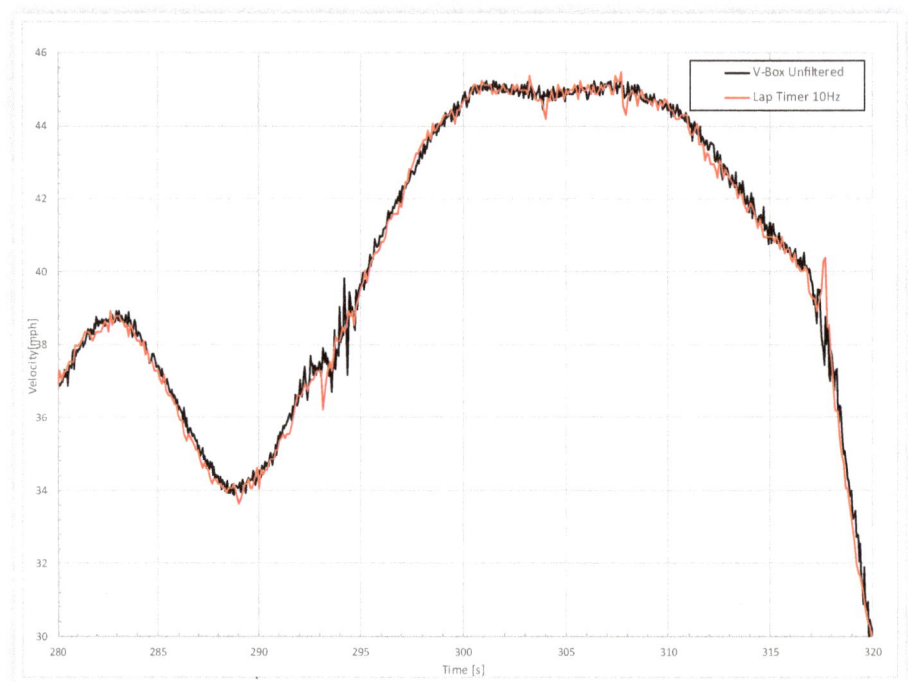

References

1. Fricke, L.B., *Traffic Crash Reconstruction*, 2nd ed., (Evanston, IL: Northwestern University Center for Public Safety, 2010), ISBN:0-912642-03-3.

2. Cossalter, V., *Motorcycle Dynamics*, 2nd ed., (2006), ISBN:978-1-4303-0861-4.

3. Rose, N.A., Carter, N., and Pentecost, D., "Analysis of Motorcycle and Rider Limits on a Curve," *Collision: The International Compendium for Crash Research* 9, no. 1, ISSN:1934-8681.

4. Policy on Geometric Design of Highways and Streets, 1990 Edition, American Association of State Highway and Transportation Officials (AASHTO), Washington, DC, ISBN 978-1560510017.

5. Baxter, A.T., *Motorcycle Crash Investigation*, (Jacksonville, FL: Institute of Police Technology and Management, 2017), ISBN:978-1-934807-18-7.

6. Carter, N., Rose, N.A., and Pentecost, D., "Validation of Equations for Motorcycle and Rider Lean on a Curve," *SAE Int. J. Trans. Safety* 3, no. 2(2015): 126-135, doi:10.4271/2015-01-1422.

7. Rose, N.A., Carter, N., and Smith, C., "Further Validation of Equations for Motorcycle Lean on a Curve," SAE Technical Paper 2018-01-0529, 2018, doi:10.4271/2018-01-0529.

8. Lambourn, R.F. and Wesley, A., "Motorcycle Tire/Roadway Friction," SAE Technical Paper 2010-01-0054, 2010, doi:10.4271/2010-01-0054.

9. Bartlett, W., "Lean Angle Selection by Motorcycle Riders," *Accident Reconstruction Journal* 21, no. 2 (March/April 2011), ISSN:1057-8153.

10. "Motorcycle Bank Angle Measurement Procedure," SAE Surface Vehicle Recommended Practice, J1168, March 2012, https://www.sae.org/standards/content/j1168_200701/.

11. Watanabe & Yoshida, "Motorcycle Handling and Performance for Obstacle Avoidance," *International Congress on Auto Safety*, San Francisco, CA, July 1973.

12. Hurt, H.H., DuPont, C.J., "Human Factors in Motorcycle Accidents," SAE Technical Paper 770103, 1977, doi:10.4271/770103.

13. Rice, R., "Rider Skill Influences on Motorcycle Maneuvering," SAE Technical Paper 780312, 1978, doi:10.4271/780312.

14. Limpert, R., *Motor Vehicle Accident Reconstruction Cause and Analysis*, 4th ed., (Michie, VA, 1994), 679, ISBN:1-55834-207-9.

15. Limpert, R., *Motor Vehicle Accident Reconstruction Cause and Analysis*, 7th ed., (Massachusetts: LexisNexis Matthew Bender, 2013), 36-36, ISBN:978-0-7698-5811-1:.

16. Daily, J., Shigemura, N., and Daily, J., *Fundamentals of Traffic Crash Reconstruction*, (Florida: Institute of Police Technology and Management, 2006), 476-479, ISBN:1-884566-63-4.

17. Bartlett, W., "Time and Distance Required for a Motorcycle to Turn Away from an Obstacle," SAE Technical Paper 2014-01-0478, 2014, doi:10.4271/2014-01-0478.

18. Shuman, K.F. and Husher, S.E., "Do I Brake or Do I Swerve – Motorcycle Crash Avoidance Maneuvering," *International Motorcycle Safety Conference*, Long Beach, CA, 2006.

19. McDonough, S., Danaher, D., and Neale, W., "Mid-Range Data Acquisition Units Using GPS and Accelerometers," SAE Technical Paper 2018-01-0513, 2018, doi:10.4271/2018-01-0513.

5

Physical Evidence from Motorcycle Crashes

This chapter describes physical evidence that may be present on the ground, on the motorcycle, or on the struck vehicle following a motorcycle crash. The first section focuses on evidence deposited at the scene, the second on damage sustained by the motorcycle, and the third on damage sustained by a struck vehicle. After these sections, this chapter covers techniques that can be utilized to document, measure, and diagram this evidence.

5.1 Scene Evidence

Scene evidence from motorcycle crashes often includes roadway markings such as tire marks, gouges, scrapes, fluid deposits, and debris. Additional evidence may appear on other scene objects that were struck, such as trees, poles, and guardrails. This evidence will typically need to be documented and preserved for later use in the reconstruction. This documentation process includes three phases: identification, documentation, and quantification. Identification involves recognizing the presence of a piece of evidence, either at the crash site or in photographs or video, and then determining if the evidence is from the subject crash or is unrelated to the crash. In the early stages of evidence preservation, it may not be apparent if a piece of evidence is from the subject crash. In such cases, it is typically better to capture the evidence and to rule it in or out during later analysis.

During the documentation phase, the investigator can record the evidence with still photography and video. The use of unmanned aerial vehicles (UAVs) or elevated cameras is becoming more common and these can provide perspectives that are useful in later analysis. Nearby bridges or hillsides can also be used to gain these elevated vantage points for taking photographs or video. During the quantification phase, the evidence is measured and located within its surroundings using tape measures, a measurement wheel, a total station, or a laser scanner or through photogrammetry using photographs or video captured with a UAV [1]. Evidence documentation typically culminates in creating a scaled evidence diagram that can be used for analysis of the vehicle motion. A sample evidence diagram for a single-vehicle motorcycle crash is included in Figure 5.1. This diagram includes tire marks, scrapes, gouges, fluid, and police paint. This evidence diagram was utilized, along with the damage to the motorcycle, to determine the motion of the motorcycle as it capsized, impacted a guardrail system, and slid along the ground. The reconstructed motion for this motorcycle is shown in Figure 5.2.

FIGURE 5.1   Sample evidence diagram.

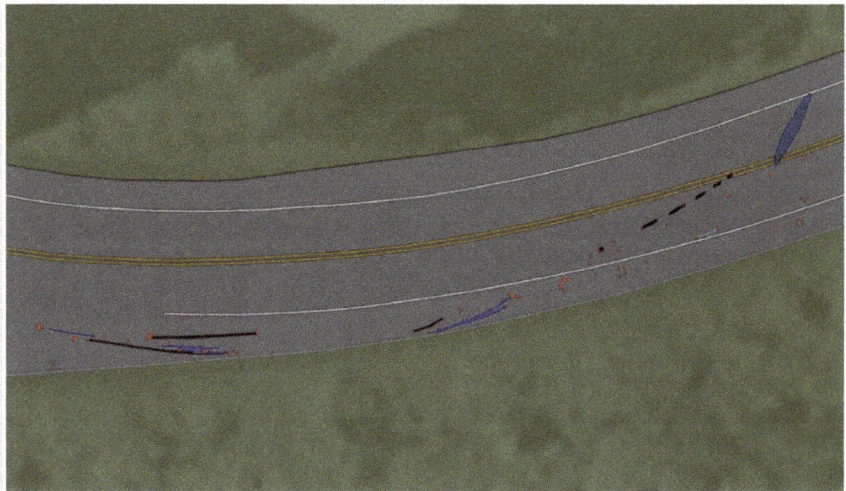

FIGURE 5.2   Evidence diagram with motorcycle positions.

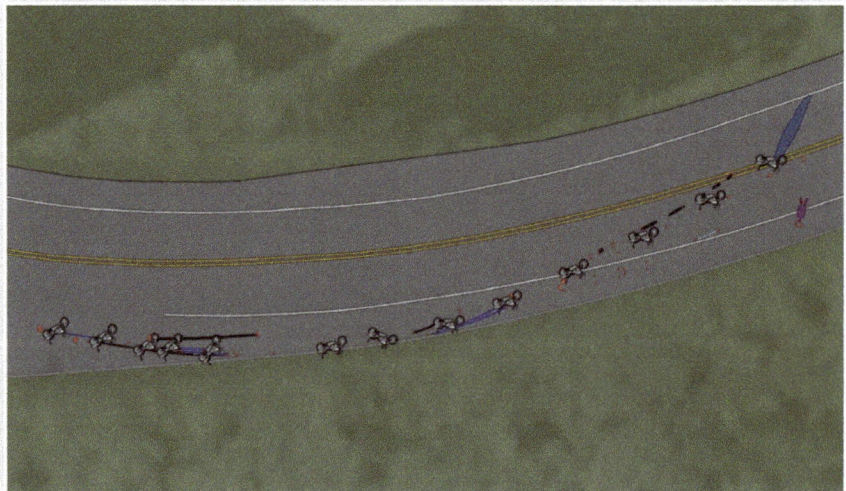

5.1.1 **Skid Marks**

A skid mark is a tire mark deposited by a locked wheel and tire. A skid mark deposited by the front wheel of a motorcycle will typically be short (say 30 ft or less), since locking the front wheel will quickly lead to capsizing. A motorcycle is inherently more stable with the rear wheel locked, and so, a skid mark deposited by the rear tire as a result of application of the rear brake can be significantly longer than one deposited by the front tire. Given that for a conventional motorcycle braking system the front and rear brakes are actuated independently, the presence of a skid mark from the rear wheel does not give the reconstructionist information about the degree to which the rider was employing the front brake.

Bartlett has observed that "there are many people who aver that one can determine if the front brake was in use by examining a rear wheel skid mark for a 'lazy-S' appearance. They claim that a straight rear skid is a clear indication of front brake use" [2, 3]. Fricke [4] falls in this camp, stating that "the use of the front brake (but not locking the wheel) provides greater braking stability, so a straight skid is more likely to have been produced using both the front and rear brakes, while a weaved/hooked skid is an indication of the rear brake being used alone." Similarly, Baxter [5] states that "if only the rear brake was applied to the point of locking the wheel, the skid mark left by the rear tire will be a long lazy S curve, trailing off in the direction of the road slope…the skid mark left during front and rear brake application…will be straight…."

Bartlett noted that "when a rider applies the rear brake only, a rearward-directed force on the tire at the contact patch acts to slow the motorcycle. This condition is inherently stable, and the rear wheel will tend to track straight. If the rear wheel is locked, it will still follow the front wheel while on level pavement (tire-roadway forces act to align the vehicle), but if the roadway is sloped, the rear wheel will tend to drift downgrade in response to gravity and the wheel's significantly reduced lateral force generation capability. By applying torque to the handlebars, the rider generates lateral forces which act on the chassis, effectively pushing the chassis to one side. A series of reversing force applications can cause the rear wheel of the motorcycle to 'weave' back-and-forth…Thus, given a locked rear wheel with no front braking, though the system is stable, lateral motions of the rear wheel can result from roadway geometry as well as from rider inputs. These motions will not necessarily occur, but they can."

Further, "if a rider applies significant front brake while the rear wheel is locked, the system may become inherently unstable. As the longitudinal force at the front contact patch exceeds the longitudinal force of the locked rear wheel, the rear wheel will try to swap places with the front. While this is easily done in a car, a motorcycle will fall over if this situation is not countered by a corrective action by the operator. The dynamic forward load transfer resulting from the increased braking action will lighten the load on the rear tire, further reducing its lateral and longitudinal force capacity. Thus, in considering only the external forces acting on the motorcycle, the tendency of the rear wheel to track in a straight line directly behind the front wheel is lowest when the front brake is in heavy use and the rear wheel is locked. This is essentially the opposite of the commonly observed nature of motorcycle skidmarks…this suggests that forces internal to the rider/motorcycle system provide a dominant influence on the shape of the skidmarks."

In addition, Bartlett conducted testing related to this issue. He concluded that "a single long straight skid mark may well be caused by a rear wheel skid generated while the front brake was used (particularly if the motorcycle was still traveling at some speed at the end of the mark), but one can NOT be confident to the level of 'more likely than not', let alone 'beyond a reasonable doubt' that this is true. The 'lazy-S' shape clearly indicates a rear brake skid mark, but without additional supporting information does not indicate 'to a reasonable degree of certainty' that the front brake was not used. Similarly, a serpentine mark can be generated with front brake use, and is dependent on the operator's 'body language'. Without testing the actual tires in use on a particular bike, or in some cases examining the tires themselves prior to their being driven on much, it may not be possible to confidently identify which tire made a particular short mark, or the vehicle's braking condition. With representative exemplar marks made under known conditions (rear only and front with rear) and using the actual tires in use on the accident unit, it would probably be possible to identify the braking condition at the time of the accident."

Dunn et al. [6] reported and analyzed braking tests and tire marks for three motorcycles—a 1995 BMW R1100RS (sport-touring with anti-lock brakes), a 2003 Buell XB9R (sport), and a 2005 Harley-Davidson XL 1200 Sportster Custom (cruising/touring). They tested three different braking strategies—best effort front braking only, best effort rear braking only, and best effort front and rear combined braking. Initial speeds for the testing were nominally 25, 45, and 60 mph and most of the tests were conducted on a flat, dry asphalt surface. One set of tests on wet asphalt were run with the BMW, a motorcycle equipped with anti-lock brakes. Skid marks documented in this study are consistent with Bartlett's findings and Dunn concluded "it is difficult to determine which brakes the rider used from only the observation of braking marks."

The skid marks generated in the testing by Peck, Deyerl, and Rose [7] are also consistent with Bartlett's findings. Figure 5.3 shows rear-wheel skid marks from all six of their braking tests. These tire marks vary in length between 52.5 and 59.5 ft. At least three of them are straight although no front-wheel braking was employed while they were being deposited. Thus, the literature does not support using the shape of a rear wheel skid mark to discern the level of front wheel braking employed by the motorcycle operator.

FIGURE 5.3 Skid marks from six rear-brake-only tests (Photo by Eric Deyerl).

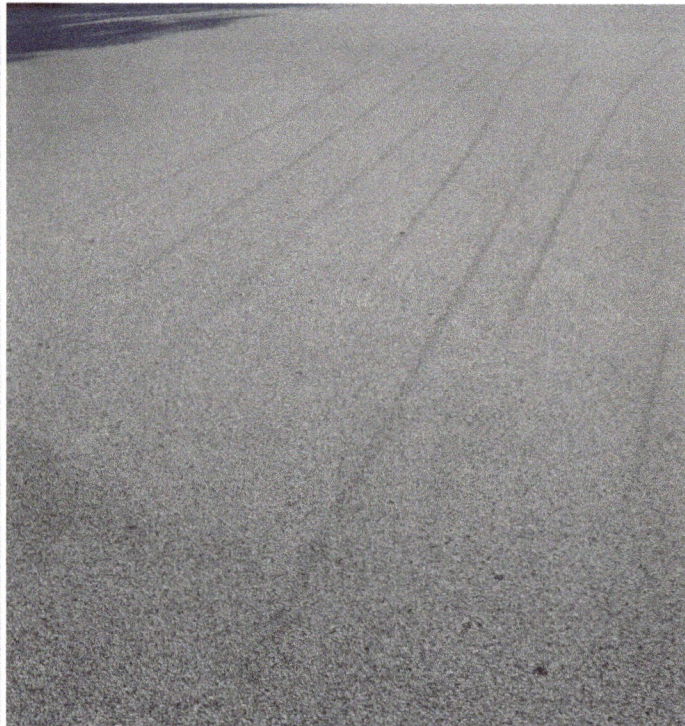

5.1.2 Gouges, Scrapes, Scuffs, and Tire Marks

When a motorcycle falls to the ground and slides or tumbles to rest, components of the motorcycle will typically gouge, scrape, or scuff the road surface. Scuff marks can be deposited along with material from the motorcycle tires, components, or the riders clothing and gear. An example of this type of marking on the roadway is shown in the photographs of Figure 5.4. Another example is shown in Figure 5.5. During scene documentation, gouges and scrapes on the road should be documented. If there is a need to understand what component of the bike or rider gear deposited specific

FIGURE 5.4 Scrapes, gouges, and tire marks from a motorcycle sliding on the roadway.

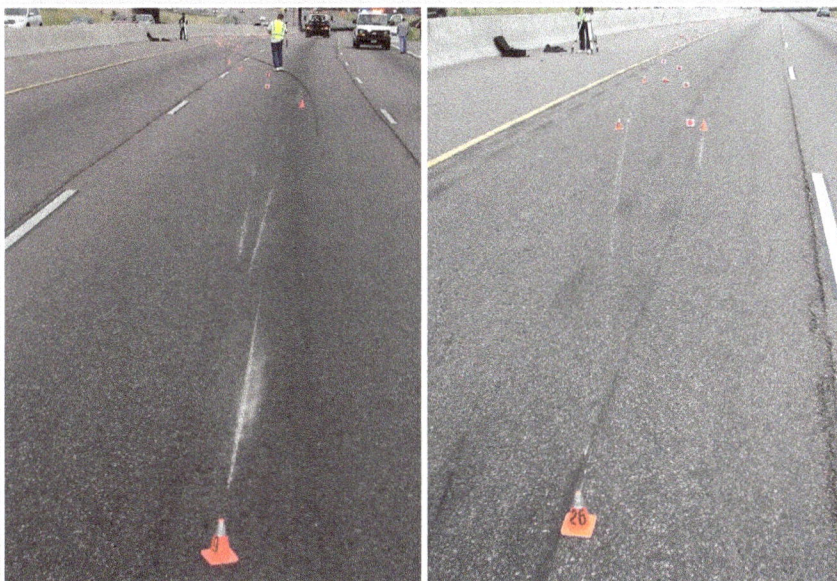

FIGURE 5.5 Scrapes, gouges, and tire marks from a motorcycle sliding on the roadway.

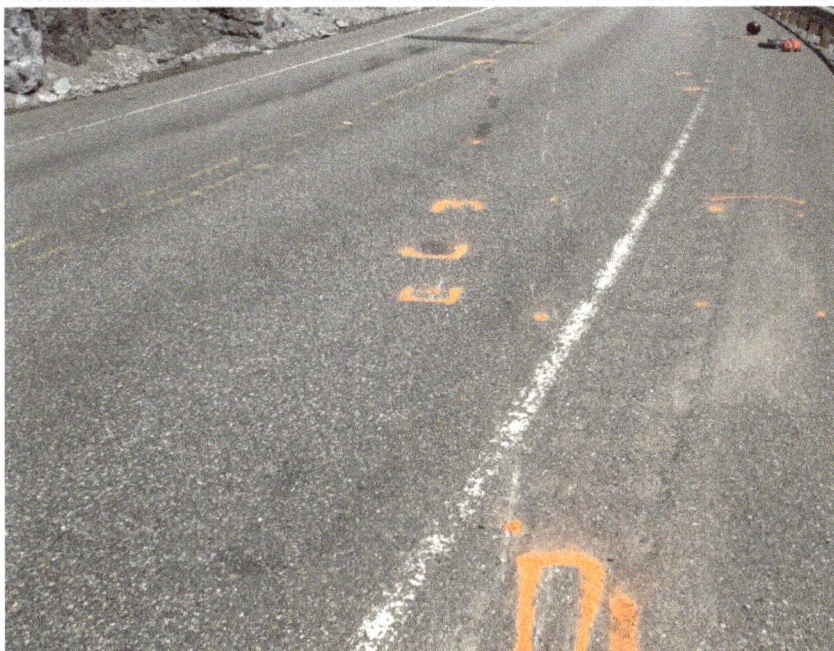

CHAPTER 5

evidence, then further documentation of the characteristics of the scrapes and gouges can be performed. These will be integral to determining the distance over which the motorcycle slid or tumbled to rest and determining what components made which marks. Also, for single-vehicle loss-of-control motorcycle crashes, the distance between the end of tire marks and the first gouging may reveal whether the motorcycle experienced a low-side or a high-side fall. Thus, the location of scrapes and gouges and the distance between them can have significance to the reconstruction. Also, the changing orientation of the scratches or gouges over the course of the path can help the reconstructionists determine the specific motion of the motorcycle along its path, particularly if specific motorcycle components can be related to specific scrapes or gouges.

As McNally observed [8], some motorcycles have "a variety of protrusions that tend to interact with the roadway surface to gouge or scrape while the motorcycle is sliding. There is only limited test information available at this time for sport motorcycles, which tend to slide more easily across the roadway due to the sleek bodywork that prevents the deep gouging on other bikes." This implies that the motorcycle type and the extent of scraping and gouging may be useful in determining a reasonable range of decelerations for the motorcycle during the sliding and tumbling on the ground. McNally continued: "Application of any particular coefficient of friction in a real-world collision should be done with consideration for the manner in which the motorcycle traveled across the roadway surface and the degree of scraping or gouging that occurred during the slide. In general, the greater the degree of roadway gouging and scraping, the higher one would expect to be the coefficient of friction."

5.1.3 Site Inspection Checklist

The evidence that is documented during a site inspection depends, in part, on what issues are being analyzing and on how much time has elapsed between the crash and the site inspection. The list that follows assumes a site inspection that is taking place before any evidence has significantly deteriorated. The items on this list are suggestions and are not intended to be a complete list:

☐ **Take photographs of the whole crash site**. Typically, this involves starting at the beginning of the physical evidence and walking along the full trajectories of the involved vehicles, taking photographs along the way. It can also be useful to walk and photograph the evidence from the end to the beginning. Aerial photography from a UAV can also be useful for overall documentation of a crash site.

☐ **Map the physical evidence from the crash**. Mapping will typically be accomplished with a total station, a laser scanner, or through image-based scanning or photogrammetry:

✓ Tire marks

✓ Gouges

✓ Scrapes

✓ Fluid deposits

✓ Debris

☐ **Map the site geometry**.

✓ Roadway striping

✓ Terrain

✓ Signage

☐ **Document site characteristics**.

✓ Speed limit

✓ Latitude and longitude

✓ Signage

✓ Note if any surveillance cameras are present

✓ Document the lighting conditions

5.2 Evidence on the Motorcycle

Evidence on the motorcycle following a crash will often include components that are scraped, scratched, and abraded, punctures and deformation to the fuel tank, wheel deformation, fork deformation, flat spots on tires from skidding, and broken forward and signal lighting. During an inspection of the motorcycle, this evidence can be documented and preserved for later use in the reconstruction. Other information about the motorcycle can also be obtained during an inspection or from manufacturer specifications or brochures. For instance, manufacturer specifications and brochures typically identify the type of braking system on a motorcycle. This can also be determined from a physical inspection of the motorcycle. As an example, Baxter and Robar [9] note that "all motorcycles that are equipped with [an integrated braking] system require the front wheel be equipped with dual disc brake calipers and rotors. The fastest way to check for this system is to follow the brake lines from each caliper. If the left and right brake hoses meet in a t-connection under the headlight area, this is a good indicator that only the front lever operates just the front brakes. Another method is to slip a piece of paper between the brake pad and face of the rotor. An assistant applies the rear brake pedal while an attempt is made to pull out the sheet of paper. If it's integrated, the front brake pad will hold the sheet in place against the rotor face."

When an upright motorcycle impacts another vehicle, there are characteristic damage patterns that will often be evident on the motorcycle. For instance, the front wheel may be deformed in the area where it first contacted the vehicle, the forks will be bent rearward and sometimes broken, and the wheel may be deformed rearward into the frame or engine components behind it. This deformation can be photographically documented and measured during an inspection or with photogrammetric analysis. The photographs of Figure 5.6 show examples of front wheel and fork deformation from motorcycle collisions with other vehicles. These photographs, which were provided by Lou Peck, are from the motorcycle collisions conducted at the World Reconstruction Exposition (WREX) held in 2016.

One issue that often comes up when a motorcycle impacts another vehicle is if the motorcyclist was braking prior to the collision. Under optimal braking, a motorcycle will not deposit skid marks, and so the analyst is left to identify other pieces of evidence that may indicate braking. Smith [10] and others have pointed out another type of evidence that may reveal pre-impact braking, noting that "because the result of a hard brake application is the transfer of weight from the rear wheel to the front wheel, this information can assist a crash investigator with understanding whether the rider was applying the brakes prior to the impact. When weight transfers to the front wheel, the front springs compress and the fork tubes slide into the shock housing. If the bend of the fork tubes occurs at the entrance to the housing, the investigator can then determine the extent to which the front wheel was loaded at the moment of impact. As an

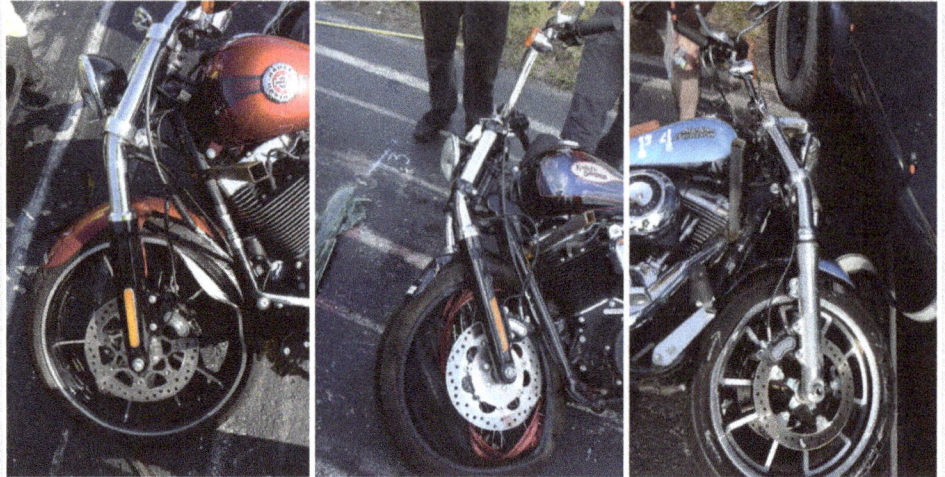

extension to this observation and based upon this test and the large number of additional motorcycle-to-car impact tests conducted by the authors, there is little or no fork compression that results from the impact itself. Therefore, evidence of fork compression observed on the motorcycle post-impact is very likely due to pre-impact weight transfer caused by braking."

When the components of a motorcycle slide along the ground scratch marks may be created on these components. Oftentimes, there are multiple families of scratches that overlap with different orientations. The orientations and order of these scratches can be documented during a post-crash motorcycle inspection. Assuming the motorcycle is not tumbling during the sliding phase of the crash, the scratches will be parallel to and opposite in direction of the motorcycle's ground plane velocity [11]. Thus, these scrapes can be used to determine the yaw orientation of the motorcycle at various times during the sliding phase. The photographs of Figure 5.7 show an example of damage to one motorcycle from sliding on the ground. The photograph on the left shows scraping and scratching on the fuel tank and the photograph on the right shows abrasions to the crash bar.

FIGURE 5.7 Motorcycle damage from sliding on the roadway.

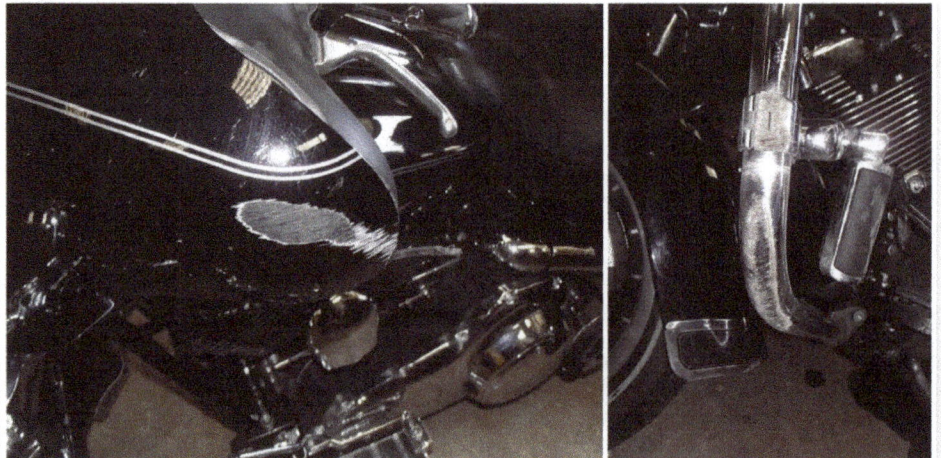

5.2.1 Motorcycle Inspection Checklist

Following is a list of guidelines and suggestions for a post-crash inspection of a motorcycle. The list below is intended for collecting basic information for reconstructing a motorcycle crash. However, this list is likely more extensive than what is necessary for many reconstructions. In some cases, not all this data is necessary or accessible. In other cases, a more detailed inspection may be necessary. In those cases, refer to the article by Kubly and Buse [12], in which they offer detailed guidelines for documenting damage to or failures of specific motorcycle components:

- ☐ **Take overall photographs of the motorcycle**. Typically, this would consist of eight photographs—one taken from each side of the vehicle and one take from each corner of the vehicle.

- ☐ **Document the motorcycle's vehicle identification number (VIN)**. The VIN istypically located on the steering head of the frame or on the frame downtube [5].

- ☐ **Document the tires and wheels of the motorcycle**.
    - ✓ Write down or photograph the tire sidewall information. This will include the manufacturer, type, size, and serial number.
    - ✓ Measure the tread depth of each tire.
    - ✓ Measure the tire pressure of each tire.
    - ✓ Photographically document damage to either of the wheels.
    - ✓ Document flat spots from heavy braking and other damage to the tires.

- ☐ **Document the braking system**.
    - ✓ Determine whether the front and rear brakes are independent or integrated.
    - ✓ Document any damage to the braking system from the crash.
    - ✓ Document the condition of the linkages, hoses, tubes, and the brake fluid level.

- ☐ **Identify any aftermarket components on the motorcycle**.

- ☐ **Document the damage to the motorcycle**, including deformation, contact markings, and fractures, taking photographs with a wide range of zoom levels:
    - ✓ Identify which components of the motorcycle exhibit wear from sliding on the road surface.
    - ✓ Determine if the damaged condition was altered when the motorcycle was removed from the crash scene.
    - ✓ Document the post-crash geometry of the motorcycle. This documentation could utilize laser scanning, photogrammetry, or hand measurements. This documentation should include documentation of the wheelbase shortening of the motorcycle.
    - ✓ Determine the height at which the front forks of the motorcycle bent. This could enable a determination of the magnitude of front suspension compression at the time of an impact.

- ☐ **Determine which gear the motorcycle is in**.

- ☐ **Determine if the motorcycle was carrying any cargo at the time of the crash**.

- ☐ **Document the condition of the headlamp assemblies and bulbs**.

5.3 **Damage to the Struck Vehicle**

Reconstructing a motorcycle collision will often involve determining the impact configuration between the motorcycle and the struck or striking vehicle. In many instances, the motorcycle will still be upright at the time of the impact, and there will be a clear indication on the vehicle of the impact configuration in the form of damage and materials transfer from the components of the motorcycle, including the wheels and tires. For example, the motorcycle will often deposit a tire mark on the struck vehicle that will make the point of first contact on the struck vehicle apparent. Several examples of such tire marks are shown in Figure 5.8. These photographs are from post-test documentation of the WREX 2016 collisions. An example from a real-world collision is shown in Figure 5.9.

In some instances, a motorcycle will capsize prior to the collision, and determining the impact configuration will be more complicated. In these instances, determining the impact configuration can still involve identifying damage from specific motorcycle components on the struck vehicle. Computer models of the motorcycle and struck vehicle can be used to determine the alignment to produce the documented damage. As an

FIGURE 5.8   Motorcycle tire marks on struck vehicles from the WREX2016 collisions.

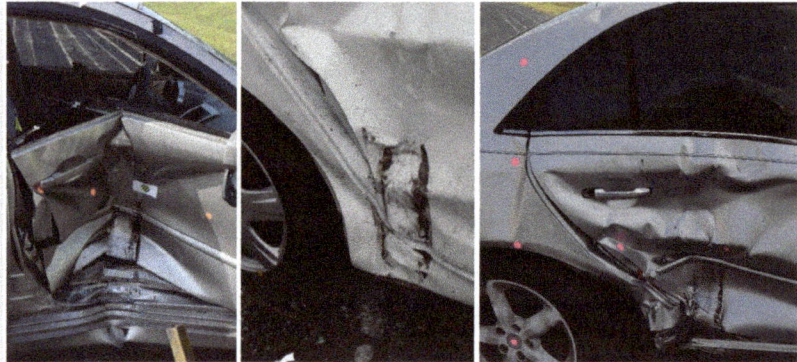

FIGURE 5.9   Motorcycle tire mark on struck vehicle from real-world collision.

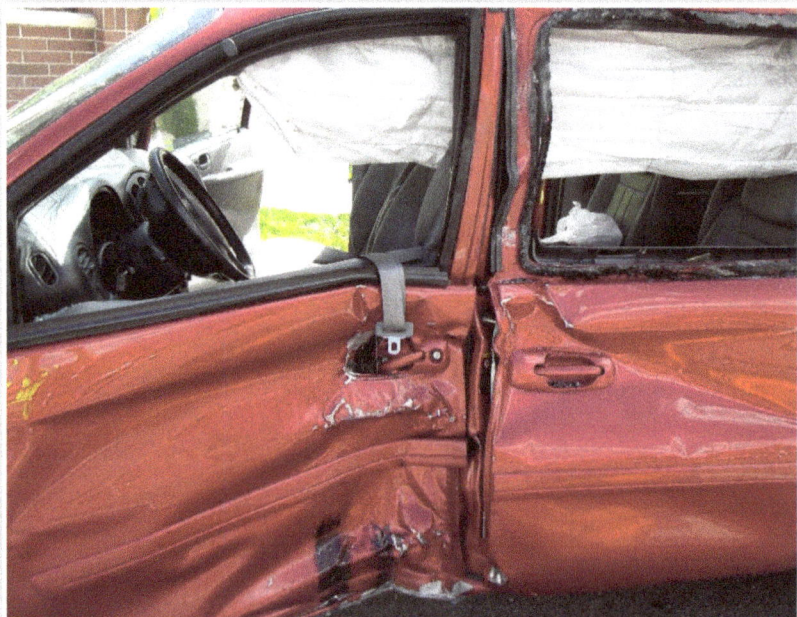

FIGURE 5.10 Crash-related damage to Plymouth Grand Voyager.

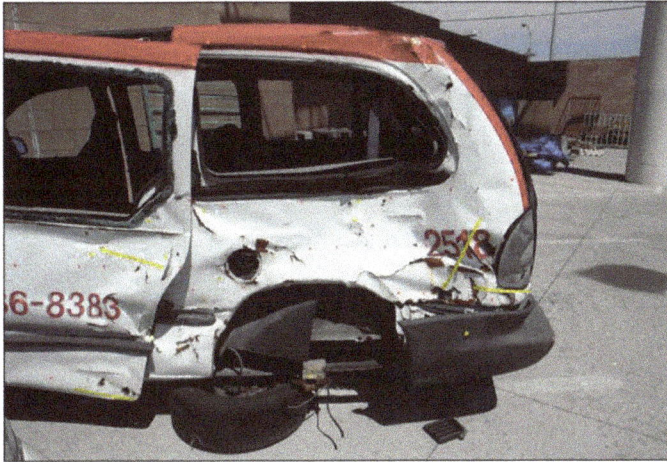

example of such analysis, consider the evidence from a collision between a Suzuki motorcycle and the driver's side of a Plymouth Grand Voyager. Figure 5.10 depicts the damage to the Plymouth that resulted from the collision. Damaged components included the driver's side sliding door, the driver's side rear quarter panel and body sheet metal, the driver's side rear wheel, the driver's side bumper fascia wrap-around, the driver's side taillight assembly, and the driver's side D-pillar and roof rail.

During an inspection of the Plymouth the following damage was identified that enabled determination of the impact configuration between the Plymouth and the Suzuki (Figure 5.11):

- An imprint from the rear Suzuki tire on the driver's side rear quarter panel of the Plymouth

- An imprint from the Suzuki chain on the driver's side rear fender and bumper fascia wrap-around

- A wheel imprint on the driver's side sliding door of the Plymouth from the front tire of the Suzuki

- A hole in the driver's side sliding door from the Suzuki's handlebar

FIGURE 5.11 Crash-related damage to Plymouth Grand Voyager.

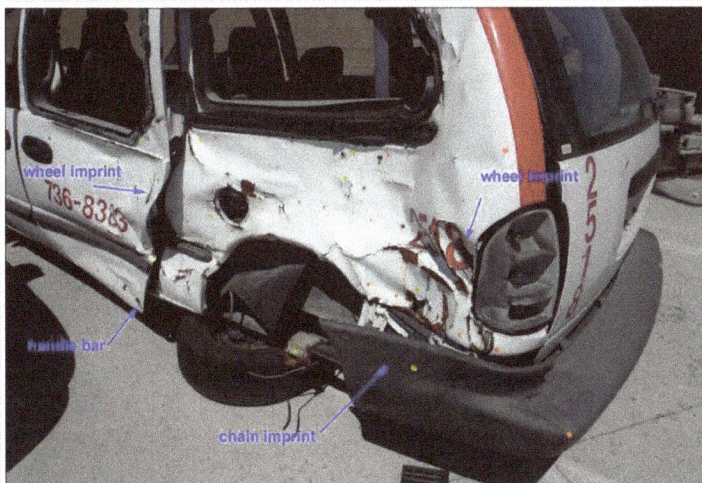

FIGURE 5.12 | Impact configuration.

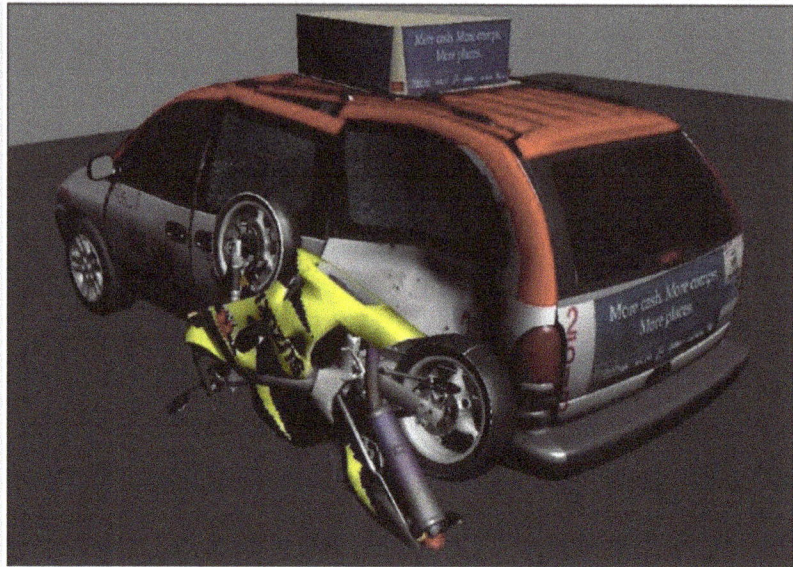

The damage to the motorcycle included the following: damage to the left-side fairing, a broken frame slider on the left side, damage to the metal frame on the left side, damage to the rearward portion of the leather seat, damage to the left side clutch lever handlebar grip, damage to left passenger foot peg, and damage to the right-side headlight fairing. The damage to the Suzuki and the corresponding imprints on the driver's side of the Suzuki imply the impact configuration shown in Figure 5.12, with the motorcycle in an inverted orientation. This collision was also captured by a surveillance camera, though the impact configuration could not be determined from the video. However, the impact configuration shown in Figure 5.12 was consistent with what was shown in the video. The vehicle damage and video together demonstrated the following sequence: (1) When the Suzuki motorcycle first entered the view of the surveillance camera, the motorcycle was pitched forward on its front wheel at an angle of approximately 12°, consistent with heavy braking. (2) As the Suzuki traversed the view of the camera, it continued to pitch forward and then rolled towards its right side. (3) The Suzuki then impacted the ground and rolled over until it impacted the Plymouth while oriented upside down relative to the ground. (4) The left side of the Suzuki impacted the Plymouth.

5.4 **Evidence Documentation Methods**

5.4.1 **Mapping with LIDAR**

Lidar, a term that is an acronym for light detection and ranging, is a method of *remote sensing* that can be used to map the geometry of an accident site or of a damaged or undamaged vehicle. Remote sensing refers to methods for the acquiring physical data and measurements of objects without physically touching them. These methods sense the physical characteristics of objects based on the characteristics and behavior of electromagnetic radiation interacting with these objects. "As [radiation from the sun] approaches the Earth, it passes through the atmosphere before reaching the Earth's surface.

Some is reflected upward from the Earth's surface; it is this radiation that forms the basis for photographs and similar images. Other solar radiation is absorbed at the surface of the Earth and is then reradiated as thermal energy. This thermal energy can also be used to form remotely sensed images, although they differ greatly from the aerial photographs formed from reflected energy. Finally, man-made radiation, such as that generated by imaging radars, is also used for remote sensing" [13]. Lidar falls in the third category of remote sensing that utilizes man-made radiation.

Campbell describes lidar as follows:

> *Lidar...can be considered analogous to radar imagery, in the sense that both families of sensors are designed to transmit energy in a narrow range of frequencies, then receive the backscattered energy to form an image of the Earth's surface. Both families are active sensors; they provide their own sources of energy, which means they are independent of solar illumination. More important, they can compare the characteristics of the transmitted and returned energy – the timing of pulses, the wavelengths, the angles – so they can assess not only the brightness of the backscatter but also its angular position, changes in frequency, and the timing of reflected pulses. Knowledge of these characteristics means the lidar data, much like data acquired by active microwave sensors, can be analyzed to extract information describing the structure of terrain and vegetation features not conveyed by conventional optic sensors.*

It is now common for crash reconstructionists to utilize a lidar (laser) scanner to map the geometry of an accident site or the post-crash condition of the motorcycle or another vehicle involved in a collision [1]. This can be particularly useful if an exemplar motorcycle or vehicle is also scanned and the damaged and undamaged scans can be compared to determine relevant measurements, such as wheelbase shortening or crush. As an example, Figure 5.13 shows the colorized scan data of an exemplar motorcycle obtained with a FARO laser scanner.

FARO is one company manufacturing and selling scanners that are widely used by accident reconstructionists [14]. When using these scanners to document accident sites where physical evidence is still present, DiTallo, Brandt, and Green recommended marking evidence with chalk or paint to make its location more evident in the resulting scan data [15]. They conducted an experiment with a FARO Focus^{3D} X 330 and offered

FIGURE 5.13 Sample scan data of an exemplar motorcycle.

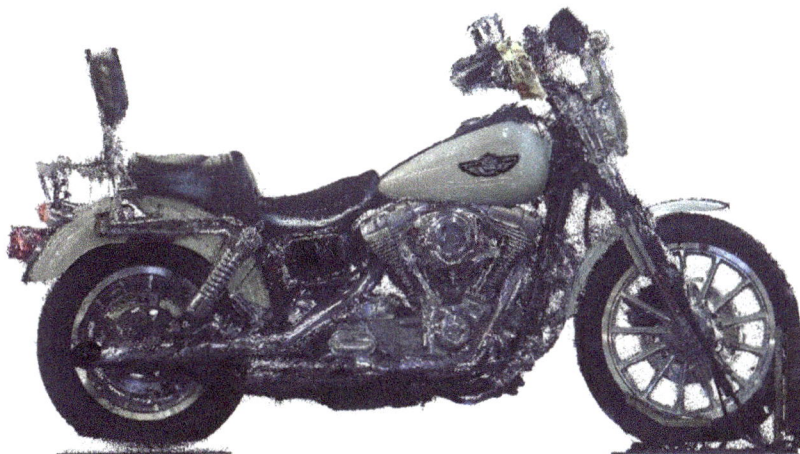

recommendations on scanner placement and settings (resolution and quality). In relationship to scanner placement, they noted that "The most effective and efficient methodology we have found is to stagger our scanner placement from one side to another, maintaining a 70-foot (21.34-meters) radius between placements…Changing the vertical height from a standard tripod (6 ft+ /1.83 m+) to an extra tall tripod (9 ft+/2.74 m+) did not gain much distance in the horizontal plane. In fact, the further the scan goes out, the more separation there is between the scan points. Your scanned data at the extremes will certainly have greater separation." In relationship to the resolution setting, they noted that "the FARO Laser Scanners provide the ability to adjust several settings which greatly affect the time required to complete a scan and the quality of the data captured. Resolution is a setting that determines the density of the scan points. Choosing a small value for resolution means there will be a larger distance between points scanned and a lower density of points in the resulting point cloud. Choosing a larger value for resolution means the distance between scanned points is smaller, so the captured points in the cloud will be dense…Choosing a higher resolution setting means each scan takes more time to complete. For most scenes, a resolution value of 1/4 or 1/5 gives good results in a reasonable amount of time." In relationship to the quality setting, they noted that "By adjusting the quality of the scan, the user is able to reduce the amount of noise (extraneous unwanted points) in the scan data. The higher the quality setting, the less noise in the scan data. You can choose from 1X to 8X depending on the resolution setting. In our experiment and demonstration for this article, we used a 3X Quality setting."

5.4.2 Photogrammetry

When the reconstructionist inspects a site after some or all the evidence has deteriorated or disappeared, that evidence can still be placed on an evidence diagram using photogrammetric analysis (if the evidence was documented through photographs or video). This situation is not at all unusual, considering that reconstructionists are often asked to analyze crashes long after they have occurred.

The term *photogrammetry* is defined by the American Society of Photogrammetry and Remote Sensing (ASPRS) as the art, science, and technology of obtaining reliable information about physical objects and the environment through process of recording, measuring and interpreting photographic images and patterns of recorded radiant electromagnetic energy and other phenomena [16]. Defined in this way, the term *photogrammetry* has considerable overlap with the term *remote sensing*. Within the field of accident reconstruction, the term *photogrammetry* has typically been defined more narrowly as mathematical and graphical techniques used for making accurate measurements from photographs [17]. Baker defined photogrammetry as the process of "obtaining reliable information about physical objects and the environment through processes of recording, measuring, and interpreting photographic images" [18]. Tumbas defined photogrammetry as "a scientific method for determining the dimensions of an object by measuring a photographic image of the object and transforming measurements of the image to the actual surface" [19]. The term *close-range photogrammetry* refers to applications of photogrammetry where the camera-to-object distances are on the order of "tens and hundreds of yards as opposed to the tens and hundreds of miles associated with aerial uses" [20].

One photogrammetric technique, referred to as *camera matching* in the more recent literature, involves reconstructing the location from which a photograph was taken and determining the field of view of the camera that took it. Once the camera location and field of view are obtained, objects (physical evidence) within the photograph can be located. This graphical technique, which is often used for diagramming scene or vehicle evidence, involves the following steps:

1. The reconstructionist selects a photograph for analysis. For a photograph to be analyzed, it needs to show objects or geometry that still exist and can be physically documented. For analysis of scene evidence, such geometry would typically be roadway striping, curbs, signs, or trees.

2. After selecting a photograph for analysis, the reconstructionist makes note of objects or geometry shown in the photographs that still exist at the scene. The reconstructionist then physically documents this geometry at the scene using a total station, a laser scanner, or by employing image-based scanning.

3. After the scene mapping data has been processed, the reconstructionist uses a computer modeling software package to create a virtual camera and to view the survey or scan data from a perspective that is visually similar to that shown in the photograph that is being analyzed.

4. Lens distortion is removed from the photograph that is to be analyzed. All camera lenses produce some level of distortion in the resulting image and this distortion can potentially introduce errors into a photogrammetric process if it is not removed. A study by Neale examined the lens distortion caused by 35 different makes and models of camera lenses and then discussed methods and software available for removing the distortion from the resulting images [21]. Neale noted that for a particular focal length, two lenses of the same make and model will produce the same distortion. Lens distortion occurs in two basic forms—barreling and pin cushioning. Barreling is distortion that squashes the edge of the image, whereas pin cushioning is distortion that stretches the edge of the image. Generally, barreling occurs from wide focal lengths and pin cushioning occurs from zoom focal lengths, although lenses can also produce a mix of barreling and pin cushioning.

5. The corrected photograph is then imported into the modeling software and is designated as a background image for the virtual camera.

6. The analyst then adjusts the location, focal length, and viewing plane of the computer-modeled camera until an overlay is achieved between the survey or scan data and the scene geometry shown in the photograph. Once a match is obtained, then the analyst has reconstructed the location, focal length, and viewing plane of the camera used to take the original photograph.

7. Once the camera location and characteristics are obtained, the evidence visible in the photograph can be traced or modeled such that it also overlays what is visible in the photograph.

A sample of the results of this technique are shown in Figure 5.14. The image in this figure shows a photograph of scene evidence from a motorcycle sliding on the roadway. This is the evidence depicted on Figure 5.1. In the image of Figure 5.14, a site survey has been overlaid on the roadway geometry, including the fog lines, the center lines, and the guardrail posts. The process through which this overlay was achieved resulted in a reconstructed position and characteristics for the camera that took the photograph.

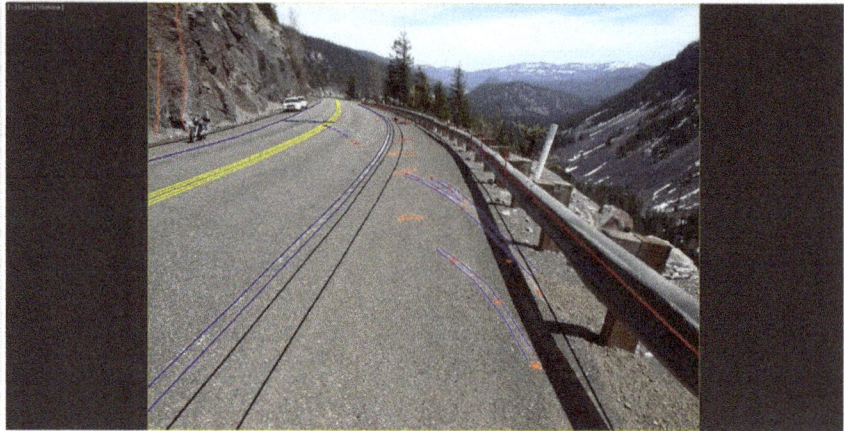

FIGURE 5.14 Sample of the camera matching photogrammetric technique.

Once this camera position and its characteristics were obtained, the geometry of the photograph becomes known and the tire marks, gouges, scrapes, and police paint could be traced in the photographs and placed on the evidence diagram.

The camera matching technique is a single-image photogrammetric method, in the sense that a single image is sufficient for its application. However, multiple photographs depicting the same evidence from different vantage points can be analyzed, and when the results are averaged, this may increase the accuracy of the technique. Campbell and Friedrich first described the camera matching technique in the accident reconstruction literature in 1993 [17]. Using a mock crash scene, they compared the positions of points obtained with the technique to the actual positions of these points. They reported a minimum position error of 0.1 ft and a maximum position error of 1.74 ft. In a 1999 study, Massa demonstrated that the technique could be applied to analyze and critique an animation [22]. In a 2001 study, Fenton described and tested the camera matching technique for obtaining dimension from another mock crash scene [23]. He compared dimensions obtained from camera matching with the same dimensions obtained with a digital survey and reported an average error of around 2%, with a range of errors between 0.48% and 8.23%. The dimensions ranged from approximately 5 ft up to approximately 140 ft.

Coleman et al. examined the accuracy of the camera matching technique when implemented with laser scan data rather than a digital survey [24]. They tested the accuracy of the camera matching technique by using it to locate evidence placed at a mock crash site, and then, comparing the obtained evidence locations to the actual locations of the evidence. They noted that "in many places the evidence location error was near zero." Their worst-case error for the camera matching technique was about 13 cm (5.1 in.).

The camera matching technique can also be applied to frames from a video. Chou et al. reported application of the technique for tracking the motion (position, roll angle, and roll velocity) of a vehicle from video of a dolly rollover crash test [25]. The tracked roll angle and calculated roll velocity were compared to the roll velocity measured with a sensor and the roll angle obtained from integration of the sensor data. Chou reported excellent agreement between the roll angles determined from camera matching and those determined from the sensor data. There were discrepancies between the roll velocities obtained from camera matching and those obtained from the sensor, though the trend of the sensor data was generally matched with the camera matching technique.

Rose and Neale reported additional application of the camera matching technique to analysis of a dolly rollover crash test, attempting to improve on the results from Chou through more extensive knowledge of the locations and characteristics of the cameras that recorded the test and the geometry of the test facility [26]. In this study, a digital survey was conducted to locate the cameras, to document the test facility geometry, and to locate targets on the vehicle. This reduced the number of unknowns in the camera matching. In addition to that, knowing the characteristics of the cameras made it easier for lens distortion to be removed from the video prior to the analysis.

Rose reported the motion of the vehicle for a 2-second segment of the test and compared the roll velocity results to sensor data. The resulting roll velocities from the camera matching were generally bracketed by the signals from the two roll velocity sensors on the vehicle. In other words, the discrepancy between the roll velocity from the camera matching and the roll velocities from either sensor were less than the discrepancy between the two sensors. Rose also reported a comparison of two separate analysts using the camera matching technique on the same 2-second segment. Around 96% of the time, the vehicle position obtained by the two analysts was different by less than an inch. This propagated to an uncertainty in the calculated over the ground and vertical speeds of 1 mph with a confidence of 96%. For the vehicle roll angle, the difference between the two analysts was less than 1 degree, approximately 85% of the time. For an analysis time step of 40 ms, this propagated to an uncertainty in the roll velocity of approximately 18 degrees per second with a confidence of 85%.

Manuel, Mink, and Kruger [27] tested the camera matching technique on frames of video from a moving camera (they referred to the technique as videogrammetry). They tracked the motion of the camera—and thus, the motion of the vehicle to which the camera was attached—and the motion of another vehicle captured by the camera. They conducted their analysis with varying levels of scene documentation to test the influence of the available scene data. These levels were as follows: (1) aerial photography as the only source of data about the site, (2) total station data defining the geometry of the site, and (3) lidar scan data defining the geometry of the site. For the vehicle carrying the camera, they reported that when aerial photography was used, "the reconstructed speed of the camera vehicle can be overestimated by 8%"; when total station data was used, "the reconstructed speed of the camera vehicle can be overestimated by 3%"; and when scan data was used, "the reconstructed speed of the camera vehicle can be underestimated by 2%." For the motion of the vehicle captured by the camera, the authors reported that when aerial photography was used, "the reconstructed speed for a moving vehicle captured by a moving camera can be underestimated by 12.8%"; when total station data was used, "the reconstructed speed for a moving vehicle captured by a moving camera can be overestimated by 10.4%"; and when scan data was used, "the reconstructed speed for a moving vehicle captured by a moving camera can be underestimated by 2.4%."

5.4.2.1 CAMERA REVERSE PROJECTION

The camera matching technique is essentially a digital implementation of a technique the earlier literature referred to a *camera reverse projection*. According to Tumbas [19], this term refers to the fact that once the location and characteristics of the camera are known, points from the photograph can be projected onto the scene. This technique followed a similar method to that described for camera matching, but the implementation did not use computer modeling programs or virtual cameras. Instead, the reconstructionist would overlay a transparency of the original photographic print, and trace geometry that was visible in the photograph that would still be visible at the site. A small version of this transparency would then be created and inserted into the viewfinder of what the Northwestern University Traffic Collision Investigation manual referred to as a "dummy" camera. While at the crash site, the reconstructionist would then change their viewing location and the camera focal length until the features traced onto the transparency overlaid on the corresponding features at the crash site. Once the viewing location, viewing plane, and focal length for the original photograph were reconstructed, the reconstructionist could then locate physical evidence that was no longer visible at the site.

One limitation in this technique is that the analyst would need to use a camera conducive to inserting a small transparency into the viewfinder. This would usually mean that the analyst would be using a different camera with different internal geometry than the camera that took the photograph. Another limitation is that the analysist would have to stand in the same place as the original photographer for an extended period. If a photograph was taken from the middle of a lane on the interstate, for example, this would not be possible without a road closure. Digital implementation of the camera matching technique does not suffer from these limitations, since the analyst has greater control over the characteristics of the computer-modeled camera and does not have to stand in the road. Another limitation of the older implementations of camera reverse projection was that there was no real way to account for or eliminate lens distortion from the photographic image. Digital implementation of the camera matching technique can correct for or eliminate distortion from many photographic images.

Despite these limitations, many reconstructionists successfully and accurately implemented the camera reverse projection technique. Breen and Anderson [28] described an implementation of reverse camera projection to determine the post-crash shape of a damaged windshield. Woolley et al. [29] applied camera reverse projection with two photographs to quantify vehicle crush. He reported average errors of less than 1 in., noting though that this level of accuracy "depends on the experience, patience, and care taken in all phases of the process. The more times camera reverse-projection is applied, either to a damaged vehicle or to a scene, the greater will become the skill of the analyst." This statement also applies to a digitally implemented camera matching process. However, what Woolley has left unsaid is the important fact that the application of the reverse camera projection and camera matching techniques typically result in a graphical output that allows others to evaluate the quality of the camera match.

Husher et al. [30] applied the camera reverse projection technique to a mock crash scene and reported that it "was able to locate the subject skid to within 20 cm (8 inches) for the least favorable camera view, and within 5 cm (2 inches) for the more favorable views. The selection of the camera view determines the accuracy of this method." They also stated that "when the results of the three [camera reverse projection] views were averaged, the determined position was almost on top of the true position for both the skid and the vehicle." This means that, though camera reverse projection is methodologically a single-image technique, applying it to multiple images and averaging the results improves the accuracy. In this study, camera reverse projection was also applied to determine vehicle crush, and the authors reported that the "longitudinal crush determined was within 2.5 cm (1 inch) of the measured value."

Husher also described an implementation of the camera reverse projection technique that involved "real time analysis with video equipment...Two video cameras view the original photo and the exemplar vehicle (or scene) simultaneously and a video mixer is used to overlay the two separate views to provide the alignment information..." Husher applied this method to determining vehicle crush and reported that "accuracy was within 2.5 cm (1 inch) of the crush." Main and Knopf [31] describe an implementation of the camera reverse projection technique using physical scale models of the crash site and vehicles. Though computer implementation of the camera matching technique began appearing in the literature as far back as 1993, the technique described by Main and Knopf is methodologically a direct precursor to the camera matching technique.

Smith [32] and Tumbas [19] noted that reverse camera projection can be accomplished analytically with two photographs. Tumbas stated this would be accomplished by "surveying selected points at the site, constructing a mathematical model of the site surfaces, mathematically locating the camera, mathematically projecting the points of interest onto the model and determining the location of the intersecting rays with the model's surface." Referring to this technique as *analytical reverse projection*, Smith described the concept of this method as follows: "This method is based on the fact that once the original position of the camera lens center, the distance from the lens center to the picture-plane (photograph), and the orientation of the photograph relative to the scene are all determined, then a vector passing from that established lens center point through any point of interest in the two-dimensional picture-plane defines the ray that passes through that same point of interest in the actual three-dimensional scene. If two or more photographs, taken from different locations, are available showing the same point of interest, then the location of that point in the scene can be determined by simply calculating the point where the two rays (on from each photograph) intersect." Tumbas reported typical accuracies for locating points with reverse camera projection of less than a foot, with maximum errors around 2 ft. For analytical reverse projection he reported typical accuracies of around a half foot, with maximum errors of less than a foot. Tumbas notes that both techniques resulted in better accuracy than methods that assume the surface containing the evidence is flat. Reverse camera projection does not require such an assumption.

These studies demonstrate that analysts could achieve levels of accuracy acceptable for accident reconstruction even though they did not necessarily utilize the same make and model camera as the one used to take a photograph, and they did not remove the lens distortion from the photographs. Given this, the importance of removing lens distortion from photographs should not be overestimated. In instances where such removal is not possible, acceptable results may still be possible. As with the application of most any technique in accident reconstruction, much depends on the level of accuracy required for the application. This will ultimately have to be judged on a case-by-case basis.

5.4.3 Removing Lens Distortion

Imperfections in the design and manufacturing processes of camera lenses cause distortion in the image captured by the sensors or by film of the camera [33]. As light is collected, focused, and transformed through the lens structure, the final collection of this light on a sensor plate or film sheet is distorted. Two common types of distortion are referred to as pin-cushion and barrel distortions.

Figure 5.15 illustrates these two types of distortion. The grid on the left of this figure shows the effect of barrel distortion and the grid on the right shows the effect of pin

FIGURE 5.15 Illustration of distortion types.

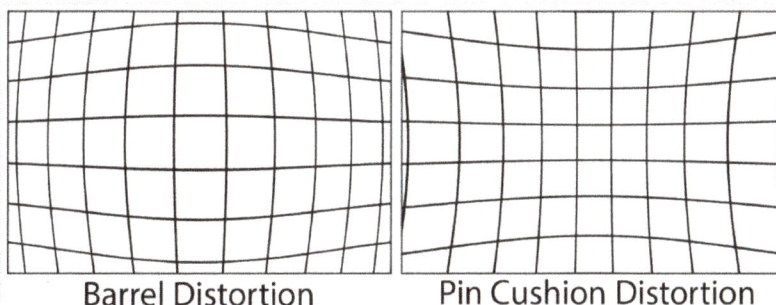

Barrel Distortion   Pin Cushion Distortion

cushioning. Barrel distortion causes the image to be expanded in a barrel shape from its center [34]. This distortion type is typically associated with wide-angle focal lengths. Pin cushioning causes images to be pinched at their center. Pin-cushion distortion is typically associated with telephoto focal lengths. Sometimes, a combination of barrel and pin-cushion distortions can be present in a photographic image. This results in a wavy distortion pattern likely to occur at the transition between wide and zoom focal lengths. Barrel and pin-cushion distortions affect the positions of pixels in an image. Since photogrammetric techniques analyze the location of objects in the image, removing distortion from an image prior to analysis can improve the accuracy of the results.

For many common camera/lens combinations, there is published data that mathematically describes the distortion they create in images. This mathematical description can be applied to remove the distortion in a digital image. There are multiple programs available that use databases of distortion coefficients to automatically correct for lens distortion. For example, Epaperpress Ptlens, Hugin, and Adobe Photoshop CS5 use the information stored in a photograph's EXIF (exchangeable image file format) data to look up the distortion coefficients from a database. These distortion coefficients are published for many camera types by the manufacturer. The EXIF data of the image is information that is stored with the image when the photograph is taken, such as the make and model of the camera, the exposure setting, f-stop, and the time and date the photograph was taken (or, at least, the time reported by the camera's clock).

Distortion correction relies on the following polynomial function that modifies the distance a pixel is from the center of the image:

$$y = ax^4 + bx^3 + cx^2 + dx \tag{5.1}$$

In this equation,
  x is the distance of the distorted pixel from the center of the image
  y is the distance of the undistorted pixel from the center of the image

The distances in this equation are typically normalized such that a value of 1 is equal to half the size of the shortest side of the image. The coefficients are determined empirically for any given camera/lens combination, and they control the transformation from the distorted to the undistorted pixel position. Coefficient a primarily affects the edges of the image, c affects the inside, and b affects the image as a whole. The d coefficient is related to the others through the following equation:

$$d = 1 - (a + b + c) \tag{5.2}$$

This equation controls the scale of the corrected image and is used to maintain the overall size of the resulting image. In addition to the published coefficients that can be obtained, image adjustment programs typically allow the user to manually enter the coefficients to perform the distortion correction.

For cameras for which coefficients are not publicly available, these coefficients can be determined with the following procedure. First, a grid is printed out and mounted on a wall as shown in Figure 5.16. Then, a photograph is taken of the grid such that the vertical and horizontal lines of the grid will be captured parallel to the digital image. The camera's make and model and the focal length for the image can then be obtained from the EXIF data. This information can be used in the image editing programs to complete the manual assessment of distortion. There can be differences between the focal length reported in the EXIF data and the actual focal length used when taking the photograph. After the photograph is taken and imported into the image processing

FIGURE 5.16   Setup for photographing a grid.

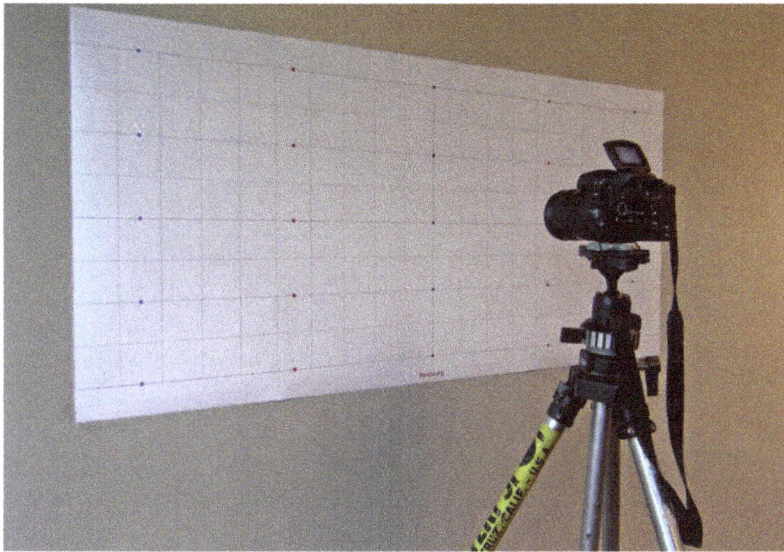

program (Photoshop, for instance), distortion correction plug-ins are used that allow the user to manually input the distortion coefficients until the distortion correction is achieved (meaning lines that are straight in the real world are also depicted as straight in the photographic image). For the case of the photograph of the grid, the coefficients would be iteratively changed until the vertical and horizontal lines match the overlaid grid lines.

Neale et al. noted a couple of trends related to lens distortion. First, the center of an image typically contains the least amount of distortion. The distortion increases moving from the center to the edges of an image. Second, the focal length at which a photograph is taken influences the resulting distortion.

5.4.4 Case Study: Photogrammetric Analysis of Video of a Motorcycle Accident

This section describes the reconstruction of an intersection collision involving a motorcycle and a station wagon. The crash was captured on video, and camera matching photogrammetric analysis was one of the methods employed in the analysis. The motorcycle was traveling straight westbound through the intersection and the eastbound station wagon turned left in front of the motorcycle. According to the police investigation, the motorcyclist entered the intersection on a red light and impacted the passenger side of the station wagon. The driver of the station wagon had reportedly initiated her turn near the end of the yellow light cycle. There was also a small bus that initiated a left turn in the lane adjacent to the station wagon. The investigating officers did not take any photographs during their investigation.

The intersection where this accident occurred is depicted in the aerial photograph of Figure 5.17. This photograph, which is oriented such that north is up on the page, shows that the east-west roadway had three westbound and three eastbound through lanes. There were two turn lanes to accommodate traffic turning left from the eastbound roadway to the northbound roadway. These are the turn lanes that the station wagon and the bus were using when this crash occurred. The station wagon was turning

FIGURE 5.17 Aerial photograph of subject intersection.

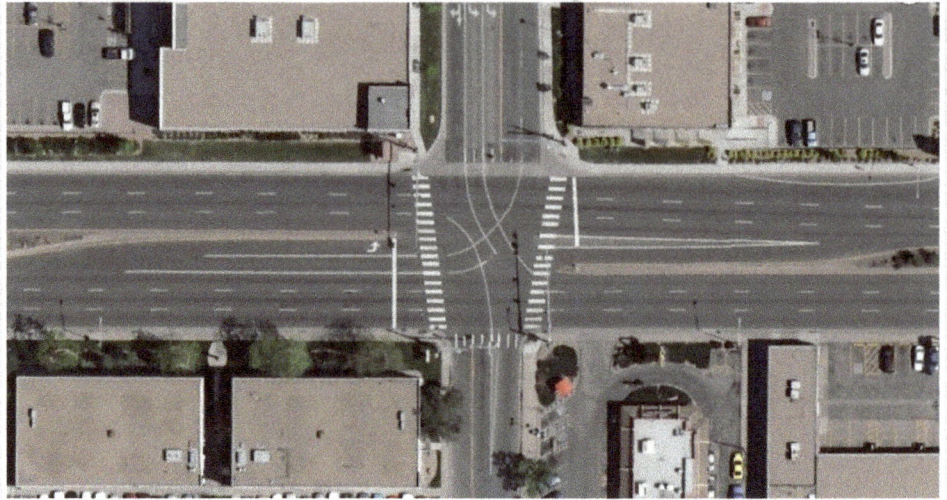

from the leftmost turn lane, and the bus was turning from the rightmost turn lane. The intersection is asphalt-paved and, at the time of this accident, the roadway was dry and there were no adverse weather conditions. The speed limit for the east-west roadway was 35 mph.

A witness that was traveling westbound behind the motorcycle stated that the motorcyclist entered the intersection when the light for their direction was red. She estimated that it had been red for 5 s when the collision occurred. She further stated that the motorcyclists "may have been traveling at an excessive speed...." Another witness, who was in a vehicle on the south side of the intersection facing north, stated that "[The station wagon] was waiting to make a left and the light for them started to turn yellow. The first left and center lane westbound started to stop. And so, [the station wagon driver] decided to make her left turn while the motorcycle was in the right lane and as soon as she got around to his lane that's when he came through trying to beat the yellow light and hit her in the front right tire."

The bus that was turning left next to the station wagon was equipped with a DriveCam system that captured portions of this accident on video. A DriveCam unit is an aftermarket, event-triggered video and data recorder that is mounted to a vehicle's windshield. DriveCam units contain accelerometers that measure longitudinal and lateral accelerations and two cameras that record video. One of these cameras looks forward through the windshield, and the other looks rearward at the vehicle occupants. If a DriveCam unit measures an acceleration that exceeds a preset threshold, it triggers an event and stores video and acceleration data. Rose [35, 36] reported research related to the accuracy of these DriveCam systems and reported that they provide reliable evidence for use in accident reconstruction.

During the subject accident, an event was triggered in the DriveCam unit on the bus because the driver of the bus braked hard as the motorcycle traveled in front of him. The DriveCam unit captured video and acceleration data for 10 s before and 10 s after this braking and the raw DriveCam data was available for analysis. This data showed that, when the bus driver braked, the bus reached a longitudinal deceleration of 0.72g. Figure 5.18 is one frame of the video from the forward-looking camera in the DriveCam unit. This frame shows the motorcyclist entering the intersection. This frame has a listed time of −0.25 s. Within the DriveCam system, time is assigned in relationship to the triggering event. The triggering event is set as time zero; times before the triggering

FIGURE 5.18   Frame of video from forward-looking camera of DriveCam unit.

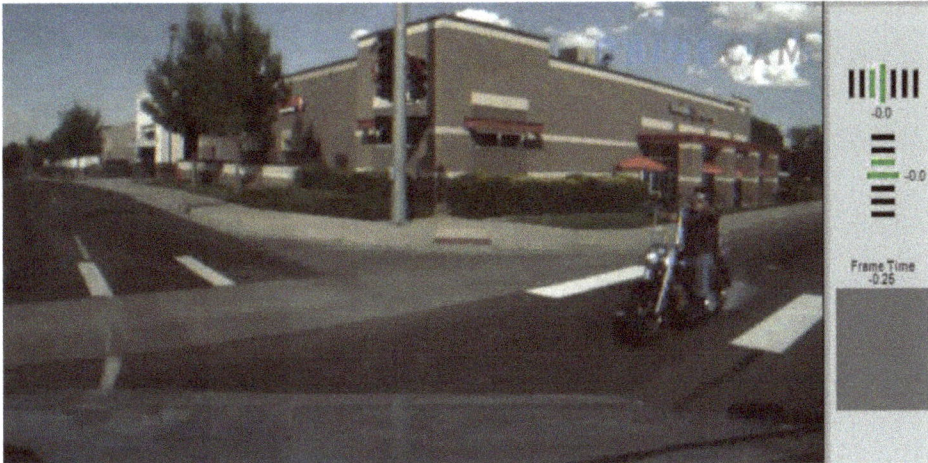

FIGURE 5.19   Colorized scan data of the northeast corner of the subject intersection.

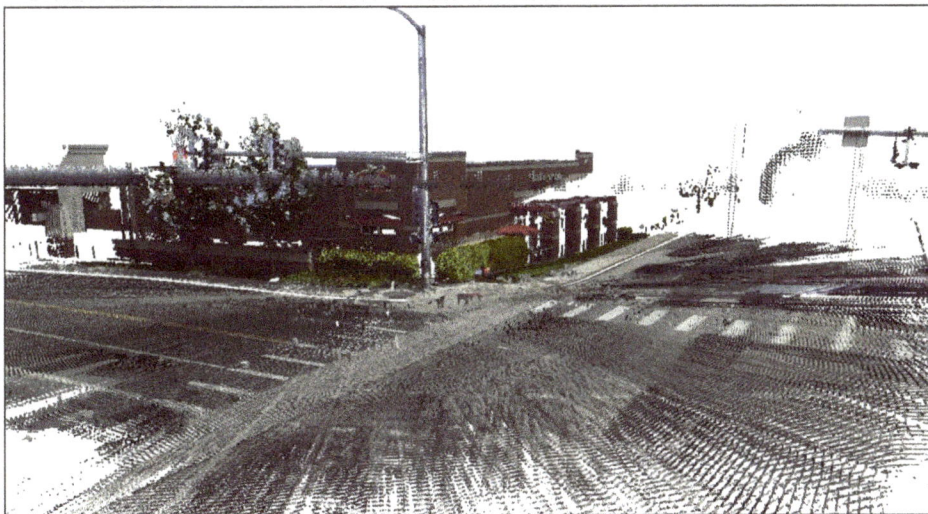

event are negative and times after the triggering event are positive. Therefore, the frame of video included below shows a point in time ¼ of a second before the DriveCam sensed the hard braking of the bus driver. This DriveCam video frame also shows smoke coming from the rear wheel of the motorcycle, indicating that this wheel locked up when the motorcyclist braked.

The intersection at which this collision occurred was inspected, documented, and mapped using a Faro Focus laser scanner. This documentation with the scanner focused on the northeast corner of the intersection because this portion of the intersection was visible in the DriveCam video. Figure 5.19 depicts some of the colorized scan data of the intersection.

Figure 5.20 is another image from the forward-facing view of the DriveCam system. In this image, the front of the bus is visible, as is a white sedan and a white van in the oncoming lanes of travel. Consistent with the witness statements, it was evident from the video that these vehicles were slowing and stopping for the westbound traffic signal that was changing to yellow and then red. The scan data was used in conjunction with camera matching photogrammetry and video tracking using a software package

FIGURE 5.20 Another frame of video from the forward-looking camera of DriveCam unit.

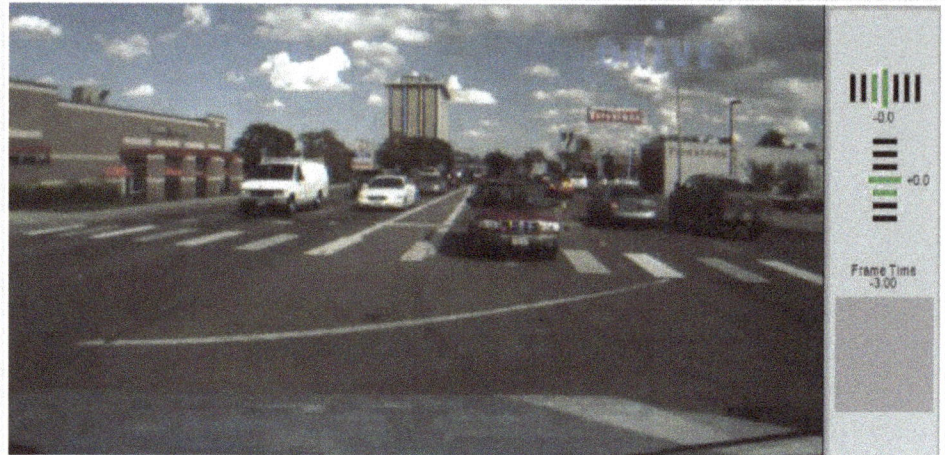

FIGURE 5.21 First frame of DriveCam video in which the motorcyclist was visible.

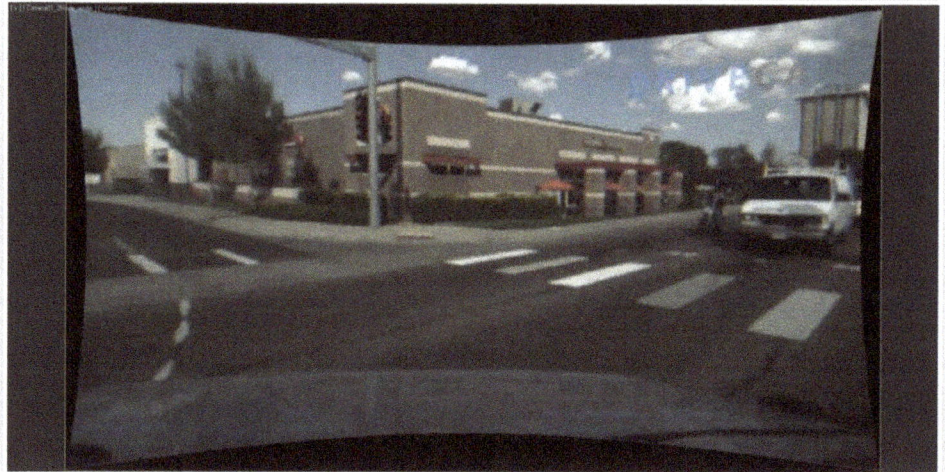

called PFTrack. The motion of the camera attached to the bus was tracked. Once this motion was known, the motions of the white sedan and white van were also tracked. Finally, the motion of the motorcyclist was tracked. The goal of this analysis was to determine the speeds and accelerations or decelerations of these vehicles and to use this data to inform a determination of when the traffic signal for westbound traffic turned yellow and red. Unfortunately, the color of these traffic signals was not visible in the video at the significant times.

The next three figures depict an example of the progression of our camera matching analysis to track the motion of the motorcycle. Figure 5.21 is the first frame from the DriveCam video in which the motorcyclist was visible (t = −0.75 s). Lens distortion has been removed from this video frame, as it was for the rest of the video frames. Figure 5.22 is the same video image with the scan data overlaid onto the corresponding intersection geometry visible in the video image. This overlay results from reconstructing the location and characteristics of the camera and mimicking those in a computer modeling software. Figure 5.22 shows the reconstructed motorcycle position for this frame. The camera matching process was repeated for two additional frames of video in which the

FIGURE 5.22 Scan data overlaid onto the video image.

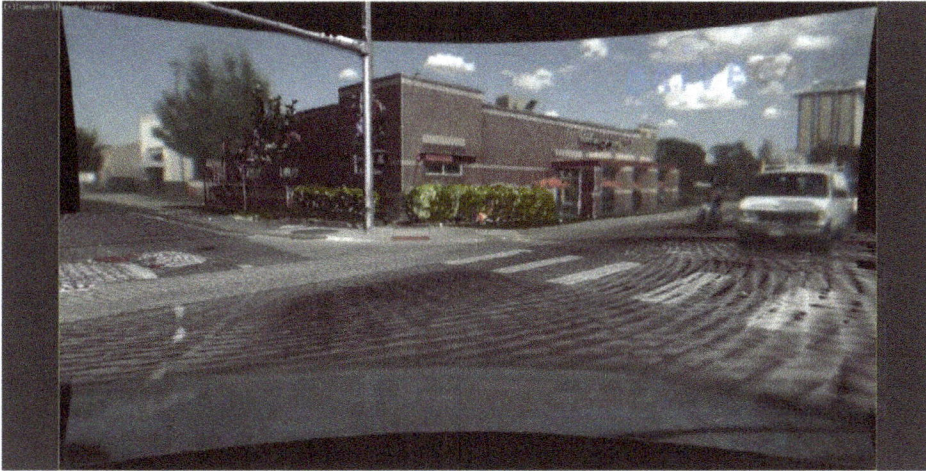

FIGURE 5.23 Reconstructed location of the motorcycle for this video frame.

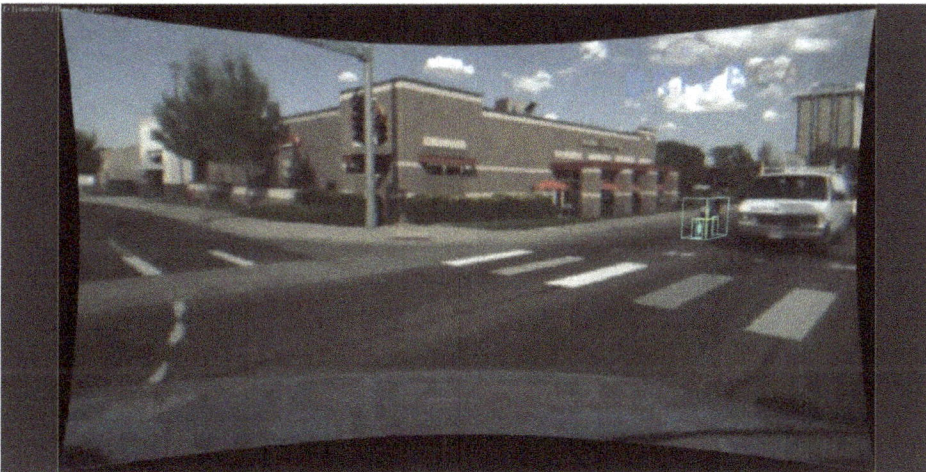

motorcyclist was visible (t = −0.50 and −0.25 s). From the resulting reconstructed positions of the motorcycle, the speed could be determined (Figure 5.23). This led to the conclusion that the motorcyclist was traveling approximately 48 mph when he entered the intersection.

When the DriveCam video depicted the motorcyclist entering the intersection (t = −0.5 s), the traffic light for the northbound roadway was visible in the video and it was red (see Figure 5.24). The color of the light for eastbound traffic is not visible in this frame. A half second later (t = 0.0 s), the traffic signals for both eastbound and northbound traffic are visible and red (see Figure 5.25). At this intersection, the traffic lights for eastbound and westbound traffic had a 4-second yellow phase and a 2-second "all red" phase. In addition to that, the two red lights illuminated and visible in the DriveCam frame at t = 0.00 s could both remain red for longer than 2 s, since these lights will remain red while the left turn arrow for southbound traffic cycles through to allow southbound drivers to turn left. During our site inspection, one instance was documented in which these two lights were both red for 12 s. Thus, there is no way to determine from one frame of the DriveCam video how long these lights had been red and how long they would continue to be red.

FIGURE 5.24 **FIGURE 5.24** Northbound traffic signal was red when motorcyclists was entering the intersection.

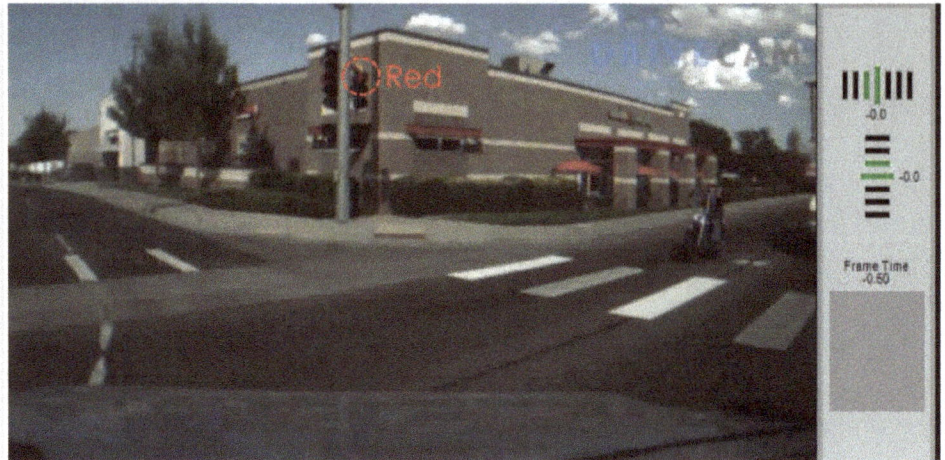

FIGURE 5.25 First video frame at which eastbound traffic signal was visible.

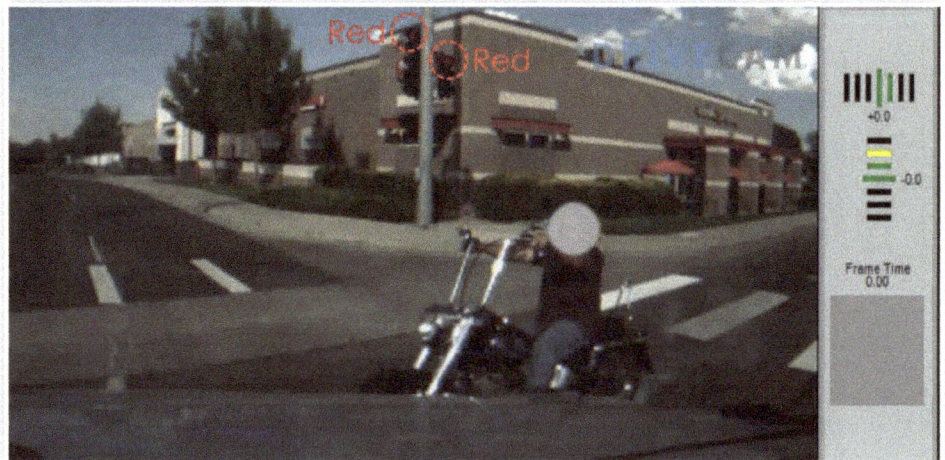

The best indication of when the traffic light for westbound traffic turned yellow and red is the actions of westbound drivers other than the motorcyclist. The graph of Figure 5.26 shows the speed of these vehicles as they approach the intersection and stop. In this graph, the time from the DriveCam video is plotted on the horizontal axis and the speed of the approaching vehicles is plotted on the vertical axis. As this graph shows, at a time of −7.0 s, the white van and sedan are approaching the intersection at a speed of around 15 mph and they are accelerating. They both begin decelerating at a time of around −5.50 s. This is an indication that, at this time, the drivers of these vehicles have seen the traffic signal turn to yellow and have begun to brake in response to that change in the light color. It would typically take a driver around 1 to 1-½ s to perceive the change in light color and begin applying their brakes [37]. That these drivers begin braking for the light at a time of −5.5 s indicates that the westbound traffic lights likely changed to yellow at a time between −6.5 and −7.0 s. This means that the light turned red at a time between −2.5 and −3.0 s. The motorcyclist was just entering the intersection at a time of −0.5 s, and so he did not enter the intersection until the traffic light had been red for between 2 and 2.5 s.

FIGURE 5.26   Results of tracking the motion of the westbound vehicles.

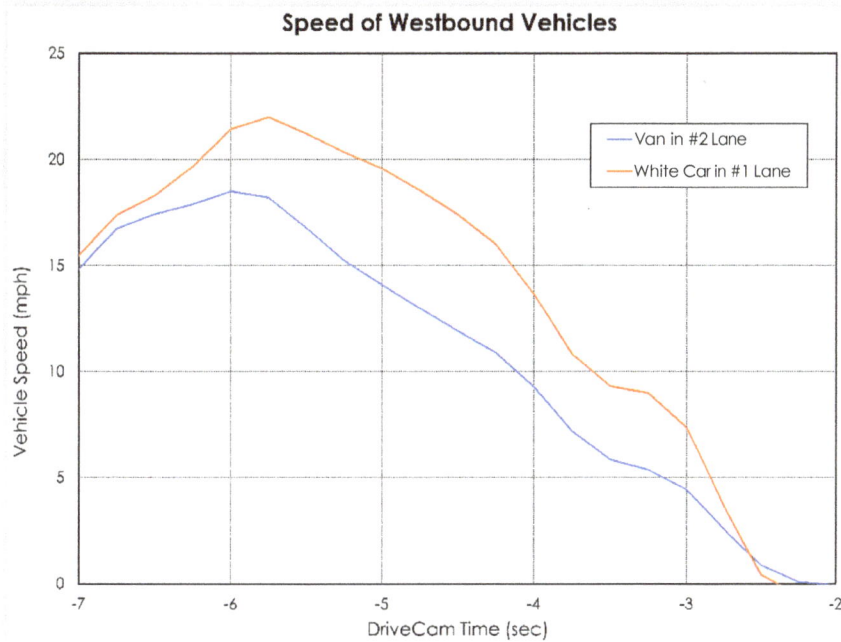

5.4.5 Case Study: Photogrammetric Analysis of Video of Another Motorcycle Accident

This section describes the reconstruction of another collision that was captured on surveillance footage and involved a motorcycle and a blue sedan. Camera matching photogrammetric analysis was again used to analyze frames from the surveillance video. The motorcycle was traveling westbound and the sedan was initially sitting in a driveway facing south. There was a surveillance camera operating near the driveway. The driver of the sedan attempted a left turn in front of the motorcyclist with the intention of traveling eastbound. The motorcyclist collided with the driver's side of the sedan. The roadway was asphalt-paved. At the time of the collision, the roadway was dry and there were no adverse weather conditions. The speed limit for the east-west roadway was 45 mph.

The driveway and roadway where this collision occurred was inspected, documented, and mapped using a Faro Focus laser scanner. This documentation focused on the portions of the driveway and roadway that were visible in the frames of surveillance footage. Figure 5.27 depicts some of the colorized scan data of the intersection. The next series of figures illustrates the progression of our camera matching analysis to track the motion of the motorcycle and the sedan. Figure 5.28 is a frame from the surveillance footage in which the driveway, the roadway, and the sedan were visible. Lens distortion has been removed from this video frame, as it was for the rest of the video frames. Figure 5.29 is the same video image with the scan data overlaid onto the corresponding driveway and roadway geometry visible in the video image. In this case, the camera was static and its position was documented during our site inspection. Thus, in this case, the purpose of this overlay was to establish the field of view and distortion characteristics of the camera lens. Once these were established, the positions of the sedan and the motorcycle could be tracked through a series of frames. Figure 5.30 shows a different frame of the video, in which both the sedan and motorcycle are visible.

FIGURE 5.27 Colorized scan data of the driveway and roadway.

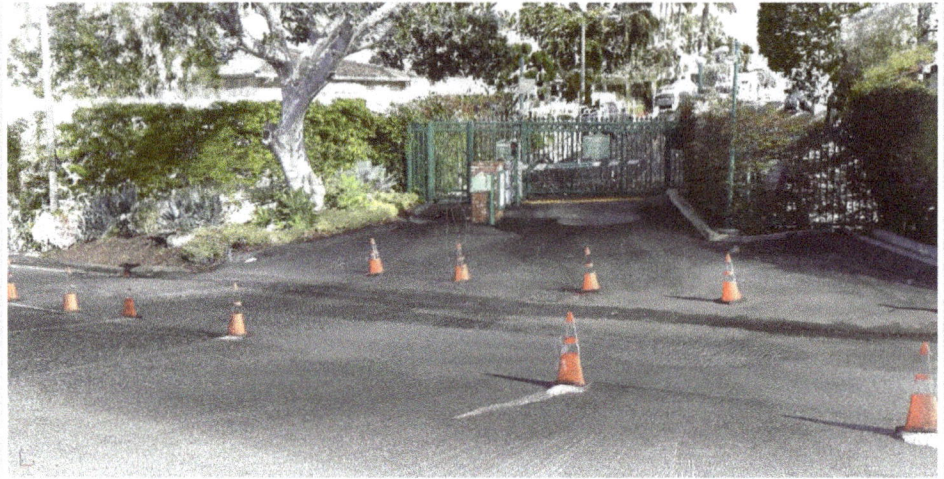

FIGURE 5.28 Frame of surveillance footage.

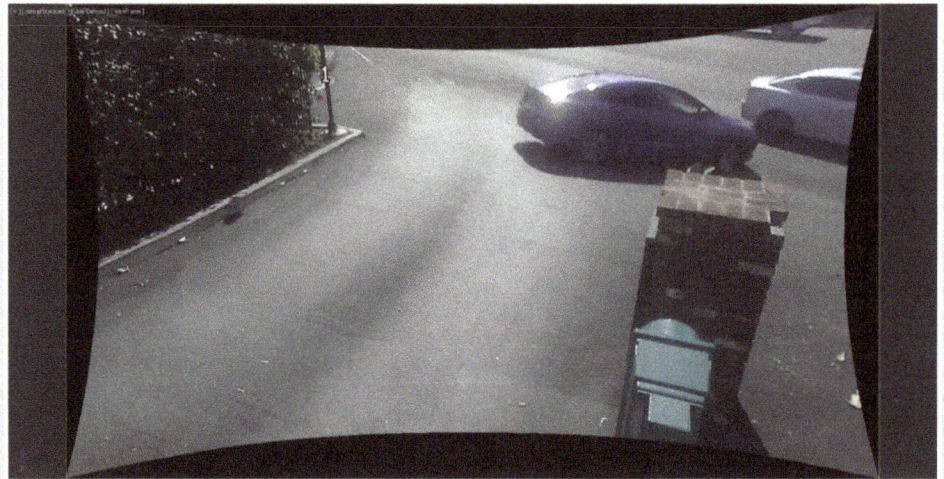

FIGURE 5.29 Scan data overlaid onto the video image.

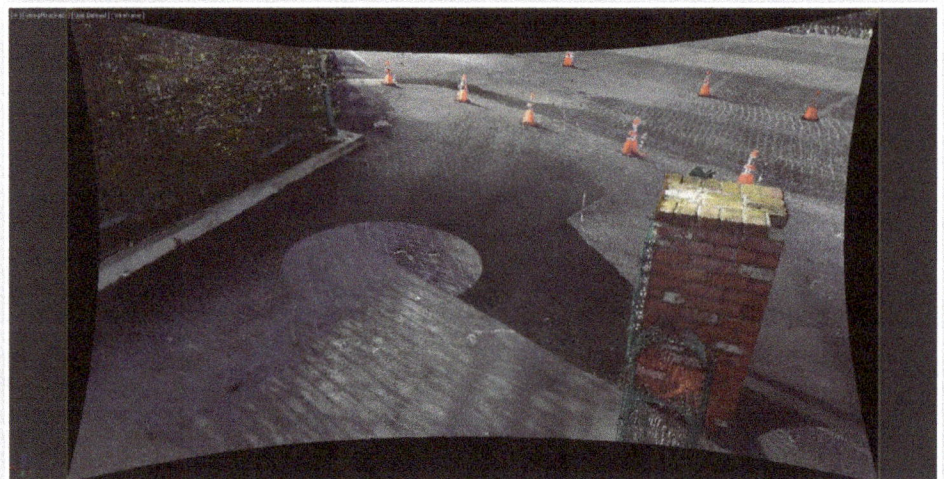

FIGURE 5.30 Reconstructed positions of the motorcycle and Chrysler for another frame.

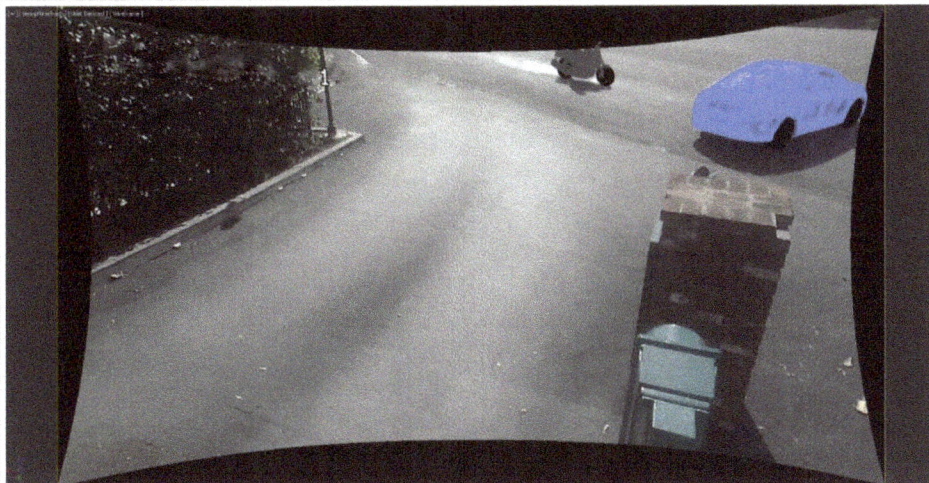

Computer models of these vehicles have been placed relative to the virtual camera such that they overlay these vehicles in the frame of video. The result is the positions of these vehicles being located within the scan of the site. This same process was completed for a series of frames showing the both vehicles, which resulted in a determination of the distances traveled by each vehicle between frames. The frame rate of the video was known (10 fps), and so the time between frames could be determined and the speeds calculated.

Five pre-collision positions were reconstructed for the motorcycle and an average speed calculated for each of the time intervals between frames. These speeds are shown in Figure 5.31. As this figure shows, the motorcycle was decelerating prior to the impact,

FIGURE 5.31 Reconstructed speeds from the camera matching video analysis.

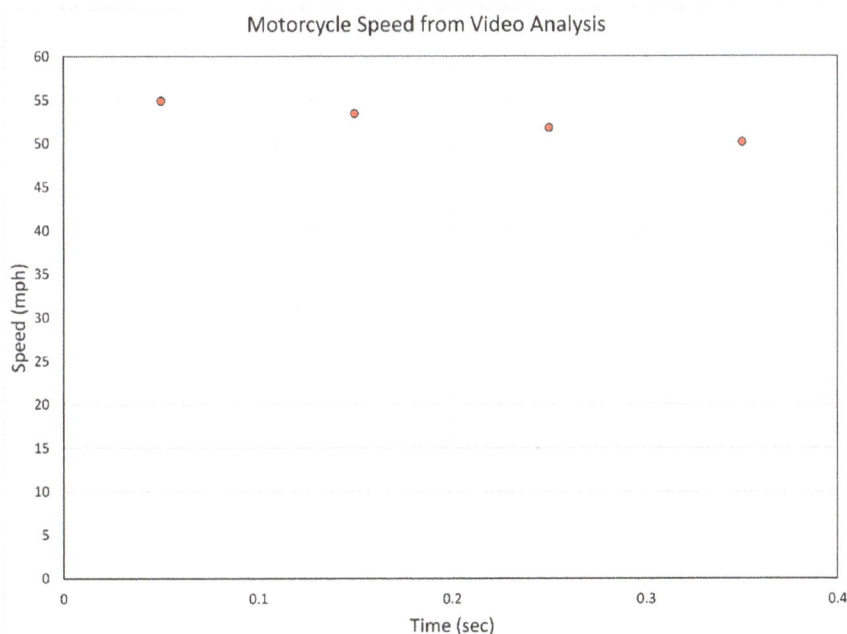

traveling a speed of approximately 55 mph when it entered the video and approximately 50 mph during the tenth of a second preceding the collision. Smoke was visible coming off the rear tire of the motorcycle in the video. The investigating officers also documented a 73-foot long tire mark from the motorcycle's rear tire leading up to the area of the collision, which was consistent with the smoke visible in the video and consistent with the speeds from the video analysis shown in Figure 5.31. The speeds from the video analysis implied a deceleration for the motorcycle of approximately 0.7g prior to the collision, implying that the motorcyclist was employing both the front and rear brakes of his motorcycle.

5.4.6 Image-Based Scanning

Photogrammetric methods can also be used to generate point cloud data for an object like what would be generated with lidar scanning. This process is referred to as image-based scanning. As an example, aerial images captured with a small unmanned aerial vehicle (sUAV) can be used in conjunction with photogrammetric software packages such as PIX4D, VisualSFM, PhotoScan, or 123DCatch to document and model accident site geometry. This software can also be used with ground-based photographs of a damaged or exemplar vehicle to generate a point cloud of the vehicle geometry.

Vergauwen presented a method to create 3D digital surface models using images without significant visual overlap [38]. Strecha examined the use of image-based modeling techniques as possible replacements for lidar-based measurement systems [39]. Dai compared spatial data collected with a Leica C10 laser scanner to various photogrammetry and videogrammetry methods and concluded that under certain circumstances, "image-based methods constitute a good alternative for time-of-flight-based methods" [40]. Erickson explored the accuracy of using 123DCatch to create 3D models of vehicles and concluded that "photo-based 3D scanning using 123D Catch® is a valid mode of reconstructing the geometry of a vehicle for the purposes of collision reconstruction" [41].

Terpstra, Voitel, and Hashemian [42] evaluated the capabilities and accuracy of four automated photogrammetry-based software programs to accurately create 3D point clouds of damaged and undamaged vehicles—Photomodeler Scanner, Photoscan, Pix4D, and VisualSFM. They compared the results produced by these software packages to the results to 3D scanning. These authors reported that all four software packages produced point clouds for which an average of nearly 60% of their points were within 0.25 in. of the LiDAR point cloud data and an average of more than 80% of their points were within 0.5 in. of the LiDAR data.

Jurkofsky explored the accuracy of using the software package Photomodeler Scanner in conjunction with images taken from an UAV to map accident scenes [43]. He created mock accident scenes and captured aerial photographs of the scenes. He then used Photomodeler Scanner software to calculate the position of objects within those scenes and compared the calculated positions to positions that he measured using a total station. Jurkofsky found that this process produced accurate results, demonstrating that UAV photography could accurately reproduce the location of physical evidence, provided the physical evidence was visible in the photographs. While this is often the case for law enforcement officials, accident reconstructionists that are not involved in law enforcement may document a scene months or years after an accident occurs. By this time, the physical evidence from an accident has often deteriorated or is no longer present.

Carter et al. published a study that examined the accuracy of camera matching photogrammetry using a point cloud of a mock accident site generated with image-based scanning using aerial images from a sUAV [44]. A mock scene was created in a parking lot with physical evidence typical of a vehicular crash. The scene was scanned with a FARO laser scanner and photographed. The evidence was then removed and video was taken of the scene from an UAV. That video footage was processed with image-based scanning software to create a point cloud, and the point cloud was used to reconstruct the positions and characteristics of the camera at the time the evidence was photographed. The evidence was then reconstructed with the camera matching technique and the position and size of the reconstructed evidence was compared to the position as documented by the FARO scanner. Some of the details of Carter's study are presented here as an example of applying image-based scanning to analyze the evidence at an accident scene.

The mock accident scene created by Carter in a parking lot is depicted in Figure 5.32. This parking lot was chosen because it featured two vertical tiers, and this would allow testing of the image-based scanning process to capture accurate changes in elevation. Tape was placed on the pavement to represent common traffic accident investigation markings: paint indicating vehicle tire rest points, a tire mark, a series of gouge marks, and paint outlining a tire mark. After the tape was placed, the mock scene was scanned using a FARO Focus^{3D} X 130 laser scanner, which is also depicted in Figure 5.32. The scan data, some of which is depicted in the graphic of Figure 5.33, consisted of 39 million points. Photographs of the scene were taken from numerous vantage points, similar to documentation of a crash scene by law enforcement officials. After the scene was scanned, the tape was removed, and video of the scene was taken from a DJI Phantom 2 sUAV equipped with a DJI Zenmuse H4-3D Gimbal and a GoPro Hero 4 camera (Figure 5.34). Video was captured at 4k resolution (3840 × 2160 pixels) at 30 fps in the GoPro "wide" setting.

The sUAV was flown in a zigzag pattern to provide overlapping video footage and was flown at low speeds to minimize motion blur. Video was taken from three different heights, approximately 3, 10, and 20 m above ground level. The video was processed using GoPro Cinema Studio to remove the camera distortion. A total of 470 frames were

FIGURE 5.32 Carter's mock accident scene [2016].

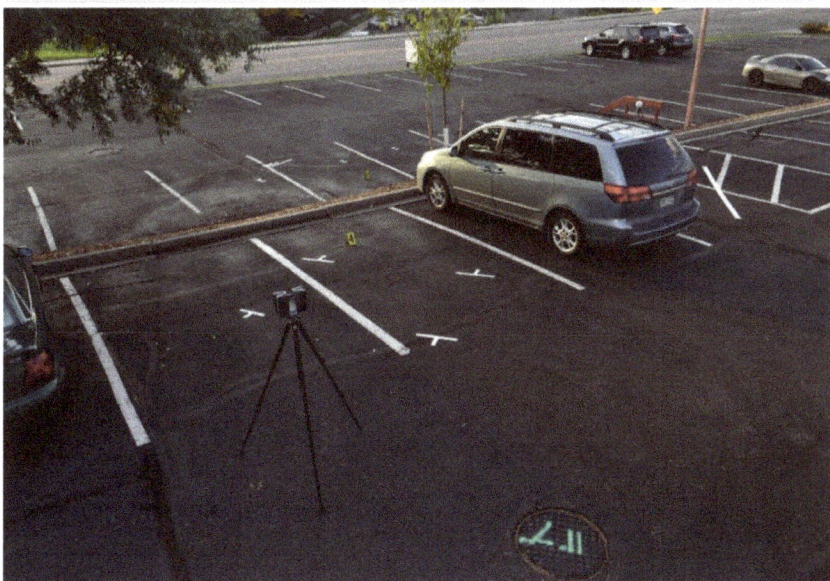

FIGURE 5.33 Scan data of the accident scene.

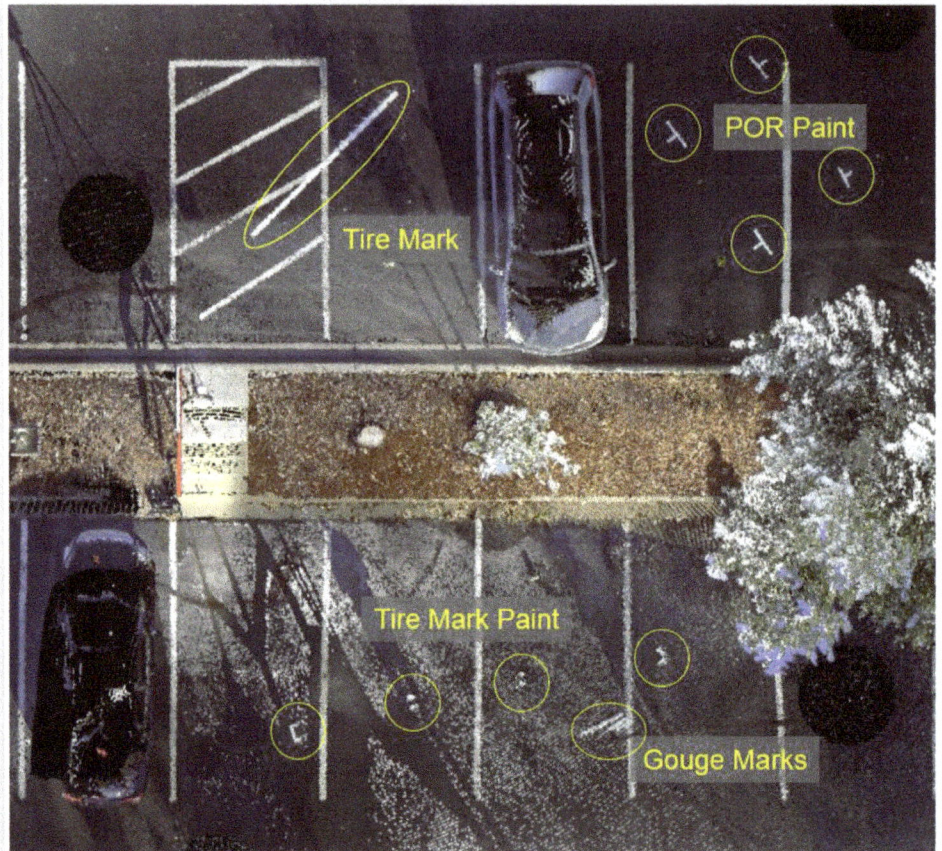

FIGURE 5.34 Phantom 2 UAV, gimbal, and camera used for documenting the scene.

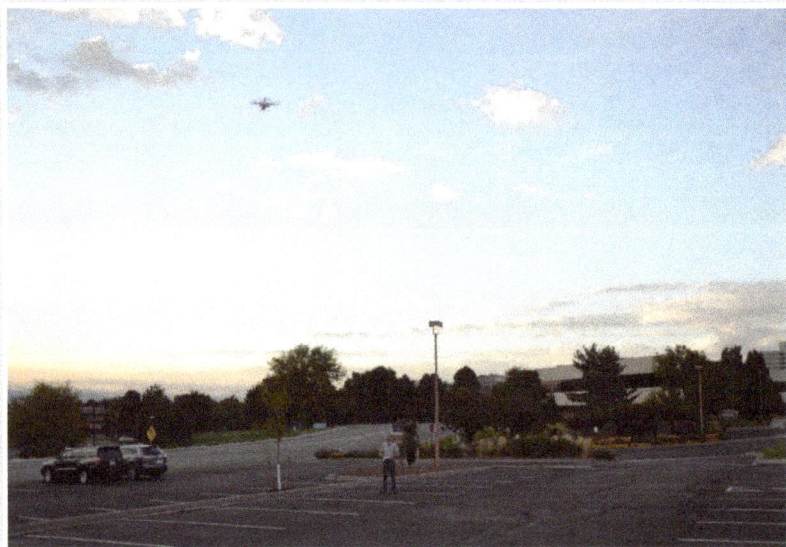

FIGURE 5.35 Photograph of mock scene.

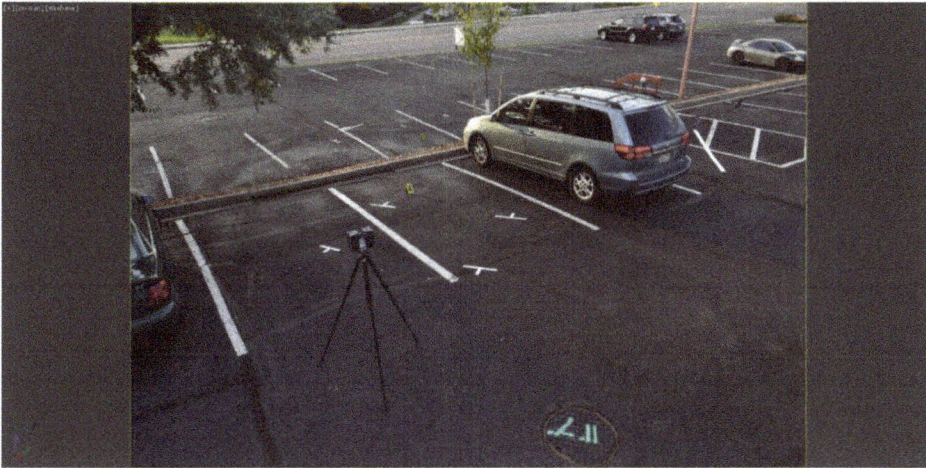

FIGURE 5.36 Point cloud of mock scene created with PIX4D.

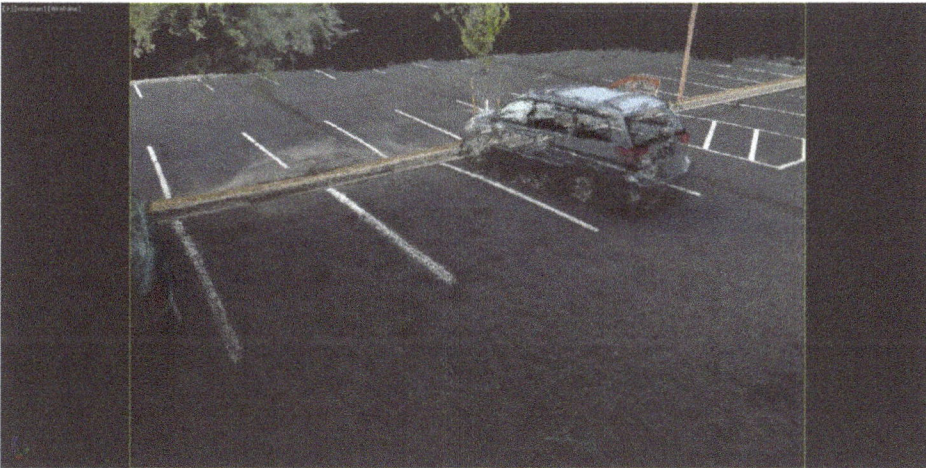

extracted from the video taken with the UAV. These frames were then processed with several photo-scanning software packages: Pix4D, VisualSFM, and PhotoScan. The resulting point clouds were visually compared to determine which software package produced the most complete point cloud. Carter chose to use the point cloud created by Pix4D for the subsequent camera matching analysis.

The camera matching process is depicted in the series of images below. Figure 5.35 is a photograph of the mock scene that was taken before the tape was removed. Figure 5.36 is a view of the point cloud created with the UAV footage and the Pix4D software. This image is taken from a perspective and location in the model similar to the perspective and location that the actual photograph was taken. Figure 5.37 depicts the image-based scanning point cloud overlaid on the photograph. Figure 5.38 then depicts the trace of the tape overlaid on an image from the FARO scan point cloud. This image visually depicts the accuracy of the evidence reconstruction.

This process was completed for four photographs of the mock scene, and a total of 32 unique points of evidence in the mock scene were reconstructed. Figure 5.39

FIGURE 5.37   Point cloud overlaid on photograph of mock scene.

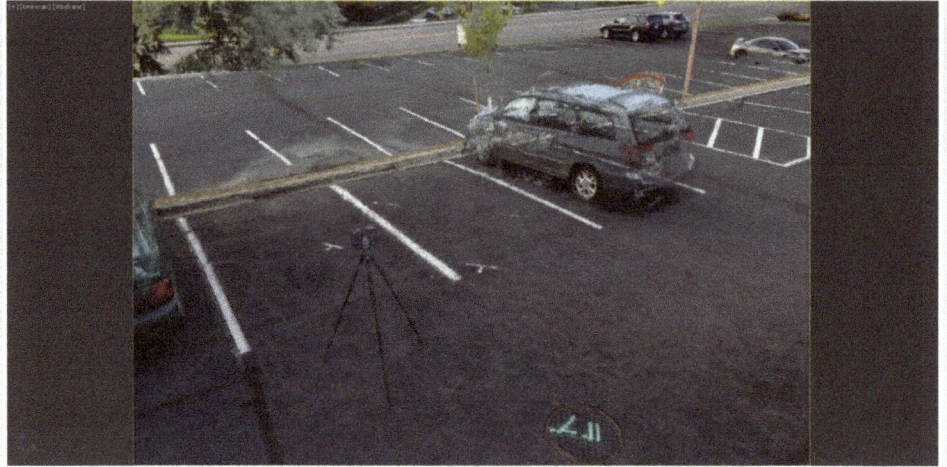

FIGURE 5.38   Reconstructed evidence overlaid on FARO scanner point cloud.

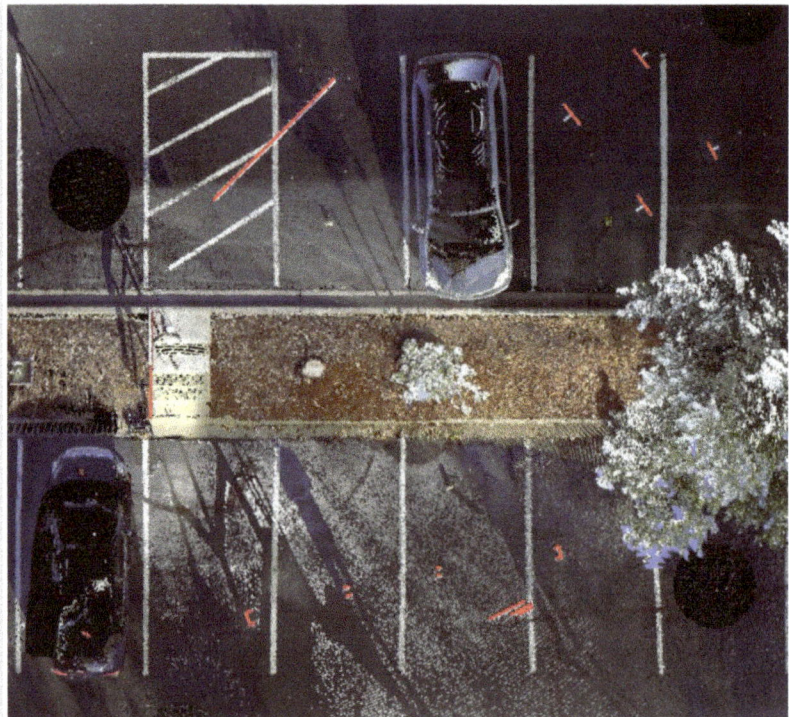

shows the individual points that were reconstructed. The accuracy of this process was analyzed by comparing the reconstructed coordinates of the tape to the coordinates of the tape as measured by the laser scanner. Table 5.1 presents the statistical results of this analysis. In this table, the "2D Distance," "Elevation," and "3D Distance" columns represent the difference between the FARO scanner points and the reconstructed points in the x-y plane, in the z-direction, and in 3D space, respectively. The average difference between position of the reconstructed evidence and the actual evidence, as measured by the FARO scanner, was approximately ½ in.

FIGURE 5.39   Points reconstructed with the camera matching analysis.

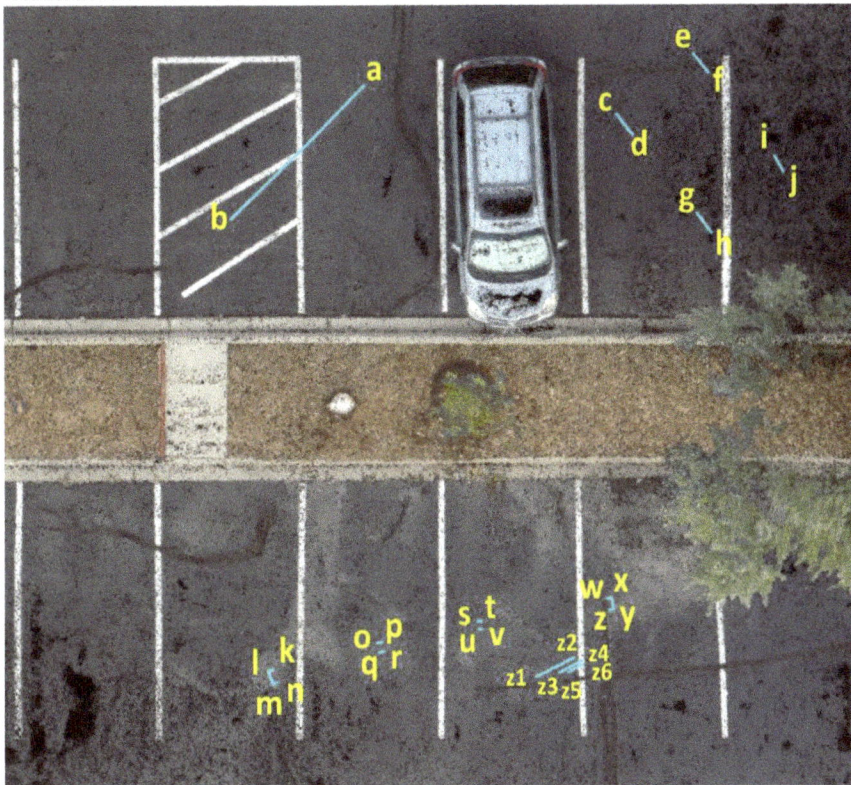

TABLE 5.1 Statistical analysis of the difference in position of reconstructed points versus their locations in the laser scan data

	2D distance (in.)	Elevation (in.)	3D distance (in.)
Average:	0.46	0.18	0.51
Standard deviation:	0.29	0.18	0.31
Maximum:	1.24	0.55	1.24

5.4.7 Mapping with Small Unmanned Aerial Vehicles

The previous section discussed the use of photographs from a sUAV with methods of photogrammetry to generate a point cloud of an accident site. Prior to the wide availability of sUAVs and photogrammetry software like PIX4D, aerial photographs had been utilized by accident reconstructionists as background images for evidence diagrams, as textures for physical models, or as background images for simulations. Fay discussed such applications of aerial imagery taken with manned aircraft [45]. Dilich and Goebelbecker described an unmanned aerial system consisting of a stabilized 35 mm camera attached to a tethered blimp that could be used to photograph vehicular accident scenes [46].

More recently, Google Earth has made high-resolution aerial photography widely available for free. Wirth examined the accuracy of aerial images from Google Earth and found accuracy levels sufficient for accident reconstruction [47]. Often, multiple aerial images of the same site will be available within Google Earth, each taken on a different date. Accident reconstructionists can often utilize these images to understand how a crash site has changed through time. These aerial images can also often be paired with historical images from Google Street View. These ground-level photographs can also help a reconstructionist determine what changes have occurred to a site through time. These images are also worth checking for physical evidence related to a crash. These authors have encountered instances in which some piece of physical evidence from a crash was not captured in the police photographs, but was captured in a Google Street View image.

Now that the U.S. government has issued rules related to the commercial application of sUAVs, accident reconstructionists have begun utilizing these devices to capture custom aerial photographs and video of accident scenes. The cameras on sUAVs are often stabilized with gimbal systems to reduce camera rotation and vibration. The use of UAV imagery as an input to the image-based scanning process for accident scenes offers many advantages over ground-level imagery. The scene can be documented from different vertical perspectives, which increases the number of images of the scene that contain overlapping geometry. The imagery is less subject to sun glare issues than ground-level images. Sun glare presents detection challenges for image-based scanning programs, since the same object will appear differently in frames where the sun is reflecting directly off the object than in frames where the sun is not reflecting off it. Ground-level imagery may also be limited by physical structures or access issues that can be overcome using an UAV. For instance, an accident scene on a bridge may only allow for a ground-level photographer to document the bridge from one end or the other. With UAVs, documentation of the entire bridge may be possible, and the resolution of the imagery would be superior to that of photographs taken from a long distance. Aerial imagery may also avoid problems with obstacles that can visually occlude key pieces of a scene.

5.4.8 Incorporating Large-Scale Lidar Data into Photogrammetry

Neale described a method for incorporating environmental features such as distant mountains into camera matching analysis. This was accomplished using digital elevation models generated with publicly available United States Geological Survey (USGS) Lidar data. The USGS formed the 3D Elevation Program (3DEP) in 2012 with the purpose of collecting and providing standardized, high-quality lidar data of the United States. The 3DEP began providing this data to the public in 2015. It is a multi-year project, and while this data is not yet available everywhere, the coverage continues to grow. A current coverage map is accessible via the USGS website.

An example of this data is shown in Figure 5.40 for a site in Colorado (a perspective view of some of this data is shown in Figure 5.41). The USGS 3DEP website offered a resolution of 0.7 to 50 m (~2.3 to 164 ft) in this area. To generate Figure 5.40, 43 individual data sets were downloaded in the LAS file format. Each file contained approximately 18 million 3D data points and covered approximately 2.25 km² (0.87 square miles). The data sets were combined within Cloud Compare 2.9 beta. Due to the large number of points, subsampling was also done within Cloud Compare to reduce the overall density of the combined point cloud. Subsampling was completed based on distance with a resulting distance of approximately 2.1 m (7 ft) between points. After combining the individual lidar data sets and subsampling, the resulting point cloud was approximately 10.5 km (6.5 miles) by 9 km (5.6 miles) and contained approximately 600 million 3D data points.

The incorporation of data like this into camera matching photogrammetry is particularly useful for instances when the number of close-range environmental features available for the analysis is limited. This was the specific situation examined by Neale et al., who found that the camera matches in which a single photograph was used without the USGS lidar were the least accurate. Using multiple photographs without the USGS

FIGURE 5.40 Planar view of sample USGS lidar data set.

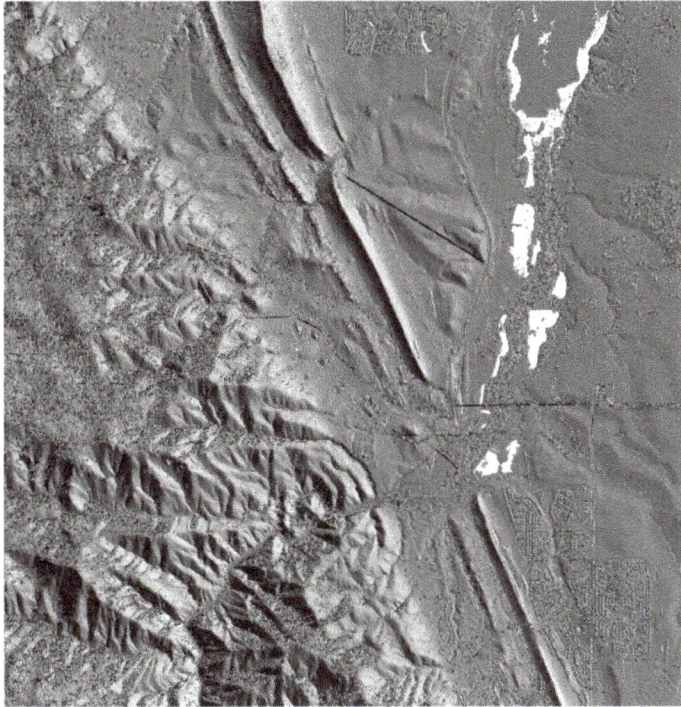

FIGURE 5.41 A perspective view of some of the lidar data of the previous figure.

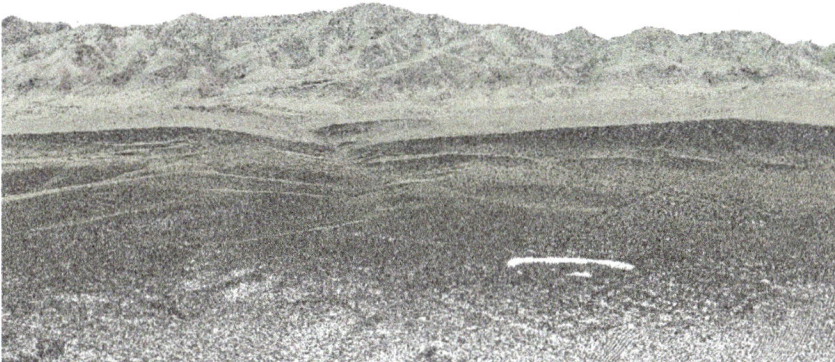

lidar improved the accuracy over using a single photograph. Utilizing the USGS lidar data, however, resulted in even greater improvements. The camera matches that utilized the lidar data and multiple photographs were found to be the most accurate.

References

1. Green, T., "3D Laser Scanners in Crash Testing," *Collision: The International Compendium for Crash Research* 12, no. 1 (September 2017), ISSN: 1934-8681.

2. Bartlett, W., "Motorcycle Braking and Skidmarks," Mechanical Forensics Engineering Services, LLC., 2000, unpublished article available at https://www.mfes.com/motorcyclebraking.html, accessed June 1, 2017.

3.   Bartlett, W., "Interpretation of Motorcycle Rear-Wheel Skidmarks for Accident Reconstruction," *Proceedings, Fourth International Conference on Accident Investigation, Reconstruction, Interpretation and the Law*, Vancouver, BC, Canada, August 2001.

4.   Fricke, L.B., *Traffic Crash Reconstruction*, 2nd ed., (Evanston, IL: Northwestern University Center for Public Safety, 2010), ISBN:0-912642-03-3.

5.   Baxter, A.T., *Motorcycle Crash Investigation*, (Jacksonville, FL: Institute of Police Technology and Management, 2017), ISBN:978-1-934807-18-7.

6.   Dunn, A., Dorohoff, M., Bayan, F., Cornetto, A. et al., "Analysis of Motorcycle Braking Performance and Associated Braking Marks," SAE Technical Paper 2012-01-0610, 2012, doi:10.4271/2012-01-0610.

7.   Peck, L., Deyerl, E., and Rose, N., "The Effect of Tire Pressure on the Deceleration Rate of a Motorcycle under Application of the Rear Brake Only," *Accident Reconstruction Journal*, July/August 2017, ISSN: 1057-8153.

8.   McNally, B., "Summary of Motorcycle Friction Tests," *Accident Investigation Quarterly* Fall (2006): 31, ISSN: 1082-6521.

9.   Baxter, A. and Robar, N., "An Examination of the Performance of Motorcycle Brake Systems," *Accident Investigation Quarterly*, no. 47 (2007): 28-31, ISSN: 1082-6521.

10. Smith, J., Frank, T., Bosch, K., Fowler, G. et al., "Full-Scale Moving Motorcycle into Moving Car Crash Testing for Use in Safety Design and Accident Reconstruction," SAE Technical Paper 2012-01-0103, 2012, doi:10.4271/2012-01-0103.

11. Bready, J., May, A., and Allsop, D., "Physical Evidence Analysis and Roll Velocity Effects in Rollover Accident Reconstruction," SAE Technical Paper 2001-01-1284, 2001, doi:10.4271/2001-01-1284.

12. Kubly, K.D. and Buse, C.R., "Motorcycle Post-Accident Inspection Techniques," SAE Technical Paper 850064, 1985, doi:10:4271/850064.

13. Campbell, J.B. and Wynne, R.H., *Introduction to Remote Sensing*, 5th ed., (The Guilford Press, 2011), ISBN:978-1-60918-176-5.

14. Voitel, T. and Terpstra, T., "Benefits of 3D Laser Scanning in Vehicle Accident Reconstruction," Technology White Paper, FARO Technologies, Inc., 2012, http://kineticorp.com/wp-content/uploads/2017/11/faro-whitepaper-benefits-of-3d-scanning-in-var.pdf.

15. DiTallo, M., Brandt, J., and Green, T.E., "Laser Scanner Basics for Public Safety – Scene Marking, Scanner Placement, and Scanner Settings," FARO White Paper, 2017, http://www.publicsafety.faro.com/assets/dynamicsafety_whitepaper_013017.pdf.

16. Wolf, P., Dewitt, B., and Wilkinson, B., *Elements of Photogrammetry with Application in GIS*, 4th ed., (New York: McGraw-Hill Professional Publishing, 2014), ISBN:978-0071761123.

17. Campbell III, A.T., "Adapting Three-Dimensional Animation Software for Photogrammetry Calculations," SAE Technical Paper 930904, 1993, doi:10.4271/930904.

18. Baker, K.S., "Chapter 9: Photogrammetry for Collision Analysis," *Traffic Collision Investigation*, 10th ed., (Evanston, IL: Northwestern University Center for Public Safety, 2002), ISBN:0-912642-09-2.

19. Tumbas, N.S., "Photogrammetry and Accident Reconstruction: Experimental Results," SAE Technical Paper 940925, 1994, doi:10.4271/940925.

20. Pepe, M.D., "Accuracy of Three-Dimensional Photogrammetry as Established by Controlled Field Tests," SAE Technical Paper 930662, 1993, doi:10.4271/930662.

21. Neale, W.T.C., Hessel, D., and Terpstra, T., "Photogrammetric Measurement Error Associated with Lens Distortion," SAE Technical Paper 2011-01-0286, 2011, doi:10.4271/2011-01-0286.

22. Massa, D.J., "Using Computer Reverse Projection Photogrammetry to Analyze an Animation," SAE Technical Paper 1999-01-0093, 1999, doi:10.4271/1999-01-0093.

23. Fenton, S., Neale, W., Rose, N.A., and Hughes, C., "Determining Crash Data Using Camera-Matching Photogrammetric Technique," SAE Technical Paper 2001-01-3313, 2001, doi:10.4271/2001-01-3313.

24. Coleman, C., Tandy, D., Colborn, J., and Ault, N., "Applying Camera Matching Methods to Laser Scanned Three-Dimensional Scene Data with Comparisons to Other Methods," SAE Technical Paper 2015-01-1416, 2015, doi:10.4271/2015-01-1416.

25. Chou, C., McCoy, R., Fenton, S., Neale, W. et al., "Image Analysis of Rollover Crash Test Using Photogrammetry," SAE Technical Paper 2006-01-0723, 2006, doi:10.4271/2006-01-0723.

26. Rose, N.A.., Neale, W.T.C., Fenton, S.J., Hessel, D. et al., "A Method to Quantify Vehicle Dynamics and Deformation for Vehicle Rollover Tests Using Camera-Matching Video Analysis," *SAE Int. J. Passeng. Cars - Mech. Syst.* 1, no. 1 (2008): 301-317, doi:4271/2008-01-0350.

27. Manuel, E.J., Mink, R., and Kruger, D., "Videogrammetry in Vehicle Crash Reconstruction with a Moving Video Camera," SAE Technical Paper 2018-01-0532, doi:10.4271/2018-01-0532.

28. Breen, K.C. and Anderson, C.E., "The Application of Photogrammetry to Accident Reconstruction," SAE Technical Paper 861422, 1986, doi:10.4271/861422.

29. Woolley, R.L.., White, K.A., Asay, A.F., and Bready, J.E., "Determination of Vehicle Crush from Two Photographs and the Use of 3D Displacement Vectors in Accident Reconstruction," SAE Technical Paper 910118, 1991, doi:10.4271/910118.

30. Husher, S.E., Varat, M.S., and Kerkhoff, J.F., "Survey of Photogrammetric Methodologies for Accident Reconstruction," *Proceedings of the Canadian Multidisciplinary Road Safety Conference VII*, Vancouver, BC, June 1991.

31. Main, B.W., "A New Application of Camera Reverse Projection in Reconstructing Old Accidents," SAE Technical Paper 950357, 1995, doi:10.4271/950357.

32. Smith, G.C. and Allsop, D.L., "A Case Comparison of Single-Image Photogrammetry Methods," SAE Technical Paper 890737, 1989, doi:10.4271/890737.

33. Goldberg, N., *Camera Technology – The Dark Side of the Lens*, (San Diego: Academic Press Inc., 1992), ISBN:0-12-287570-2.

34. Taylor, J.T., *The Optics of Photography and Photographic Lenses*, (Adamant Media Corporation, 2005), ISBN:1-4212-4851-4.

35. Rose, N.A., Carter, N., Pentecost, D., Voitel, T. et al., "Using Data from a DriveCam Event Recorder to Reconstruct a Vehicle-to-Vehicle Impact," SAE Technical Paper 2013-01-0778, 2013, doi:10.4271/2013-01-0778.

36. Rose, N.A., Neale, W.T.C., and Carter, N., "Using Data from a DriveCam Video Event Recorder to Reconstruct a Hard Braking Event," *Collision: The International Compendium for Crash Research* 7, no. 1 (Spring 2012), ISSN: 1934-8681.

37. Gates, T.J., "Analysis of Dilemma Zone Driver Behavior at Signalized Intersections," *2007 Annual Meeting*, Paper No. 07-3351, Transportation Research Board, https://doi.org/10.3141/2030-05.

38. Vergauwen, M., "Wide Baseline 3D Reconstruction from Digital Stills," *ISPRS Workshop on Visualization and Animation of Reality-Based 3D Models*, Tarasp-Vulpera, Engadin, Switzerland, February 2003.

39. Strecha, C., von Hansen, W., Van Gool, L., and Thoennessen, U., "Multi-view Stereo and Lidar for Outdoor Scene Modelling," *International Archives of Photogrammetry, Remote Sensing and Spatial Information Science*, 2007, https://pdfs.semanticscholar.org/ac1b/7b3c7b687a8cb2e4fed9a3a896653356a1aa.pdf.

40. Dai, F., Rashidi, A., and Brilakis, I., Vela, P., "Comparison of Image-Based and Time-of-Flight-Based Technologies for 3D Reconstruction of Infrastructure, *Construction Research Congress 2012: Construction Challenges in a Flat World*, ISBN:9780784412329.

41. Erickson, M., Bauer, J., and Hayes, W., "The Accuracy of Photo-Based Three-Dimensional Scanning for Collision Reconstruction Using 123D Catch," SAE Technical Paper 2013-01-0784, 2013, doi:10.4271/2013-01-0784.

42. Terpstra, T., Voitel, T., and Hashemian, A., "A Survey of Multi-View Photogrammetry Software for Documenting Vehicle Crush," SAE Technical Paper 2016-01-1475, 2016, doi:10.4271/2016-01-1475.

43. Jurkofsky, D., "Accuracy of SUAS Photogrammetry for Use in Accident Scene Diagramming," *SAE Int. J. Trans. Safety* 3, no. 2 (2015): 136-152, doi:10.4271/2015-01-1426.

44. Carter, N., Hashemian, A., Rose, N., and Neale, W., "Evaluation of the Accuracy of Image Based Scanning as a Basis for Photogrammetric Reconstruction of Physical Evidence," SAE Technical Paper 2016-01-1467, 2016, doi:10.4271/2016-01-1467.

45. Fay, R., Robinette, R., and Larson, V., "Engineering Models and Animations in Vehicular Accident Studies," SAE Technical Paper 880719, 1988, doi:10.4271/880719.

46. Dilich, M. and Goebelbecker, J., "Accident Investigation and Reconstruction Mapping with Aerial Photography," SAE Technical Paper 960894, 1996, doi:10.4271/960894.

47. Wirth, J., Bonugli, E., and Freund, M., "Assessment of the Accuracy of Google Earth Imagery for Use as a Tool in Accident Reconstruction," SAE Technical Paper 2015-01-1435, 2015, doi:10.4271/2015-01-1435.

6

Sliding and Tumbling of the Motorcycle and Rider

When performing speed calculations, one approach is to assume that a motorcycle decelerates at a constant rate as it slides and tumbles along the roadway. This assumption is adequate for most crash reconstruction applications, though there will be some variability in the deceleration along the slide distance, depending on which motorcycle components are engaging the road surface at any point in time. If the motorcycle slides across multiple surfaces, different decelerations may need to be assigned for each different surface. In practice, the reconstructionist would determine the slide distances based on the physical evidence, and then a range of decelerations would be selected from physical tests reported in the literature for similar type motorcycles sliding on similar surfaces. A number of these studies are reviewed in this chapter.

6.1 Typical Decelerations for a Sliding Motorcycle

Day and Smith [1] reported a study of motorcycle sliding deceleration in 1984, analyzing the behavior of two downed motorcycles on various surfaces—a 1967 Honda CB305 and a 1973 Yamaha 550 Special. They towed the motorcycles using a rope (see Figure 6.1) with an in-line force gauge and documented the forces required to pull the motorcycles at 1 and 40 kph (25 mph). For pavement, Day and Smith found a sliding friction factor range of 0.45 to 0.58 during the 25 mph tests. For gravel, the friction

FIGURE 6.1   Day and Smith's setup for towing motorcycles across the pavement [1].

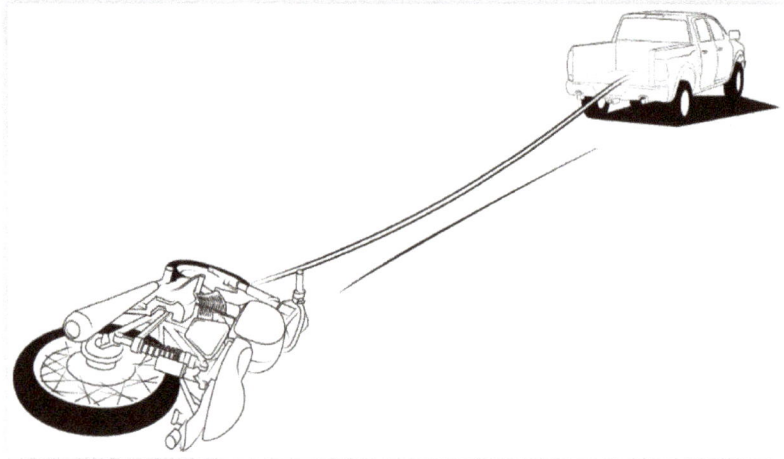

factor was 0.68 to 0.79 and for grassy earth, 0.79. Day and Smith noted that "during the testing, it was observed that projecting elements, such as the foot pegs and handle bars, would tend to plow into the soil at low speeds, creating momentary high drag factors." In this testing, the motorcycle started in a capsized position on the ground, and so deceleration from a fall was not a part of the friction factors reported by Day and Smith.

Lambourn [2] explored how sliding decelerations experienced by motorcycles differed between tests where the vehicle was dragged at low speeds and tests where the motorcycle was dropped at a higher speed and allowed to slide to rest. For the higher-speed tests, motorcycles were dropped from a low platform (already on their side) or allowed to fall to their side from an upright position. The photographs of Figure 6.2 depict the test setup for the upright drops and one of the tests from this setup. In his literature review, Lambourn noted that some studies had reported a speed dependence on the sliding deceleration, with the rate decreasing with increasing speed. He also examined this issue of speed dependence of the deceleration in his testing.

Lambourn reported that the decelerations (what they termed as a *friction factor*) measured "in the low-speed drag tests gave a value close to the high-speed sliding value. The friction was affected by the road surface texture, the presence of prominent side

FIGURE 6.2   Setup and sample test using the upright drop method [2]. (Much thanks to Richard Lambourn for his efforts digging these photographs up from his archives and for giving us permission to use them.)

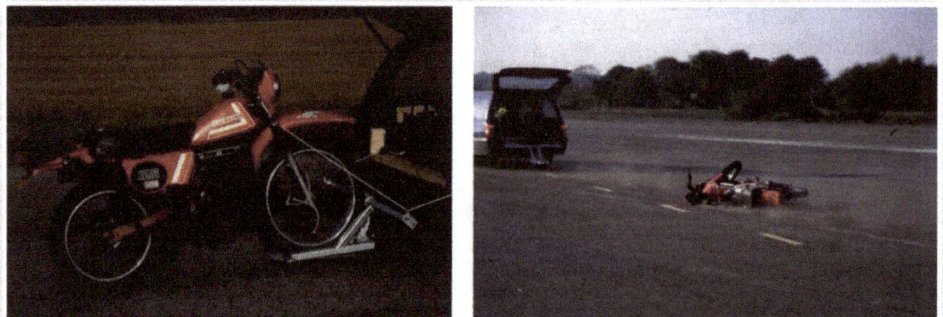

projections, and the wearing away of these projections during the slide. Some speed dependence was noted in the upright-launch tests which appears to be due to the 'digging-in' of the machine as it falls to the road, rather than an effect of the sliding friction itself." He also concluded that "the reason for there being a clear speed dependence in the results of Becke and of Ashton, but not in the tests reported here, is almost certainly due to the fact that in both their experimental methods the motorcycles were dropped a distance onto the road surface. This would subject the machines to a large decelerating impulse as they struck the ground, which would considerably increase the average deceleration in low speed tests but be relatively unimportant in high speed runs." Lambourn concluded that the sliding deceleration of a motorcycle was dependent on the roughness characteristics of the road surface.

Other authors have suggested that differences in test methodology—if the motorcycle drops to the ground in the test and from what height—account for some of the variability in the deceleration for sliding motorcycles and the apparent speed dependence in the decelerations. For instance, Baxter [3] stated: "One word of caution; read the test methodology as to how the friction values were obtained. In some drop tests, the motorcycle was pre-positioned laterally a few inches/centimeters above the road surface. [Friction values obtained] using this method are generally lower than a motorcycle falling from vertical (normal position) onto its side on the road." Hague [4], Wood [5], and Walsh [6] also discussed the influence of the fall (capsize) on the deceleration. Hague stated: "The methodology of a motorcycle slide test can significantly affect the measured deceleration rate, apparently due to the speed lost in the initial ground impact. Those tests in which motorcycles were dropped from an increased height resulted in increased deceleration rates. During a road traffic accident, the motorcycle will also lose speed upon ground impact and testing should therefore try to mimic this process. Bearing this in mind, the most appropriate tests for the majority of collisions would be those in which an upright motorcycle was allowed to capsize from a normal height." This is different than the approach proposed by Wood and Walsh. They proposed splitting the speed calculations into separate phases for the capsize and the slide. Thus, within their method, the ideal test procedure for the sliding phase would not include a fall of the motorcycle. Walsh presented a method for incorporating the speed loss from a fall into the calculation of the deceleration from a test or the calculation of the motorcycle's initial speed in a reconstruction.

Donohoe reported sliding decelerations for a 1982 Kawasaki KZ1000 Police Special. Testing with this motorcycle, which was conducted at the Los Angeles Police Department's Specialized Collision Investigation Detail, utilized a flatbed truck with a lift gate on the rear [7]. The lift gate was positioned parallel to the roadway and approximately 6 inches above the road surface. The motorcycle, which was facing along the direction of travel, was dropped an upright position with its front tire on the lift gate and its rear tire on the roadway. The roadway was a residential, asphalt roadway adjacent to Dodger Stadium. The initial speed of the motorcycle was measured with radar. Donohoe reported five tests with sliding decelerations between 0.38 and 0.50.

In 1995, Raftery slid an unknown motorcycle wearing Suzuki Katana fairings from an initial speed of 85 kph (53 mph) and reported an average deceleration of 0.26g [8]. Another test, seemingly from a similar speed, resulted in the same 0.26g. As a control test, Raftery took the same motorcycle, removed the fairings, and performed another test. The resulting deceleration was 0.33g. The deceleration was calculated using the initial drop speed and the documented sliding distance. Raftery's methodology involved suspending the motorcycle from a boom at the rear of a tow truck, driving the tow truck up to the test speed, and releasing the motorcycle from the boom. It appears from Raftery's description of his tests that he suspended the motorcycle from the boom with

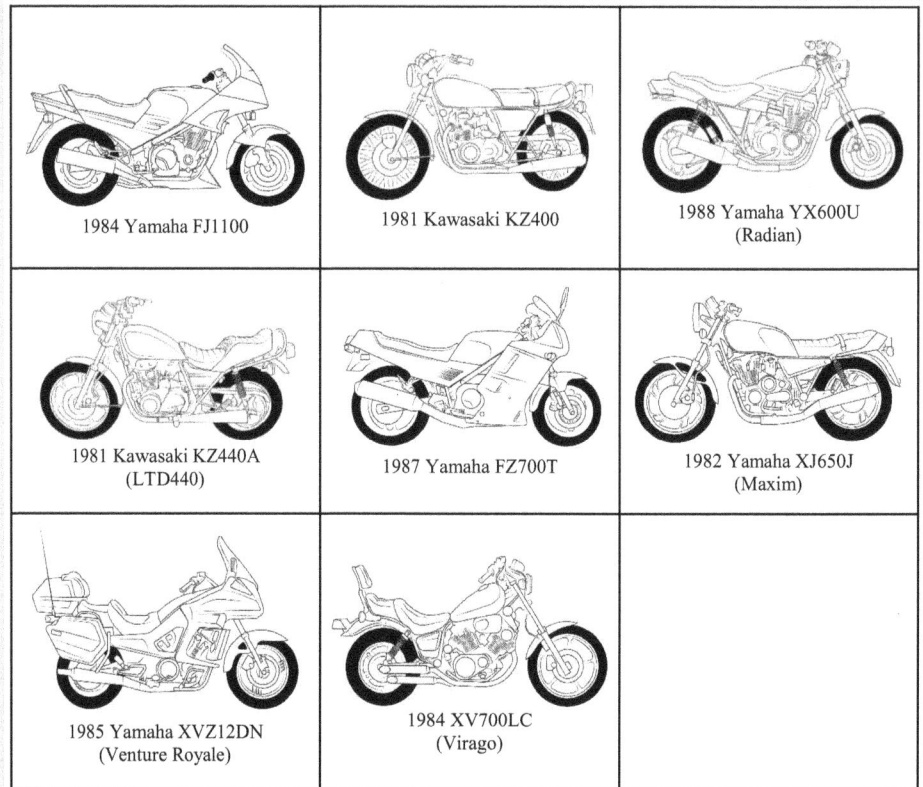

FIGURE 6.3 Motorcycles tested by Carter [1996].

the wheels rolling on the ground and when the motorcycle was released it fell to the road surface. Raftery's deceleration rates appear to be low compared to many other studies reviewed here.

Carter [9] tested eight different motorcycles (see Figure 6.3) on three different surfaces (asphalt, dirt, and gravel) to determine their sliding decelerations from target speeds of 48 and 97 kph (30 and 60 mph). All of the tests run on off-road surfaces utilized a target speed of 48 kph (30 mph). The motorcycles that Carter tested included the following motorcycle types: standard, cruiser, sport, and touring. In all, Carter reported 50 tests. Carter reported that "some speed effects were observed, i.e., for higher speeds, the slide coefficient was lower (likely due to heat softening of structure contact points with the pavement)." Also, "for full fairing equipped motorcycles the slide coefficient was consistently lower than for non-fairing equipped motorcycles" and "deep gouges left by the motorcycle in the surfaces corresponded with higher slide coefficients."

Carter attempted to improve on prior studies by developing a test rig that allowed for consistent positioning and release of the motorcycles. The motorcycles were positioned front wheel forward and on their left or right sides. The motorcycles were released from a position with the lowest point on the side of the motorcycle approximately 5 centimeters above the ground. As Carter noted, "this release height was chosen to minimize the impact forces upon release, therefore restricting (to the extent possible) the tests only to energy dissipated during sliding."

Medwell [10] performed four motorcycle sliding tests using a fully faired 1992 Kawasaki ZX-7 Ninja. Medwell stated that "the tests were designed to approximate, as closely as possible, the motion of a motorcycle falling over from an upright position. The motorcycle was positioned upright on a fabricated platform mounted on the right side of a pickup truck…The height of the platform was adjusted so that its underside was as close as possible to the roadway surface. This test setup resulted in the motorcycle tire contact surface being approximately 90mm above the roadway. The motorcycle was held upright by an assistant riding in the bed of the pickup truck. The truck was accelerated to the test speed, then the motorcycle was released and allowed to fall over sideways onto the road surface." In two of the tests, the Kawasaki initially slid along the pavement but then traveled into a nearby area of grass, making them difficult to analyze. However, two of the tests were confined to the asphalt. Both had a release speed of approximately 80 kph (50 mph). The motorcycles slid for 69.5 and 86.3 meters (228 and 283 feet) before coming to rest. The calculated decelerations were 0.36 and 0.29g. The 0.36 value was obtained during the test involving the right side of the motorcycle, which is the exhaust side. Like those reported by Raftery, Medwell's decelerations appear to be low relative to other studies reviewed here.

Bartlett [11] reported motorcycle drop tests from Motorcycle Crash Reconstruction classes conducted at the Institute for Police Technology and Management (IPTM) from 1987 to 2006. These tests were conducted on asphalt or concrete, but the surfaces varied from class to class. The drop techniques also varied from class to class. Bartlett observed: "The results are a chaotic mix of sliding and tumbling, not unlike real motorcycle crashes." Bartlett's dataset initially consisted of 237 drop tests using 107 different motorcycles. Twenty tests were discarded because the reported drop speed, slide distance, and deceleration were inconsistent with each other. Additional tests were excluded in which the motorcycle was dropped from a pickup bed or in which the motorcycle slid off the road surface onto the off-road terrain. The final dataset included 162 tests with 99 different motorcycles. Bartlett reported that the decelerations trended slightly higher with increasing speed and that the overall average deceleration for all the tests was 0.521 ± 0.140g. Bartlett also combined his dataset with other available datasets. This resulted in 386 tests for which Bartlett reported decelerations of 0.480 ± 0.134g.

In 2003, McNally and Bartlett slid a fully faired Suzuki Katana at IPTM's Special Problems and analyzed the results via frame-by-frame video and field data (known initial speed and measured slide distance) [12]. Video analysis yielded a deceleration of 0.42g while the sliding distance and known initial speed yielded a result of 0.39g. Bartlett has also reported nine additional tests performed using fully faired motorcycles during IPTM classes over the years [11]. The individual results were not detailed in the paper, but combined with the data from Raftery, Medwell, and McNally, the total set of 14 tests had an average coefficient of friction of 0.37g with a standard deviation of 0.08g.

In 2004, Hague compiled data from prior studies where motorcycles capsized and then slid to rest [4]. Hauge concluded that "the analysis shows that a more accurate estimation of deceleration rate can be made if the motorcycles are split into two different categories, based on the presence of fairing, crash bars and/or panniers." He noted that, while "one might expect partially faired motorcycles to have lower deceleration rates than unfaired machines…the two categories exhibit similar deceleration rates. Perhaps also initially surprising is that fully faired machines equipped with panniers gave similar results to the partially/unfaired motorcycles." In relation to crash-bar-equipped motorcycles, the only available tests were those conducted by Lambourn [2], in which the decelerations varied between 0.25 and 0.35. Hague noted that, "As expected, fully faired and crash bar equipped motorcycles decelerated at relatively low rates. The crash bar equipped results are probably artificially low because they were all dropped from a very low height. If they had capsized from an upright position, they would have lost additional speed on striking the ground which would increase the average deceleration rate, more so at lower speeds. Although deceleration rates as low as 0.2 have been suggested for crash bar equipped machines there appears to be no published data to support such low values." Hague reported an average deceleration for partially faired and unfaired motorcycles of 0.39 and for fully faired motorcycles of 0.27.

Peck worked with several members of CA2RS (California Association of Accident Reconstruction Specialists) to perform 14 sliding tests using modern GPS data acquisition technology, which captured the motorcycle speed at 10 Hz. In 2014, Peck reported this data, which included two tests with fully faired motorcycles, a 1989 Suzuki GSX-R750 and a 1991 Suzuki GSX600F [13]. These tests yielded sliding decelerations of 0.42 and 0.47g, respectively.

Missing from the literature cited so far is documentation of the sliding deceleration for motorcycles equipped with frame sliders, a common sport bike modification. Frame sliders, usually comprised of a plastic composite, are mounted to the sides of motorcycles to mitigate damages during a fall. Over the course of 2 years, Peck collected data from track crashes at track days and racing events at New Hampshire Motor Speedway and New Jersey Motorsports Park. All analyzed crashes involved motorcycles equipped with a QSTARZ GPS data acquisition system (5 or 10 Hz). In total, data from 15 crashes were collected and analyzed. All 15 crashes involved faired motorcycles equipped with plastic composite frame sliders. The average coefficient of friction was 0.45 with a standard deviation of 0.09. These numbers are more consistent with data from non-faired motorcycles, indicating that frame sliders increase the sliding deceleration for sport motorcycles. In addition, these crashes involved the potential interaction between the motorcycle and the operator that could occur in the real world.

DiTallo [14] examined three different test methods for determining the drag factor for motorcycles sliding on their sides. This testing utilized 26 motorcycles sliding on an asphalt roadway in North Las Vegas, Nevada. The following three methods were utilized: (1) dragging an already capsized motorcycle across the pavement, (2) releasing a motorcycle from the rear hydraulic lift of a box truck and allowing it to fall to the pavement and slide to rest, and (3) towing a motorcycle behind a moving vehicle with its front tire held in a pneumatic clamp until its release. After release, the motorcycle would fall to the ground and slide to rest. DiTallo noted that many of the motorcycles had been previously utilized in impact testing at the 2016 ARC-CSI conference. These motorcycles included sport, touring, and motocross motorcycles along with mopeds. One of the sport motorcycles had frame sliders.

A total of 36 pull tests (Method 1) were conducted with 9 motorcycles. The motorcycles were pulled in varying orientations. This series of tests resulted in a range of drag factors between 0.36 and 0.64 and an average of 0.51. DiTallo also noted that the tests with tires leading exhibited an average drag factor of 0.54 and the tests with the tires trailing exhibited an average drag factor of 0.51. Drop tests (Method 2) were conducted with 12 motorcycles at speeds ranging from 30.7 to 41.1 mph. These tests produced drag factors between 0.28 and 0.70. Clamp tests (Method 3) were conducted with five motorcycles at speeds ranging between 29 and 43.9 mph. These tests resulted in average drag factors between 0.28 and 0.43. This group contained the sport motorcycle with frame sliders. In addition to parsing his data by test methodology, DiTallo also considered motorcycle type. He found that the sport motorcycles had drag factors between 0.28 and 0.61, the touring motorcycles had drag factors between 0.28 and 0.60, the mopeds had drag factors between 0.35 and 0.54, and the motocross motorcycle had a drag factor of 0.43.

Data from many of the studies reviewed here was compiled in a spreadsheet and illustrative decelerations were calculated for various motorcycle types on asphalt and concrete road surfaces. Means and standard deviations of these decelerations are reported in Table 6.1.

TABLE 6.1 Average sliding deceleration for motorcycles (asphalt/concrete)

Motorcycle type	Average sliding deceleration on asphalt/concrete (g)
Standard	0.47 ± 0.13
Cruiser/Touring	0.47 ± 0.10
Sport	0.48 ± 0.11
Dirt/Enduro	0.52 ± 0.12
Scooter/Moped	0.49 ± 0.13

These decelerations do not appear to exhibit a strong dependence on motorcycle type. The values in this table were calculated using the decelerations as they were reported in the published studies. All test types were combined and no attempt was made to adjust for the various test procedures. This table does not address motorcycle-to-motorcycle differences that could be relevant on specific cases (whether the motorcycle was fully or partially faired and what components were present to scrape and gouge the road surface, for instance). The decelerations reported here are consistent with those reported by Bartlett for a large dataset [11].

6.2 Average Decelerations for a Sliding or Tumbling Rider

Often, when a motorcycle capsizes, the rider will separate from the motorcycle and will also slide or tumble along the ground. Typically, the rider will decelerate at a different and higher rate than the motorcycle. If the point of separation between the rider and the motorcycle can be determined, along with the rest positions of both the rider and the motorcycle, the rider's slide/tumble distance can be used as further confirmation of the calculated speed of the motorcycle at the point of separation. As with the motorcycle, the assumption will typically be made that a sliding or tumbling rider decelerates at a constant rate. Again, this assumption is adequate for most crash reconstruction applications, though there will be some variability in the deceleration along the slide distance. As with the motorcycle, if the rider slides across multiple surfaces, different decelerations may need to be assigned for each different surface. The reconstructionist can determine the slide distance based on the physical evidence and then use a range of decelerations for the rider selected from physical tests reported in the literature.

Severy [15] observed that a sliding and/or tumbling person "has a higher effective drag coefficient than the automobile undergoing emergency braking...." In making this statement, Severy was including the speed loss that occurred when the person first struck the ground, along with the speed loss that occurs during the sliding following that initial impact. Referencing the CRASH2 User's Manual, Warner [16] reported a range of decelerations for a "motorcycle skidding on [its] side" of between 0.55 and 0.7g. He reported a deceleration for a "human body skidding" of 1.1g and for a "human body tumbling" of 0.8g. Haight and Eubanks [17] reported decelerations between 0.8 and 0.95g for ATDs sliding on the ground after being involved in vehicle versus bicycle collisions. These decelerations also include the initial collision with the ground. In discussing motorcycle/vehicle collisions where the rider is thrown through the air, Collins [18] stated that "a rider launched from a motorcycle may fall to the ground or be slammed into the pavement, so on paved surfaces the ejected rider's friction coefficient will range between 0.8 and 1.2."

Fricke [19], on the other hand, reported the following drag factors for people sliding on various surfaces: grass, 0.45 to 0.70; asphalt, 0.45 to 0.60; and concrete, 0.40 to 0.65. Contrary to those in the previous paragraph, these drag factors exclude the speed loss the pedestrian experiences from landing on the road surface. Thus, if these drag factors were utilized for speed analysis, the additional speed loss would need to be accounted for separately.

Happer [20] observed that the literature contains decelerations (drag factors) for people that are defined in several different ways: (1) a simple sliding coefficient of friction between the person and the ground, (2) a drag factor that includes the speed loss from when the person first impact the ground, or (3) an average drag factor for the entire trajectory of the person, including the airborne phase. The first two of these are, of course, similar to the issues that arise in the different test procedures used to obtain the decelerations of sliding or tumbling motorcycles. Happer conducted an extensive literature review and found that "regardless of the ground surface (i.e. asphalt, grass, wet or dry), the drag factor for a pedestrian sliding along the ground ranges from about 0.40 to 0.72. The drag factor for a tumbling pedestrian [meaning the impact with ground is included] ranges from 0.7 to 1.22. The drag factor significantly increases for the tumbling pedestrian as the pedestrian will lose speed from impacting the ground after being vaulted through the air. The effective pedestrian drag factor for the full trajectory ranges from 0.37 to 0.79."

Wood [21] noted that the deceleration of a person sliding on the ground is decreased if the surface is wet. Happer noted that "if the road surface is not level and has a substantial grade, then this slope should be considered. In addition, the reviewed data did not include a significantly slippery road surface (e.g. ice); thus, a very slippery surface may also significantly affect the pedestrian drag factor." Brach and Brach [22] listed the following formula that can be used to adjust a flat-ground deceleration (f) for application to a sloped surface ($f_{adjusted}$). In this equation, θ is the angle of the slope in degrees. This angle is positive for an upgrade and negative for a downgrade:

$$f_{adjusted} = f \cdot \cos\theta + \sin\theta \qquad (6.1)$$

Fugger [23] reported a series of 160 pedestrian crash tests utilizing high-fronted vehicles that would generate forward projection trajectories. An Alderson Research Labs CG-95 dummy was utilized to represent the pedestrians in these tests (75.5 inches tall, 169 pounds). The dummy was clothed in a wetsuit covered by coveralls and standard athletic footwear. The following vans were used in this test series: a 1976 Ford Econoline 250, a 1971 Dodge B200, a 1982 Dodge B250, a 1980 Plymouth D100, a 1982 Chevrolet G20, and a 1977 Dodge Sportman. The leading edge of the hood of each of these vehicles was above the center of gravity of the dummy such that they would produce forward projection trajectories. Of the 160 tests, 56 were conducted on dry asphalt and 84 on wet asphalt. Impact speeds varied between 4 and 60 kph, with most of the tests conducted at speeds below 32 kph. He reported average decelerations of the sliding pedestrians of 0.43 for the dry asphalt and between 0.31 and 0.41 for the wet asphalt, depending on the water depth. These decelerations excluded the initial impact with the ground.

Baxter [3] states that "the occupants of a motorcycle thrown to a highway surface will decelerate quite rapidly, tumbling or rolling at first, then sliding to a stop. Various test by Hurt and Baird [24], using cadavers or specialized instrumented dummies, show a sliding friction range of 0.90g to 1.2g. Clothing worn does have an effect on the value. Leather clothing and a full coverage helmet reduce the friction value to a level of 0.60g to 0.70g…Values for other clothing, such a polyester (0.70g) and cotton or wool (0.70g to 0.85g), were also established." In reviewing the Hurt and Baird study, Baxter appears to be citing incorrect values. That study actually states that "when the rider or passenger falls to the pavement, the deceleration to the point of rest will usually be rapid. When the rider is wearing soft cloth apparel, the deceleration will be on the order of 0.9 to 1.2g, with the mode including violent tumbling and rolling. Such violent motion and high abrasion may tear the soft clothing from the downed rider. Only when the rider is clad with full leathers, boots, and protective headgear is the mode of deceleration likely to change. Then the lower friction of the leather clad body will reduce the tumbling and rolling tendency and also reduce the deceleration to the range of 0.7 to 0.9 g." Thus, the deceleration for a rider clothed in leather clothing and a full coverage helmet was 0.7 to 0.9g, not 0.6 to 0.7g.

6.3 Determining the Initial Speed for a Sliding Motorcycle or Rider

The slide distance should be measured from the initiation of sliding evidence on the roadway to the rest position of the motorcycle or rider and should include any gaps in the visible marks [4]. Once the slide distance has been determined and a range of decelerations assigned, the speed of the motorcycle or rider at the beginning of the slide (v_{slide}) can be determined with the following equation:

$$v_{slide} = \sqrt{2gf_{slide}d_{slide}} \tag{6.2}$$

In this equation, d_{slide} is the slide distance, f_{slide} is the deceleration during the slide, and g is the gravitational constant. Equation (6.2) can be applied with decelerations that already include the speed loss from capsizing. However, if the reconstructionist wants to account for this speed loss separately, the following equation can be used [6, 25, 26]:

$$v_{land} = f_{slide}v_z + \sqrt{2gf_{slide}d_{slide}} \tag{6.3}$$

In Equation (6.3), v_z is the vertical impact velocity of the motorcycle's center of gravity. If this equation was being utilized, then the selected deceleration rates should not already include the speed loss from capsizing. Walsh [6] presented the following equation for estimating the downward velocity of motorcycle that capsizes under the influence of gravity without a rider:

$$v_z = \sqrt{\frac{2gh_{cg} - gf_w}{1 + \left(\dfrac{k_r}{h_{cg}}\right)^2}} \tag{6.4}$$

This equation could be applied to calculate the downward velocity of the motorcycle in motorcycle drop tests, but it may not apply to many real-world crashes, where the motorcycle motion will also be influenced by tire forces and interaction with the rider. Also, in the real world, not all capsizes are the same. A low-side fall of a motorcycle, for example, is likely to be associated with less speed loss from the landing than a high-side fall. These two types of falls are considered in the next chapter.

6.3.1 Example Calculation of Motorcycle Speed at Onset of Sliding

As an example, consider a standard motorcycle that capsizes on an asphalt roadway and then slides for 150 feet. The speed of this motorcycle at the onset of sliding can be calculated with Equation (6.2), as follows. The range of deceleration rates used in this sample calculation utilized the mean and standard deviation reported in Table 6.1 for standard motorcycles on asphalt and concrete to calculate a low and high value. This results in a relatively wide range of approximately 13 mph. For a real-world case, it is possible that features of the motorcycle or the physical evidence could enable the reconstructionist to further limit this range:

$$v_{slide} = \sqrt{2gf_{slide}d_{slide}} = \sqrt{2 \cdot 32.2 \cdot \begin{bmatrix} 0.34 \\ 0.60 \end{bmatrix} \cdot 150} = \begin{bmatrix} 57.3 \\ 76.1 \end{bmatrix} \text{fps} = \begin{bmatrix} 39.1 \\ 51.9 \end{bmatrix} \text{mph}$$

CHAPTER 6

References

1. Day, T. and Smith, J., "Friction Factors for Motorcycles Sliding on Various Surfaces," SAE Technical Paper 840250, 1984, doi:10.4271/840250.

2. Lambourn, R., "The Calculation of Motorcycle Speeds from Sliding Distances," SAE Technical Paper 910125, 1991, doi:10.4271/910125.

3. Baxter, A.T., *Motorcycle Crash Investigation*, (Jacksonville, FL: Institute of Police Technology and Management, 2017), ISBN:978-1-934807-18-7.

4. Hague, D., "Calculation of Speed from Motorcycle Slide Marks," *Impact: The Journal of the Institute of Traffic Accident Investigators* (Spring 2004).

5. Wood, D.P., Alliot, R., Glynn, C., Simms, C.K. et al., "Confidence Limits for Motorcycle Speed from Slide Distance," *Proc. IMechE, Part D: J. Automobile Engineering* 222 (2008).

6. Walsh, D.G., Wood, D.P., Alliot, R., Glynn, C. et al., "Motorcycle Capsize Mechanisms and Confidence Limits for Motorcycle Capsize Speeds from Slide/Bounce Distance," *18th EVU Conference*, Hinckley, UK, 2009.

7. Donohue, M.D., "Motorcycle Skidding and Sideways Sliding Tests," *Accident Reconstruction Journal* 3, no. 4 (1991), ISSN: 1057-8153.

8. Raftery, B., "Determination of the Drag Factor of a Fairing Equipped Motorcycle," SAE Technical Paper 950197, 1995, doi:10.4271/950197.

9. Carter, T., Enderle, B., Gambardella, C., and Trester, R., "Measurement of Motorcycle Slide Coefficients," SAE Technical Paper 961017, 1996, doi:10.4271/961017.

10. Medwell, C., McCarthy, J., and Shanahan, M., "Motorcycle Slide to Stop Tests," SAE Technical Paper 970963, 1997, doi:10.4271/970963.

11. Bartlett, W. et al., "Motorcycle Slide-to-Stop Tests: IPTM Data through 2006," *Accident Investigation Quarterly* (Spring 2007), ISSN: 1082-6521.

12. McNally, B. and Bartlett, W., "Motorcycle Sliding Coefficient of Friction Tests," Presentation at *IPTM Special Problems in Accident Reconstruction*, 2003.

13. Peck, L., Focha, W., and Gloekler, T., "Motorcycle Sliding Friction for Accident Investigation," *Proceedings of the 10th International Motorcycle Conference*, Institute for Motorcycle Safety, Essen, Germany, 2014, 62-67.

14. DiTallo, M. et al., "3 Different Methodologies for Determining the Drag Factor for Motorcycles Sliding on Their Sides," *Collision: The International Compendium for Crash Research* 12, no. 1 (September 2017), ISSN: 1934-8681.

15. Severy, D. and Brink, H., "Auto-Pedestrian Collision Experiments," SAE Technical Paper 660080, 1966, doi:10.4271/660080.

16. Warner, C., Smith, G., James, M., and Germane, G., "Friction Applications in Accident Reconstruction," SAE Technical Paper 830612, 1983, doi:10.4271/830612.

17. Haight, W. and Eubanks, J., "Trajectory Analysis for Collisions Involving Bicycles and Automobiles," SAE Technical Paper 900368, 1990, doi:10.4271/900368.

18. Collins, J.C., *Accident Reconstruction*, (Springfield, IL: Charles C Thomas Publisher, 1979), ISBN:0-398-03907-0.

19. Fricke, L.B., "Vehicle-Pedestrian Accident Reconstruction," *Accident Reconstruction Journal* (January/February 1992), ISSN: 1057-8153.

20. Happer, A., Araszewski, M., Toor, A., Overgaard, R. et al., "Comprehensive Analysis Method for Vehicle/Pedestrian Collisions," SAE Technical Paper 2000-01-0846, 2000, doi:10.4271/2000-01-0846.

21. Wood, D., "Application of a Pedestrian Impact Model to the Determination of Impact Speed," SAE Technical Paper 910814, 1991, doi:10.4271/910814.

22. Brach, R.M. and Brach, R.M., *Vehicle Accident Analysis and Reconstruction Methods*, (Warrendale: SAE International, 2005), ISBN:0768007763.

23. Fugger, T., Randles, B., Wobrock, J., and Eubanks, J., "Pedestrian Throw Kinematics in Forward Projection Collisions," SAE Technical Paper 2002-01-0019, 2002, doi:10.4271/2002-01-0019.

24. Hurt, H.H. and Baird, J.D., "Accident Investigation Methodology Peculiar to Motorcycles and Minibikes," *Second International Congress on Automotive Safety*, Paper No. 73051, 1973.

25. Searle, J.A., "The Trajectories of Pedestrians, Motorcycles, Motorcyclists, etc., Following a Road Accident," SAE Technical Paper 831622, 1983, doi:10.4271/831622.

26. Searle, J., "The Physics of Throw Distance in Accident Reconstruction," SAE Technical Paper 930659, 1993, doi:10.4271/930659.

7

Motorcycle Falls

The previous chapter provided data and methods for analyzing the sliding and tumbling phase of a motorcycle crash. This phase is always preceded by a fall of the motorcycle and rider to the ground, either due to a collision or a loss of control. This chapter discusses the dynamic processes that lead to the motorcycle and rider falling to the ground. The previous chapter discussed a simple capsize, a fall that would be most likely to occur in a parking lot or in a laboratory setting. This chapter analyzes types of falls that are more frequent in real—world crashes-low-side falls, high-side falls, and impact-induced capsizing.

7.1 **Low-Side Falls**

Low-sides typically occur during acceleration or braking. The sequence of events that lead to these falls begins when the longitudinal force at the rear tire, from either acceleration or braking, consumes enough of the available traction to leave insufficient traction available for maintaining lateral stability. This can occur during cornering, when the motorcycle needs lateral traction to maintain stability around the curve. It can also occur during straight-line braking if the rider brakes with sufficient force to lock the rear wheel. In either instance, the rear wheel begins sliding laterally, the motorcycle develops a yaw rotation, and the motorcycle and rider roll to the inside of the yaw and fall to the ground. In this type of fall, the rider will slide upstream of the motorcycle and, since the rider typically decelerates at a higher rate during sliding than the

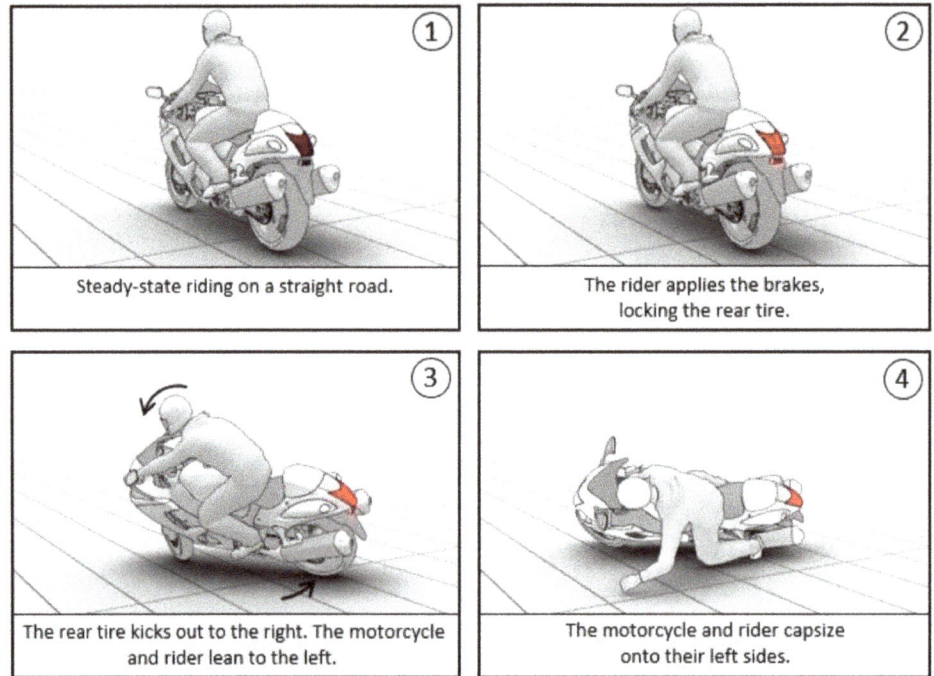

①	②
Steady-state riding on a straight road.	The rider applies the brakes, locking the rear tire.
③	④
The rear tire kicks out to the right. The motorcycle and rider lean to the left.	The motorcycle and rider capsize onto their left sides.

motorcycle, will usually come to rest upstream of the motorcycle. Figure 7.1 illustrates the motorcycle and rider motion that would be typical of a low-side that results from the rider locking the rear wheel of the motorcycle.

7.1.1 Case Study: A Low-Side Fall

To further introduce the dynamics of a typical low-side fall, consider a motorcycle crash that occurred in the Santa Monica Mountains of California on a curve of the Mulholland Highway called Edwards Corner. This crash, which was captured on video by Ken Snyder, shows a low-side fall. Ken Snyder is a videographer who captures video at Edwards Corner and posts footage of crashes on his YouTube channel under the name RNickeymouse. To aid in this analysis, we mapped Edwards Corner using both a Sokkia total station and a Faro laser scanner. This enabled determination of the initial speed of the motorcycle, identification of rider actions, quantification of the motion of the motorcycle and rider, and characterization of the roadway radius and superelevation throughout the curve.

The images below depict the geometry and characteristics of Edwards Corner. Figure 7.2 is an aerial image showing the curve and is oriented such that north is up. Figure 7.3 is a photograph that shows the overall geometry of the curve from the vantage point of a nearby hillside. Riders traveling westbound through the curve would be traveling toward the viewer of this image. Figure 7.4 is another photograph of the ascent into the curve from the westbound direction. Motorcyclists traveling westbound around Edwards Corner would be traveling into this photograph and traversing a leftward curve, whereas motorcyclists traveling eastbound would be coming toward the viewer of this photograph and would be traversing a rightward curve. Figure 7.5 shows the combined survey and scan data collected by the authors.

FIGURE 7.2 Aerial photograph of Edwards Corner.

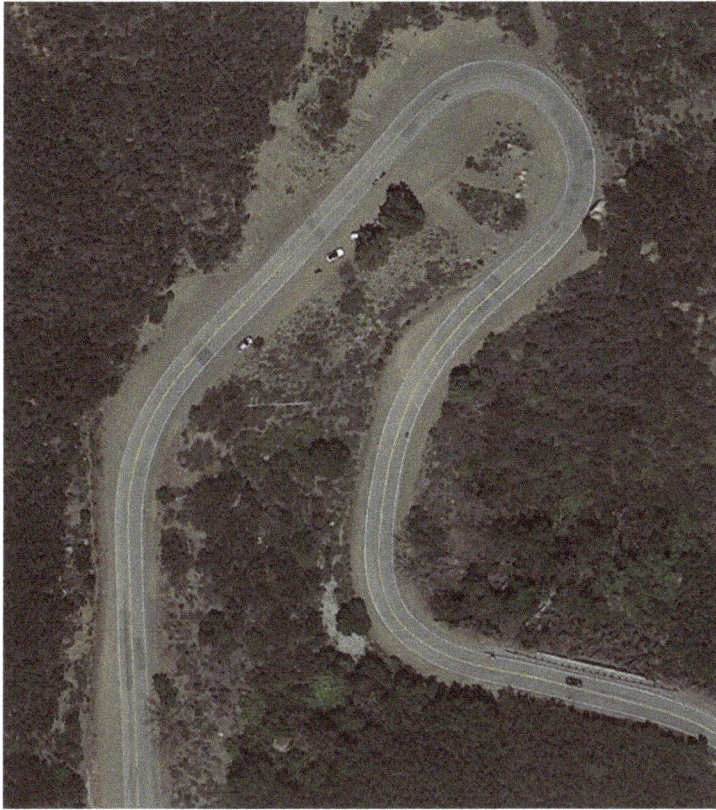

Map data © 2018 Google

FIGURE 7.3 Photograph of Edwards Corner.

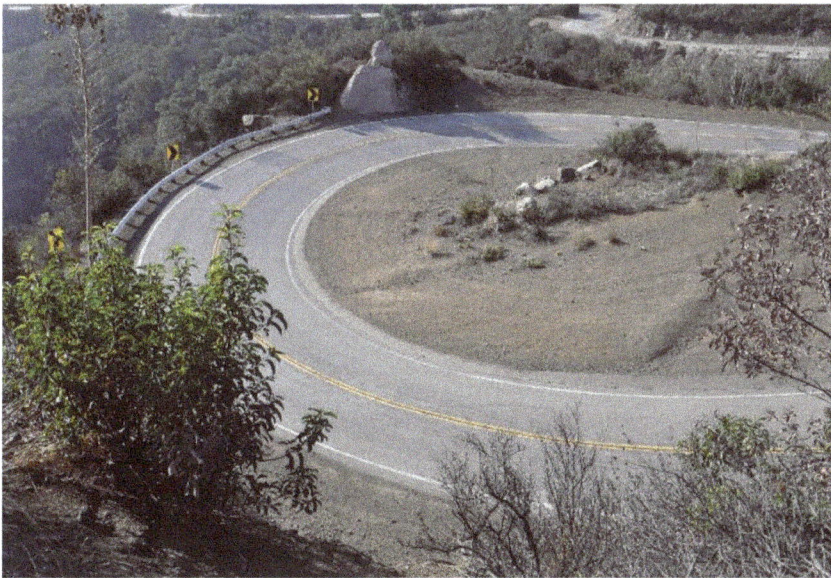

FIGURE 7.4   Photograph of the ascent into Edwards Corner.

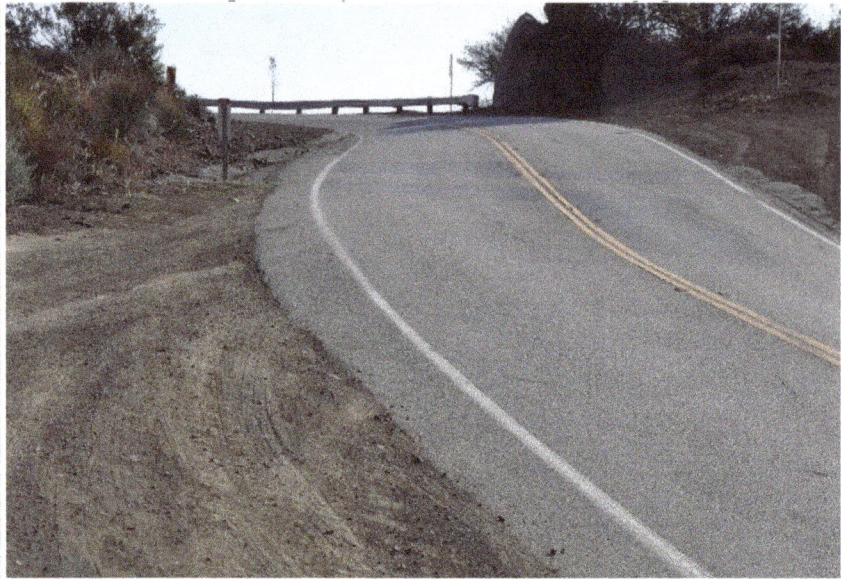

FIGURE 7.5   Survey and scan data of Edwards Corner combined.

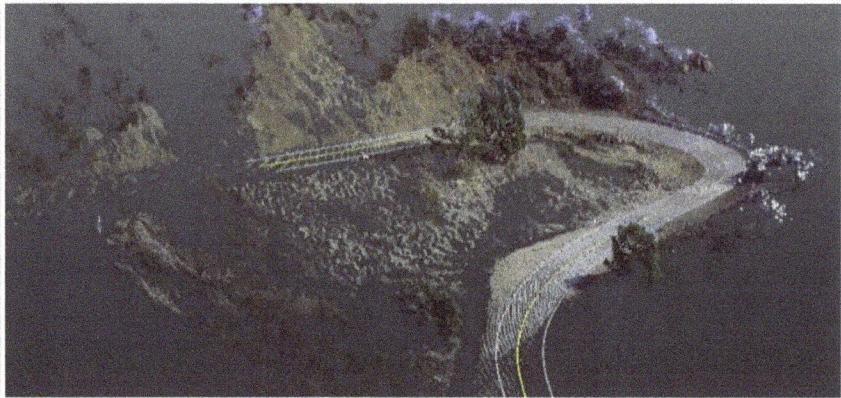

Survey and scan data from this site inspection was used to quantify the geometry of the curve, in terms of its radius, slope, and cross-slope. Riders traveling westbound through Edwards Corner encounter a left-hand curve with an upslope. During the first half of the curve, the upslope is approximately 3.2°, and during the second half it is 4.9°. There is a total elevation gain of 27.6 ft over a 390.8 ft travel distance. At the westbound entry to the curve, the cross-slope is negligible. It increases to a maximum cross-slope of 5.7° (with the inside of the curve being lower than the outside). The cross-slope then begins to decrease again, reaching a value of 1.9° at the exit of the curve. The radius of the curve in the center of the westbound lane is approximately 82 ft. Given the radius and cross-slope, a rider traveling through this curve at a speed in the range of 35 to 45 mph would need a leftward lean angle of approximately 40° to 55° relative to the roadway while traversing the curve [1, 2].

Figure 7.6 contains a series of video frames from the previously mentioned low-side video. This crash involved a Kawasaki Ninja ZX-10R traveling westbound through Edwards Corner. The frames of Figure 7.6 begin after the motorcyclist has entered the curve and developed maximum lean. The frames end after both the rider and motorcycle have begun sliding on the ground. Note, the motorcycle and rider are still in motion at the end of these video frames.

FIGURE 7.6 Video sequence (low-side fall).

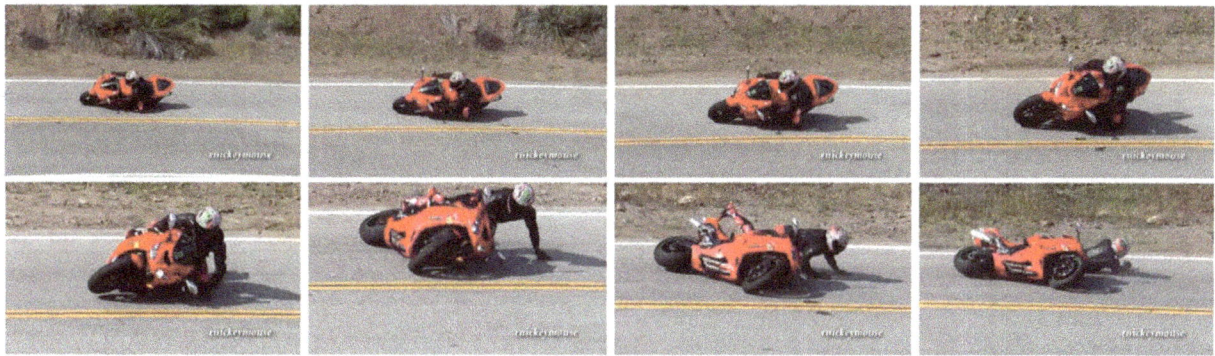

The development of a right-side leading sideslip at the rear tire becomes evident by the second frame of video in Figure 7.6. The motorcycle begins yawing in a counterclockwise direction. During this yaw, the rear tire of the motorcycle generates a tire mark. Eventually, the rider and the motorcycle go down onto their left sides and begin sliding along the roadway. Oftentimes, motion like this will result in the motorcycle depositing at least one tire mark on the roadway prior to capsizing and scrapes or gouges on the roadway during the slide. For a low-side fall, there will typically be little distance between the end of the tire mark(s) and the beginning of scrapes and gouges on the roadway. Also, for a low-side fall, the motorcycle will typically lead in the slide, with the rider following behind.

In addition to the low-side demonstrated in this case study, low-side falls can also be caused by the rider "tucking the front." This occurs when a rider enters a turn going too fast for their comfort and while in a lean, applies the front brake, thereby taking the front tire beyond its friction limit. The tire saturates, losing the ability to maintain lateral traction. The dynamics in this situation would be like the above dynamics, with the exception that it would have been precipitated by "losing" the front end. This can also occur at the entry of the turn. If a rider is braking heavily as approaching a turn and begins to turn while still braking (trail braking), the front may tuck.

7.2 **High-Side Falls**

This section describes the dynamics of high-side falls. Like low-sides, high-sides typically occur during acceleration or braking. The sequence of events that lead to these falls begins identically to a low-side fall. The longitudinal force at the rear tire, from either acceleration or braking, consumes enough of the available traction to leave insufficient traction available for maintaining lateral stability. This typically occurs during cornering, when the motorcycle needs lateral traction to maintain stability. It can also occur during straight-line braking if the rider brakes with sufficient force to lock the rear wheel. In either instance, the rear wheel begins sliding laterally, the motorcycle develops a yaw rotation, and the motorcycle and rider begin to lean to the inside of the yaw. If the rider does not release the throttle or brake, the motorcycle and rider will continue to fall to the inside of the yaw until they strike the ground, resulting in a low-side. High-sides, on the other hand, occur if the rider releases the throttle or rear brake. This allows the rear tire to regain traction and therefore generates a sudden increase in the available lateral traction. This sudden spike in lateral force at the rear tire can lead to the motorcycle and rider rolling to the opposite direction of the initial lean. The rider is then often projected upward and thrown ahead of the motorcycle [3, 4].

High-side fall from locking the rear wheel.

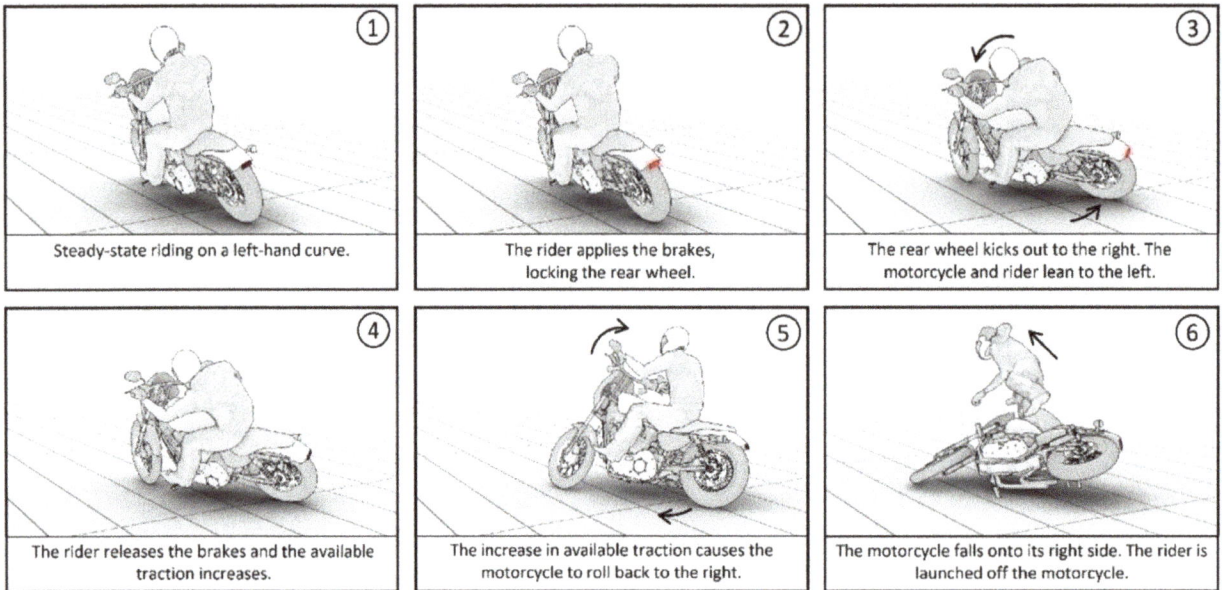

① Steady-state riding on a left-hand curve.

② The rider applies the brakes, locking the rear wheel.

③ The rear wheel kicks out to the right. The motorcycle and rider lean to the left.

④ The rider releases the brakes and the available traction increases.

⑤ The increase in available traction causes the motorcycle to roll back to the right.

⑥ The motorcycle falls onto its right side. The rider is launched off the motorcycle.

Figure 7.7 illustrates the motorcycle and rider motion that would be typical of a high-side fall that results from the rider locking the rear wheel of the motorcycle. Several observations can be made based on the prior discussion and on this graphic. First, for a high-side fall, there will be a gap between a tire mark deposited by the rear wheel of the motorcycle and the scraping and gouging that results from the motorcycle impacting and sliding on the ground. For a low-side fall, there will not be such a gap [5]. The tire mark will be immediately followed by the scraping and gouging. In addition to that, the rider will initially be thrown out ahead of the motorcycle. That said, because the rider will typically decelerate at a higher rate than the motorcycle, the motorcycle may ultimately pass the rider and come to rest downstream of the rider.

7.2.1 Case Study: A High-Side Fall

This section examines another motorcycle crash that Ken Snyder captured on video at Edwards Corner. This crash involved a Honda CBR1000RR (MY 2006 or 2007) traveling westbound through Edwards Corner. Figure 7.8 contains a series of frames from the video of this crash showing the motorcycle and rider motion. Snyder provided the video for this crash, which was captured at 59.94 fps. The time intervals between the frames shown in Figure 7.8 are not constant but instead were chosen so that the sequence of images would give the reader a sense for the motion of the motorcycle and rider during the loss of control and fall. The frames of this figure begin after the motorcyclist has entered the curve and developed maximum lean, which developed over approximately 1 second. The sequence of frames in this figure concludes with the rider and motorcycle having struck the ground but before coming to final rest.

Tar marks and dark asphalt patches on the roadway, visible in Figure 7.8, were used as reference points to determine travel distances of the motorcycle and rider across a series of video frames. Calculations based on the distances traveled by the motorcycle between reference points and the known frame rate established that the motorcycle was traveling at a speed of 43 mph as he approached the exit of the curve. Prior to this, the

FIGURE 7.8 Video sequence (high-side fall).

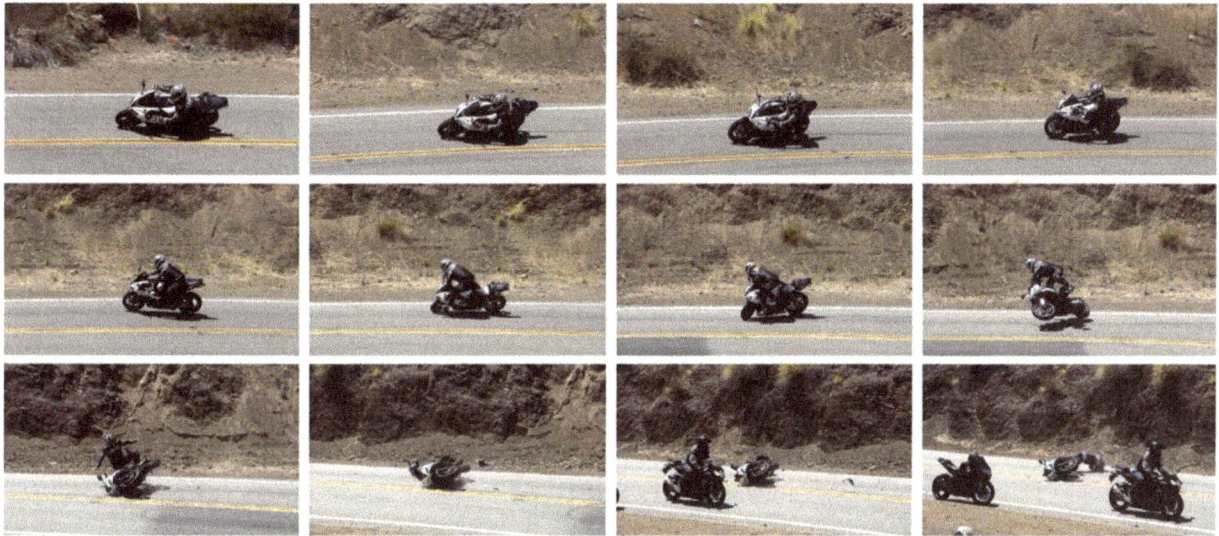

rider had been applying throttle to increase his speed, as was indicated by the audio of the video. Beyond this point, the speed began to decrease, as expected.

The development of a right-side leading sideslip at the rear tire becomes evident in the video, and the motorcycle begins yawing in a counterclockwise fashion. During this yaw, the rear tire of the motorcycle generates a tire mark on the roadway. As the yaw progresses, the rider steered the front wheel to the right and decreased the throttle input. When the rider rolled off the throttle, the longitudinal force demand on the rear tire decreased, and the available lateral traction increased. This caused the rear tire to seek alignment with the front tire, and the leftward lean of the motorcycle began to decrease. Eventually, the counterclockwise yaw ceased, and the motorcycle yawed clockwise as the motorcycle righted itself. The rear tire mark terminated as the motorcycle came back to vertical.

As the heading of the motorcycle came into alignment with its velocity direction and the motorcycle righted itself, the rider steered the front tire to the left. The momentum of the motorcycle initially continued to carry it toward a leftward lean/fall with a clockwise yaw rotation. A left leading sideslip developed. As this occurred, the rider's buttocks separated from the motorcycle. Eventually, the leftward steer input reversed the yaw direction, and the motorcycle again developed a right-side leading sideslip. The rear tire of the motorcycle generated a tire mark on the roadway, and the lateral tire forces throw the motorcycle into a rightward lean. As the motorcycle transitioned from a leftward lean to a rightward lean, the rider's groin and left thigh impacted the fuel tank of the motorcycle. The tires lost contact with the roadway, and the rider was projected upward, out ahead of, and to the right of the motorcycle.

In the subject accident, the motorcycle landed on its right side, and then the rider landed in a seated posture facing rearward, opposite his initial direction of travel. The rider was launched in the air approximately 54 ft. The motorcycle stayed on its right side throughout its entire slide on the ground and did not tumble. It decelerated at an average rate of approximately 0.4 g and then came to rest on its right side facing opposite its initial direction of travel. As the rider traveled to rest, his torso and head rotated toward the ground and ultimately struck it. He then tumbled to rest. The rider decelerated at a rate of approximately 1.07 g, a rate significantly higher than the rate at which the motorcycle decelerated. This includes the speed loss from the rider impacting the ground. Because of this high deceleration of the rider, the motorcycle came to rest further down the road than the rider.

The video footage included some documentation of the motorcycle after it had been removed from the roadway and revealed abrasions to the following components of the motorcycle due to interaction with the roadway: the end of the right handlebar, broken front brake lever, the right-side cowling, fuel tank cover, right-side engine crash protector and the right-side passenger seat cowling. The video footage did not show the entire motorcycle, so other components may also have been damaged. The rear tire also showed scuffing consistent with high slip angles. The rider's helmet was also documented and showed striated abrasions to its rear.

Rose [6] reported the analysis of three additional high-side crash videos captured by Snyder. These four crashes had several common features, including the following: (1) The loss of control in each case began with a loss of lateral stability at the rear tire. This loss of stability was caused either by a throttle application while cornering or by a braking force at the rear wheel of sufficient severity. (2) A yaw developed, the motorcycles and riders leaned to the trailing side of the yaw, and the riders steered to counteract the yaw. (3) As this yaw developed, the riders released the throttle or the brake. (4) Because of the throttle or brake release, the available lateral traction quickly increased. (5) At this point the rear tires were operating with a large sideslip angle, and thus, the increase in traction caused an overturning moment to be generated that was not adequately countered by the lean of the motorcycles and riders. This induced a roll of the motorcycle toward the leading side of the yaw. There are differences between the four crashes as to what happens next, differences that are discussed in the next paragraph. (6) Ultimately, though, the riders were projected upward and out ahead of the motorcycle. The riders were also projected to the side of the motorcycle paths, toward the outside of the final yaw. (7) The motorcycles landed on their leading sides and slid to rest, remaining on that side without losing contact with the ground. They did not tumble. (8) The riders landed and tumbled to rest.

There were distinct differences between the motorcycle motion in crashes where the loss of lateral stability was a result of accelerating excessively in a curve versus a crash where the loss of lateral stability was due to locking of the rear wheel. In all the cases, the rider counter-steered to the right during the initial yawing of the motorcycle. However, in the acceleration cases, the increase in lateral traction that accompanied the throttle release was less significant than in the locked rear wheel case. This is because, in the locked rear wheel case, all the available traction was consumed. Thus, there was no available lateral traction before the brake was released. In the acceleration cases, on the other hand, the throttle application consumes some, but not all, of the available traction. Therefore, the difference in lateral force when the rear brake is released is greater than the force difference in the acceleration cases. Because of this, the riders' counter-steer inputs were more effective in the acceleration cases, and the motorcycles yawed side-to-side several times before falling on their sides. In the locked rear wheel case, the motorcycle fell directly onto its side after the initial sideslip developed. In the acceleration cases, between 0.87 and 1.13 s elapsed from the time when the motorcycles were at maximum sideslip to the time that they impacted the roadway. For the braking case, this time was about 0.33 s.

7.2.2 Case Study: A High-Side Fall

This section describes the reconstruction of a motorcycle crash involving a high-side fall. This accident occurred on a rural, two-lane highway, and the motorcyclist was driving in a westbound direction when his motorcycle capsized. According to a witness, a westbound pickup that was three cars ahead of the motorcyclist had slowed down and made a U-turn. This required an SUV traveling behind the pickup to "slam on his brakes." The witness, who was traveling behind the SUV in a sedan then, applied her brakes "pretty hard" but did not have to use "emergency braking or drive off the road to avoid a collision." The motorcyclist was behind this sedan, and he applied his brakes. The witness "heard brakes squealing from behind her and saw the motorcycle crash on the road." The witness stated that, prior to the accident, she was traveling 60 mph and that when she braked she slowed to a speed of 5 mph. There was no contact that occurred between the witness's vehicle and the motorcycle. When the accident occurred, the weather was clear and the asphalt roadway was dry. The posted speed limit was 60 mph.

Prior to capsizing, the motorcycle deposited a 106 ft long skid mark on the roadway. The motorcyclist came to rest 184 ft west of the beginning of this skid mark, and the motorcycle came to rest on its right side approximately 204 ft west of the beginning of the skid mark. Given the length of the skid mark, it was deposited by the rear tire of the motorcycle. There was a 31 ft gap between the end of the tire mark and the beginning of these scrapes. This gap is an indication that the motorcycle and rider experienced a high-side fall during this crash. The scrapes from the motorcycle were 67 ft long and led up to the point of rest. The motorcycle exhibited scrape marks on the left and right-side crash bars, the left side of the gas tank, and the right side of the windscreen. The motorcycle came to rest on its right side. The diagram of Figure 7.9 depicts the evidence from this crash, along with relevant dimensions of that evidence.

Equation (6.2) was used to evaluate the speed the motorcycle was traveling when it began sliding on the roadway. The inputs into this analysis were the distance traveled by the motorcycle from the time it began sliding on the road surface until the time it came to rest, the slope of the roadway, and the motorcycle's deceleration rate while it was sliding. The motorcycle slid on the road for approximately 67 ft, and the section of roadway along which this sliding occurred was essentially flat. The motorcycle's deceleration rate while sliding was estimated using the data summarized in the previous chapter. In evaluating these studies, tests involving motorcycles and road surfaces like those involved in this accident were utilized. The motorcycles in these tests decelerated at an average rate of approximately 0.47 g, with a standard deviation of approximately 0.10 g.

Utilizing this range of decelerations, Equation (6.2) yielded a speed range for the motorcycle at the beginning of sliding of between 27.2 and 33.8 mph. These calculations are illustrated below for both the low and high end of this range:

$$v_{slide} = \sqrt{2 g f_{slide} d_{slide}} = \sqrt{2 \cdot 32.2 \cdot \begin{bmatrix} 0.37 \\ 0.57 \end{bmatrix} \cdot 67} = \begin{bmatrix} 40.0 \\ 49.6 \end{bmatrix} \text{fps} = \begin{bmatrix} 27.2 \\ 33.8 \end{bmatrix} \text{mph}$$

If the motorcyclist was initially traveling the same speed as the witness (60 mph), which she indicated he was, the motorcyclist applied the brakes of his motorcycle at a sufficient rate to decelerate from 60 mph down to a speed in the range of 27.2 to 33.8 mph

FIGURE 7.9 Physical evidence diagram.

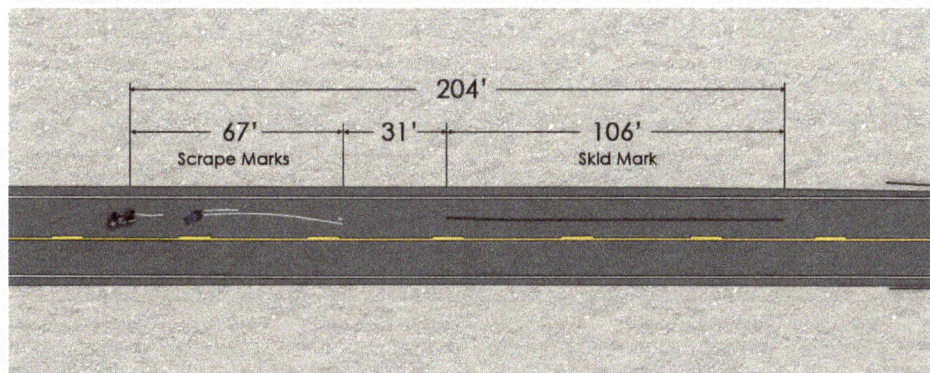

204'

67' ——— 31' ——— 106'

Scrape Marks   Skid Mark

before his motorcycle began sliding on the ground. This implies that when his motorcycle was upright and he was braking (depositing a rear wheel skid), Mr. Baca was braking with sufficient force to decelerate his motorcycle at a rate between 0.77 and 0.9 g. This level of deceleration implies that the motorcyclist employed both the front and rear brakes. This implied deceleration rate is on the high end of what a typical motorcyclist would be able to achieve. It is possible that the range of deceleration employed for the sliding phase is too low, since this was a high-side fall and the motorcycle may have lost significant speed when it impacted the pavement. Shifting the deceleration range up higher for the sliding phase would result in a lower implied braking deceleration. However, this would be unlikely to change the conclusion that the motorcyclist was employing both his front and rear brake.

7.3 Impact-Induced Capsize

So far, this chapter has addressed capsizing of a motorcycle that occurs due to the rider losing control of the motorcycle. Capsizing of the motorcycle can also occur due to the motorcycle and/or rider being struck by another vehicle or object. In these instances, the motorcycle and rider will typically end up separating and falling. The specific motion that the motorcycle and rider experience will depend on many factors, including the degree to which they interact with the struck vehicle or object and the direction of travel between them. As an example, if a motorcycle strikes the front fender of a passenger car, the rider may be thrown forward over the hood of the vehicle with minimal interaction with the vehicle. On the other hand, if a motorcycle strikes the front door of a sport utility vehicle, the rider may be thrown forward and experience full engagement with the vehicle. These two different interactions would result in significantly different postimpact motion for the riders and significantly different rest positions. Additionally, these two different interactions would call for different ways of handling the rider's weight in mathematical analysis of the collision.

7.4 Analyzing the Motion of Projected Riders

Determining the speed at which a rider was thrown from a motorcycle can sometimes be helpful in a reconstruction. Several theoretical models for making this determination have been presented in the literature, and these are described in the sections that follow.

7.4.1 Collins Model

Collins [7] developed the following equation for calculating the launch speed of a person first undergoing an airborne trajectory and then landing and sliding to rest. The model assumed a horizontal launch (no launch angle). In this equation, v_{proj} is the throw speed of the person, h is the height of the person's center of gravity prior to the collision, g is the gravitational acceleration, μ is the coefficient of friction between the person and the road surface, and d_t is the throw distance (the total distance from the beginning of the projection to rest). This equation would have to be applied iteratively to determine the projection velocity from the throw distance. This would be accomplished by iteratively changing the throw speed of the rider until the measured throw distance was matched:

$$d_t = v_{proj}\sqrt{\frac{2h}{g}} + \frac{v_{proj}^2}{2\mu g} \qquad (7.1)$$

There will be some speed loss from air resistance during the airborne trajectory. However, air resistance is often neglected in modeling a person's airborne trajectory. Collins stated that speed loss from air resistance could be neglected at projection speeds below 25 mph (40 kph). At projection speeds exceeding 25 mph, he stated that the calculated speed in his model should be corrected to account for speed loss due to air drag by adding a correction to the calculated speed. Collins proposed the following table of correction factors for apogee heights of 5 and 7 ft (Table 7.1).

TABLE 7.1 Corrections for initial projection velocity of airborne person

Uncorrected speed (mph)	Correction for 5 ft apogee (mph)	Correction for 7 ft apogee (mph)
25	3	3
30	4	5
35	5	6
40	6	8
45	8	10
50	10	13

7.4.2 Searle Model

Searle [8, 9] derived the following formula for determining a pedestrian's projection velocity, based on the conceptual model depicted in Figure 7.10. In this equation, μ is the coefficient of friction between the pedestrian and the ground, g is the acceleration due to gravity, s is the throw distance, including the airborne and sliding/tumbling phases, and θ is the projection angle. Searle reported a typical coefficient of friction for a person sliding on asphalt of 0.66. This model improved on the Collins model by incorporating a launch angle and incorporating the ground plane speed loss due to the person landing on the ground after vaulting through the air:

$$v_{proj} = \frac{\sqrt{2\mu gs}}{\cos\theta + \mu\sin\theta} \tag{7.2}$$

Searle observed that the projection angle is often not known, and so, he derived a version of this equation that would yield the lowest possible value and one that would yield the highest possible value. These equations are as follows:

$$v_{impact,min} = \sqrt{\frac{2\mu gs}{1+\mu^2}} \tag{7.3}$$

$$v_{impact,max} = \sqrt{2\mu gs} \tag{7.4}$$

Application of Equation (7.4) requires the analyst to ensure that the maximum projection angle could not have been greater than a critical projection angle calculated with the following equation:

$$\theta_{crit} = 180° - 2\arctan\frac{1}{\mu} \tag{7.5}$$

FIGURE 7.10 Searle's model.

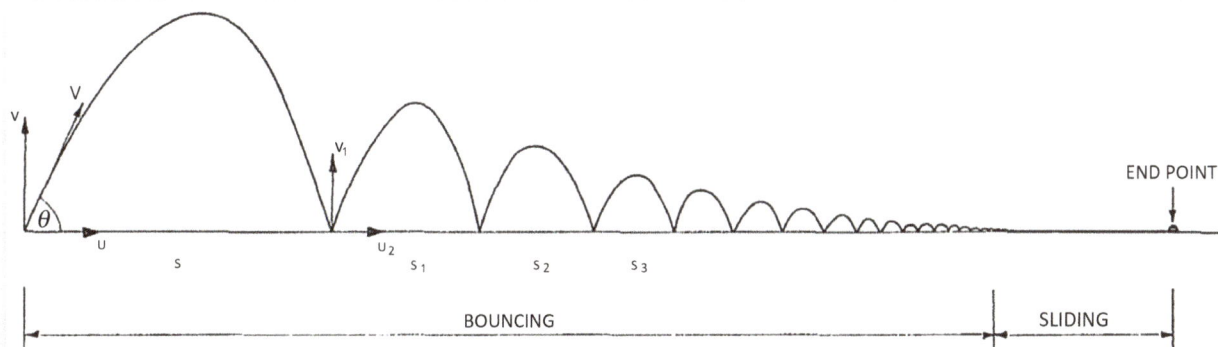

If projectile analysis is being applied to analyze the motion of a motorcycle rider that was thrown from their motorcycle due to an impact with another vehicle, then it is important to keep in mind that these formulas (like the Collins model) would yield the speed of the rider upon separation with that other vehicle, not the initial impact speed of the rider. The analyst would need to consider the degree to which the rider interacted with the struck or striking vehicle and how that would have altered the rider's speed before separation.

7.4.3 Aronberg Model

Aronberg [10] derived another alternative to the Collins model. His model differed from the Collins model by utilizing "the time of the body in the air, at the launch velocity, to determine the adjustment necessary to the launch velocity to account for air drag. In addition, the component of velocity corresponding to total horizontal distance traveled is limited to the horizontal velocity component of the body following the airborne trajectory. Collins' method incorrectly includes both the vertical and horizontal components." Aronberg's model is shown graphically in Figure 7.11, along with the meaning of the variables within the model.

The vertical velocity through time is given by the following equation. In this equation, V_y is the vertical velocity, V_0 is the total initial projection velocity, θ is the launch angle, g is the gravitational acceleration, and t is time:

$$V_y = V_0 \sin \theta - gt \tag{7.6}$$

Integrating Equation (7.6) yields the vertical position through time, as follows:

$$y = h_0 + V_0 t \sin \theta - \frac{gt^2}{2} \tag{7.7}$$

At the apogee of the airborne trajectory, $y = h$ and $V_y = 0$. Thus, the elapsed time and trajectory height at the apogee can be calculated with the following equations:

$$t_{apogee} = \frac{V_0 \sin \theta}{g} \tag{7.8}$$

$$h = h_0 + V_0 t_{apogee} \sin \theta - \frac{gt^2_{apogee}}{2} \tag{7.9}$$

When the body strikes the ground, $y = 0$. In this equation, t_{land} is the time at which the body lands on the ground:

$$0 = h_0 + \left(V_0 \sin \theta\right) t_{land} - \frac{g}{2} t^2_{land} \tag{7.10}$$

FIGURE 7.11   Aronberg model.

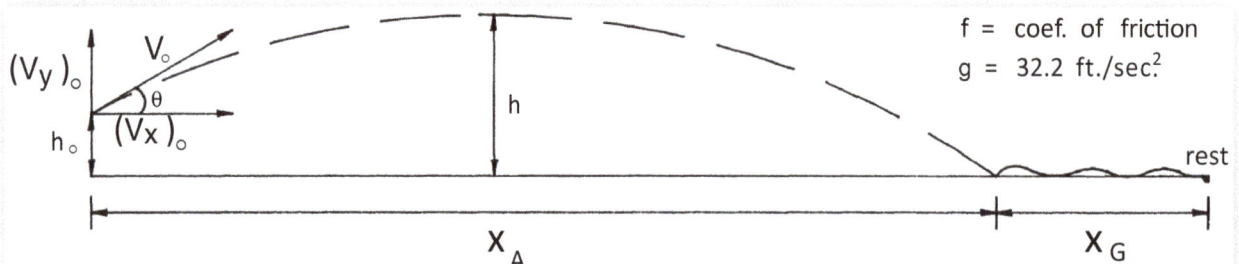

Applying the quadratic equation to calculate t_{land} yields the following:

$$t_{land} = \frac{V_0 \sin \theta + \sqrt{\left(V_0 \sin \theta\right)^2 + 4\frac{g}{2}h_0}}{g} \quad (7.11)$$

The ground plane distance traveled by the pedestrian during the airborne trajectory can now be calculated with the following equation:

$$x_A = V_0 \cos \theta \cdot t_{land} \quad (7.12)$$

In addition, to the airborne distance, the pedestrian will also typically slide and tumble upon landing. The slide/tumble distance can be calculated with the following equation. In this equation, f is the coefficient of friction (or drag factor) of the pedestrian for the sliding and tumbling phase. Since Aronberg's model does not incorporate a separate term for the speed loss due to landing, the drag factor in Equation (7.13) would be one that incorporates this speed loss:

$$x_G = \frac{\left(V_0 \cos \theta\right)^2}{2gf} \quad (7.13)$$

The total throw distance, d_t, is therefore given by the following equation:

$$d_t = x_A + x_B = \frac{V_0^2 \cos \theta \sin \theta + \sqrt{\left(V_0 \sin \theta\right)^2 + 4\frac{g}{2}h_0}}{g} + \frac{V_0^2 \cos^2 \theta}{2gf} \quad (7.14)$$

Aronberg recognized that his model neglected speed loss due to air resistance. To incorporate this speed loss, he examined published data on skydiving free fall velocity with respect to time. Aronberg used this data to produce the graph of Figure 7.12.

FIGURE 7.12 Speed loss due to air resistance.

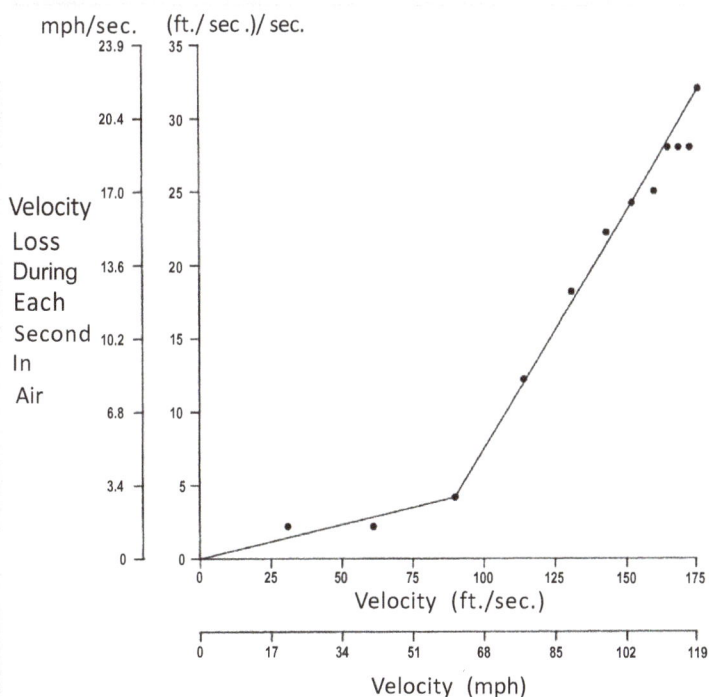

This graph shows that the speed loss due to air resistance generally increases linearly up to a speed around 60 mph. At a speed of 61 mph, air resistance would cause just under 3 mph of speed loss for every second the pedestrian is in the air. Above 61 mph, the air resistance continues to increase but at a greater rate than at speeds below 61 mph. Aronberg notes that "the free fall data presented and air drag derived are for humans in a spread position. Therefore, this graph represents the maximum expected air drag." Aronberg observes that the data he obtained yields corrections significantly lower than what Collins suggested and that Collins methods overestimates the speed loss due to air resistance. Like the Collins and Searle models, Aronberg's model also yields the projection velocity of the rider, not necessarily the speed of the rider and motorcycle at the time of a collision. Again, the analyst would need to account for any speed loss of the rider due to the collision itself.

References

1. Rose, N., Carter, N., and Pentecost, D., "Analysis of Motorcycle and Rider Limits on a Curve," *Collision: The International Compendium for Crash Research* 9, no. 1 (Spring 2014), ISSN: 1934-8681.
2. Carter, N., Rose, N., and Pentecost, D., "Validation of Equations for Motorcycle and Rider Lean on a Curve," *SAE Int. J. Trans. Safety* 3, no. 2 (2015): 126-135, doi:10.4271/2015-01-1422.
3. Cossalter, V., Bellati, A., and Cafaggi, V., "Exploratory Study of the Dynamic Behaviour of Motorcycle-Rider During Incipient Fall Events," *Proceedings of the 19th International Technical Conference on the Enhanced Safety of Vehicles*, June 2005, Paper Number 05-0266.
4. Cossalter, V., *Motorcycle Dynamics*, 2nd ed., (2006), ISBN:978-1-4303-0861-4.
5. Baxter, A.T., *Motorcycle Crash Investigation*, (Jacksonville, FL: Institute of Police Technology and Management, 2017), ISBN:978-1-934807-18-7.
6. Rose, N., Carter, N., Pentecost, D., and Hashemian, A., "Video Analysis of Motorcycle and Rider Dynamics During High-Side Falls," SAE Technical Paper 2017-01-1413, 2017, doi:10.4271/2017-01-1413.
7. Collins, J.C., *Accident Reconstruction*, (Springfield, IL: Charles C Thomas Publisher, 1979), ISBN:0-398-03907-0.
8. Searle, J.A., "The Trajectories of Pedestrians, Motorcycles, Motorcyclists, etc., Following a Road Accident," SAE Technical Paper 831622, 1983, doi:10.4271/831622.
9. Searle, J., "The Physics of Throw Distance in Accident Reconstruction," SAE Technical Paper 930659, 1993, doi:10.4271/930659.
10. Aronberg, R., "Airborne Trajectory Analysis Derivation for Use in Accident Reconstruction," SAE Technical Paper 900367, 1990, doi:10.4271/900367.

Motorcycle Collisions with Vehicles and Roadside Barriers

In 1970, Severy and his colleagues reported seven collision experiments involving motorcycles [1]. The motorcycles were carrying rider dummies, and they struck either the front door or fender of a stationary passenger car. Three different motorcycle models were tested (Honda CL-90, Honda CB-350, Honda CB-750) with impact speeds of 20, 30, and 40 mph. Table 8.1 summarizes these tests, including the vehicles involved, the motorcycle impact speed, the total motorcycle deformation, and the motorcycle wheelbase reduction.

Severy used these tests to make observations that continue to be examined and developed by the crash reconstruction community. For example, Severy observed that "the permanent shortening of the motorcycle wheelbase as a result of collision varied linearly with the speed of collision and did not appear to be significantly affected by variations in size of the motorcycle or in location of impact." This concept has been further developed and refined over the past five decades, and this chapter covers these developments. Another observation that emerged from this testing relates to the deformation that occurred to the spoked wheels of the motorcycles in these tests. Figure 8.1 is a series of photographs included in Severy's article that show the postcrash condition of each motorcycle.

Severy reported that the test at 20 mph produced 4.7 in. of wheelbase reduction due to fork deformation and no wheel deformation. The tests at 30 mph, on the other hand, exhibited varying levels of wheel deformation, in addition to the wheelbase reduction that occurred. These different levels of wheel deformation with the same impact speed can be attributed to the different stiffnesses of the vehicle structures impacted by these motorcycles. Stiffer passenger vehicle structures produced greater deformation to the wheel than softer ones, given the same impact speed. Similar trends emerge from additional tests that have been reported since the time of Severy's tests.

Severy's testing also enables observations related to the motion of the riders on motorcycles that impact passenger vehicles. First, the rider and the motorcycle are not

TABLE 8.1 Summary of the motorcycle-to-vehicle tests reported by Severy et al. [1]

Experiment number	Motorcycle	Motorcycle weight (lb)	Passenger vehicle	Impact speed (mph)	Impact location	Motorcycle deformation (in.)	Wheelbase reduction (in.)
127	Honda CL-90	200	1964 Plymouth Fury	30	Driver's door	17.0	9.2
128	Honda CB-350	350	1964 Plymouth Fury	30	Driver's door	15.0	8.5
129	Honda CB-350	350	1964 Plymouth Fury	20	Passenger's side front door	4.7	4.7
130	Honda CB-350	350	1964 Plymouth Fury	30	Passenger's side front door	16.7	9.5
131	Honda CB-350	350	1964 Plymouth Fury	30	Right front wheel	9.5	9.5
132	Honda CB-750	480	1964 Plymouth Fury	30	Passenger's side front door	16.7	9.3
133	Honda CB-350	350	1964 Plymouth Fury	40	Driver's door	21.0	13.0

FIGURE 8.1 Wheel deformation from the Severy et al. collisions [1].

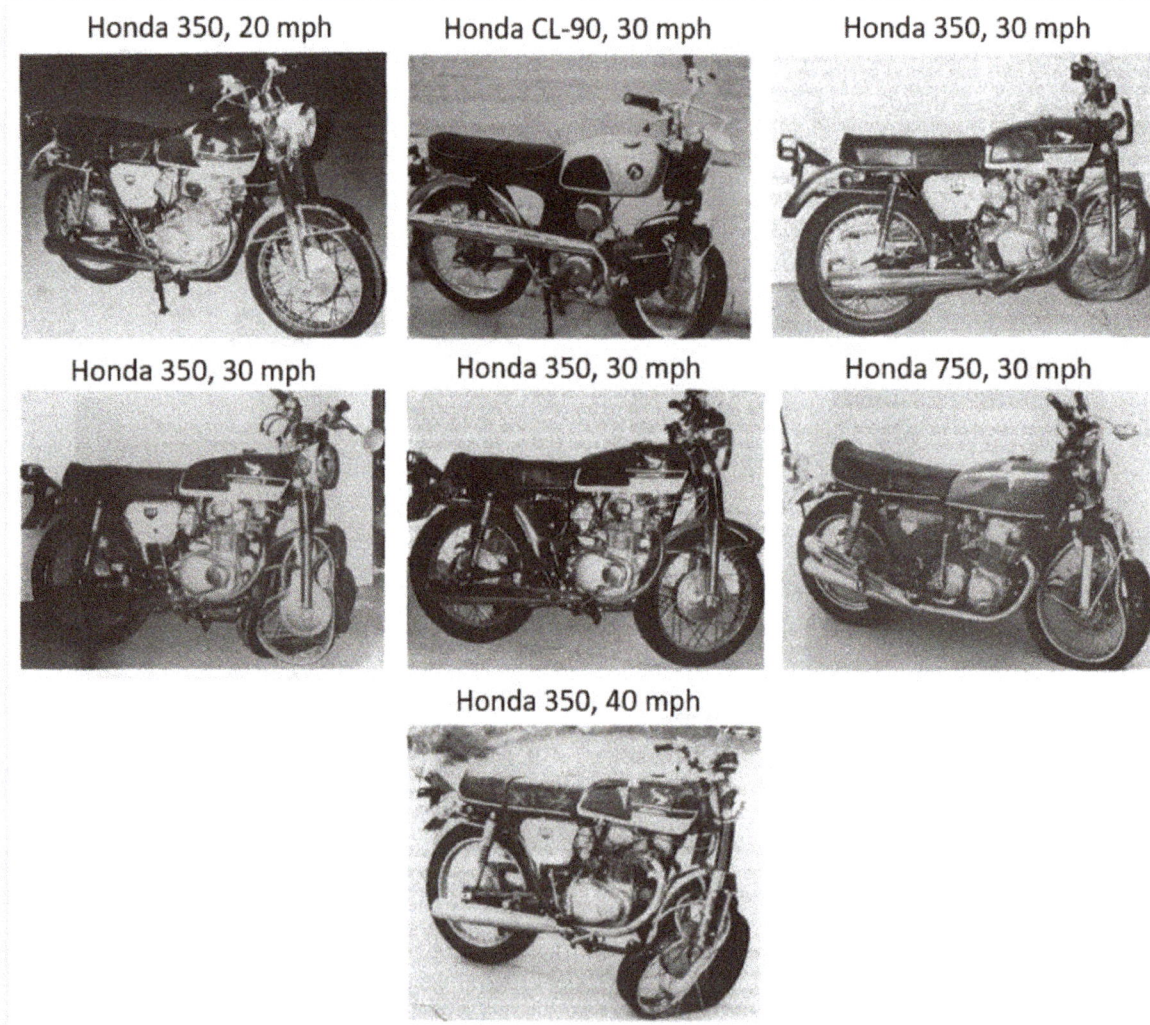

Honda 350, 20 mph

Honda CL-90, 30 mph

Honda 350, 30 mph

Honda 350, 30 mph

Honda 350, 30 mph

Honda 750, 30 mph

Honda 350, 40 mph

TABLE 8.2 Timeline for the tests reported by Severy et al. [1]

Experiment number	First contact (ms)	Motorcycle forward movement stopped (ms)	First contact of rider with vehicle (ms)	Rider's body impacts vehicle (ms)
127	0	55	75	130
128	0	55	75	120
129	0	53	185	195
130	0	UNK	70	195
131	0	80	90	160
132	0	55	120	125
133	0	63	55	80

coupled in the same way that a passenger car and its belted occupants would be. During an impact, the rider interacts with the motorcycle to a degree but can ultimately separate from the motorcycle entirely. Second, there is typically a much smaller weight disparity between a motorcycle and its rider than between a passenger car and its occupants. These facts become relevant when modeling collisions between motorcycles and passenger cars since, for some analysis methods, the analyst will have to decide how much of the weight of the rider participated in the collision and thus, what effect, if any, that weight has on the wheelbase reduction of the motorcycle, the damage to the car, and the post-impact motion of the car. These issues are illustrated in Table 8.2, which is a timeline of the Severy collisions. As this table demonstrates, the collision between the motorcycle and the car is essentially complete prior to the occurrence of the collision between the rider and the car. Another important observation given the event data recorders now present on many passenger cars, the separation in time between the motorcycle and rider collisions with the struck vehicle could result in an event data recorder on the struck vehicle not capturing the effects of the collision between the rider and the vehicle. When interpreting EDR data, the analyst may need to recognize this possibility.

8.1 Analysis Based on Motorcycle Wheelbase Reduction

Since the introduction of Severy's work, many additional tests have been conducted, and numerous researchers have worked to further develop speed analysis methods that utilize the reduction in motorcycle wheelbase. Some of these methods also consider the crush to the struck vehicle. In 2002, for example, Adamson reported analysis of 17 crash tests that involved 1989–1993 model year Kawasaki 1000 police motorcycles [2]. These tests were conducted at the World Reconstruction Exposition in September of 2000 (WREX 2000).

In the first seven WREX2000 tests, the motorcycles impacted a concrete block at speeds varying between 10 and 42 mph. The concrete block was 120 in. wide, 24 in. thick, and 39 in. high, had a steel bottom surface, and weighed 11,080 lb. The reported static and dynamic coefficients of friction between the runway and the concrete block were 0.46 and 0.40, respectively. The block was non-deformable but was light enough that it moved during most of the tests. In the remaining 10 crash tests, the motorcycles impacted 1 of 2 stationary 1989 Ford Thunderbirds, both weighing just under 3600 lb, at various locations. Motorcycle impact speeds for these tests varied between 25 and 49 mph and were measured with a handheld Stalker radar gun. All tests were run on an abandoned concrete runway with a reported coefficient of friction for vehicle tires of 0.72.

Adamson published a graph showing the wheelbase reduction experienced by each of the 17 motorcycles (vertical axis) plotted against the impact speed of each motorcycle (horizontal axis). Once these points were plotted, Adamson used linear regression to obtain a best-fit line describing the relationship between the impact speed and the wheelbase reduction. Separate linear fits were obtained for the motorcycle-to-concrete block impacts and the motorcycle-to-vehicle impacts. These best-fit lines were then displayed on the graph. For the motorcycle versus concrete block impacts, a reasonably strong linear fit ($R^2 = 0.87$) was obtained. However, for the motorcycle versus vehicle impacts, the linear fit was weak ($R^2 = 0.47$).

This weak correlation between the wheelbase reduction and the impact speed for the motorcycle-to-car impacts is expected, since the magnitude of the wheelbase reduction depends not only on the motorcycle's impact speed but also on the stiffness of the impacted object (among other factors). A strong linear correlation would only be expected if the tests were grouped according to the portion of the vehicle they struck. For example, motorcycles striking a door would need to be categorized separate from impacts where the motorcycle strikes a wheel. In the 10 motorcycle-to-car collisions reported by Adamson, different regions of the vehicles were impacted, and thus, the stiffness varied from collision to collision. There are too few tests in the Adamson data set to parse them by impact location.

To illustrate these issues with the data from the Adamson publication, consider the graph of Figure 8.2, which contains seven filled diamonds, each representing the wheelbase reduction (horizontal axis) and impact speed (vertical axis) for one of the seven motorcycle-to-barrier impacts reported by Adamson. A best-fit line through these points is also shown on the graph. This line, which exhibits an R^2 value of 0.87, has the following equation:

$$S = 2.4545 \cdot WBR + 5.935 \tag{8.1}$$

In this equation,

S is the motorcycle's impact speed
WBR is the wheelbase reduction that resulted from the impact

FIGURE 8.2 Linear fit to barrier impact wheelbase reduction data from Adamson [2].

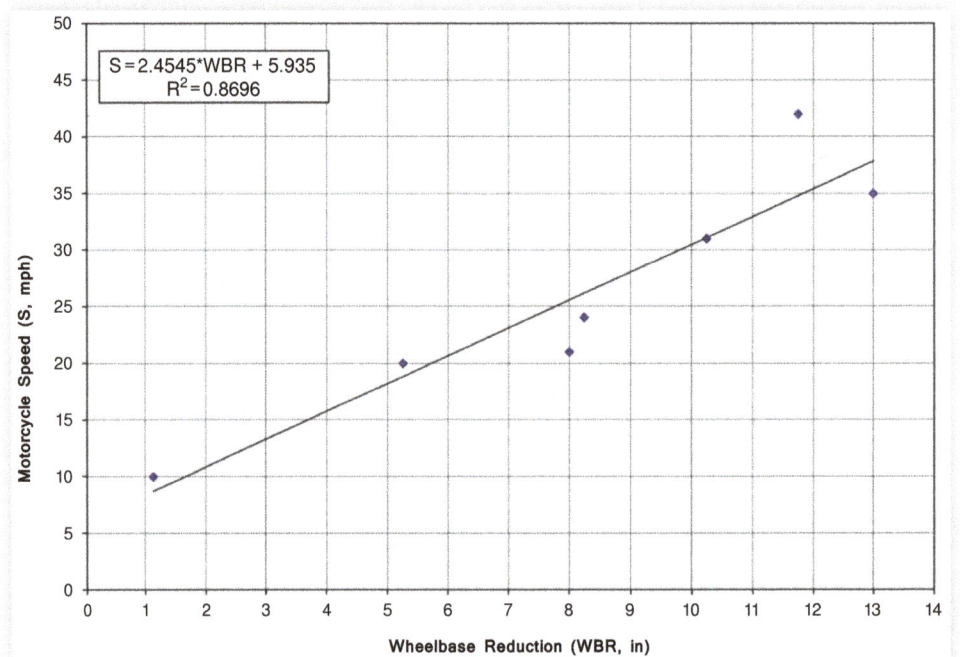

FIGURE 8.3   Wheelbase reduction versus speed graph for motorcycle-to-vehicle tests.

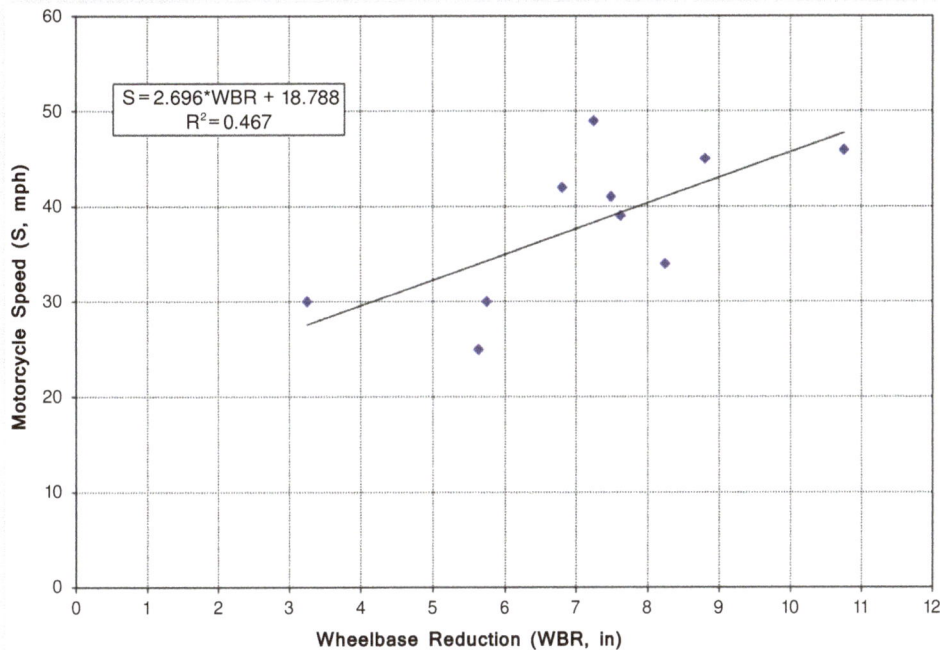

Equation (8.1) is in a different form than the one reported by Adamson because the wheelbase reduction (*WBR*) has been treated as the independent variable and the motorcycle's speed (*S*) as the dependent variable. Arranging the data like this is more consistent with how it would be utilized in practice.

Now, consider the graph of Figure 8.3, which contains 10 filled diamonds, each representing the wheelbase reduction and impact speed for 1 of the 7 motorcycle-to-vehicle impacts reported by Adamson. A best-fit line through these points is also shown on the graph. This line, which exhibits an R^2 value of 0.47, has the following equation:

$$S = 2.696 \cdot WBR + 18.788 \tag{8.2}$$

The weakness of the correlation in this instance is due to variability in the stiffness of the different structures on the vehicles that were impacted by the motorcycles. Baxter [3] noted this issue and observed: "Depending on the area of the automobile that is struck, the wheel and fork will begin to deform. If a stiff portion of the car is struck (a wheel for example), the motorcycle will collapse more severely than if contact had been made with a softer sheet-metal area." Interestingly, given the narrowness of the motorcycle front wheel, for impacts involving the front wheels of a passenger vehicle, even the location of the impact on that wheel can influence this wheelbase deformation. This is because an impact to the wheel forward or rearward of the wheel centerline can cause the wheel to steer to the left or to the right. This effectively makes the wheel less stiff, since up to a point, it gives way to the motorcycle.

In a 2009 article, Bartlett also considered this variability in stiffness of the impacted structures [4]. He began by collecting the published crash test data relating wheelbase deformation and struck vehicle crush to the motorcycle impact speed. When the available data was analyzed without consideration of what portion of the vehicle was struck, he found a weak correlation between wheelbase reduction and impact speed. Bartlett made the following observation: "This [weak correlation] is certainly influenced by the variety of vehicles tested, and the variety of impact locations on the car sides: body panels such as fenders and doors do not have the same crush characteristics as axles and wheels. Another limitation of the analysis is its relative insensitivity at higher speeds: after the front wheel and fork have collapsed to the frame and engine block there is little additional motorcycle deformation possible."

Bartlett proceeded to parse the available data into two categories—(1) motorcycles striking a door or fender and (2) motorcycles striking at a pillar or within a foot of an axle. He noted that "the pillar/axle tests produced 3 to 5 inches less total crush [motorcycle wheelbase reduction plus maximum car crush], supporting the notion that pillar/axle locations were stiffer." Bartlett presented the following two equations for when the motorcycle strikes the door or fender:

$$S = 2L + 1.8C + 2 \tag{8.3}$$

$$S = 1.4534(L + C) + 10.124 \tag{8.4}$$

In these equations:
    L is the motorcycle wheelbase reduction in inches
    C is the maximum crush to the struck vehicle
    S is the impact speed of the motorcycle in miles per hour

Bartlett noted that the functional form of Equation (8.3) was originally derived based on testing conducted by the California Association of Accident Reconstruction Specialists (CAARS) in 2004. He updated the coefficients to the equation by adding additional data. This equation will be referred to as the modified CAARS equation for doors and fenders. The functional form of Equation (8.4) was originally presented by Eubanks in 1991 [5]. Bartlett used the same form but again updated the coefficients by adding additional data. This equation will be referred to as the modified Eubanks equation for doors and fenders.

For instances where the motorcycle struck a pillar or within 1 ft of an axle, Bartlett presented the following two equations:

$$S = 2.5L + 1.9C + 4.5 \tag{8.5}$$

$$S = 1.5875(L + C) + 14.72 \tag{8.6}$$

Again, Equation (8.5) follows the form of the original CAARS equation but Bartlett updated the coefficients by adding additional data. This equation will be referred to as the modified CAARS equation for pillars and axles. Equation (8.6) follows the form of the Eubanks equation, and again, Bartlett updated the coefficients with additional data. This equation will be referred to as the modified Eubanks equation for pillars and wheels. When compared to the available data, Bartlett reported that modified Eubanks equations yielded "slightly more accurate" predictions than the modified CAARS equations. He reported that, for the modified Eubanks equations, "the door/fender collision speeds were found to be predicted with a 95% confidence range of plus or minus 20% of the nominally calculated value, while the pillar/axle speeds were predicted with a range of plus or minus 28%."

Two other observations by Bartlett are worth mentioning. First, "evaluating the crush energy or wheelbase reduction of just the motorcycle does show a slight variation based on the type of wheel, with the cast-wheeled motorcycles typically experiencing 5 to 2 inches less crush at a given impact speed. The variation goes down as the speeds increase. However, when the total crush experienced by both the motorcycle and the car is evaluated this differentiation disappears, and the wheel type becomes less relevant…It appears that while the stiffer cast wheels deform less, they produce additional crush in the cars they are striking." Second, "collisions involving cars moving at high enough speeds to affect the motorcycle's trajectory appear to reduce the total measured crush, such that using the relationships developed here will underpredict speeds, typically by 15%. The additional complication of a moving target vehicle also increases the data spread significantly."

The equations covered so far have recognized the link between the severity of an impact and the deformation that results from that impact. They have also recognized that the stiffness of the colliding vehicle structures will determine how the total deformation is split between the two vehicles involved in the collision. However, these concepts have not been formulated in the way they are traditionally formulated for vehicle-to-vehicle collisions. For car-to-car collisions, the collision reconstruction literature has often formulated the relationships between impact severity, impact force, deformation level, and stiffness in terms of the crush analysis equations used in the CRASH algorithm and its derivatives [6, 7, 8, 9, 10, 11, 12, 13, 14, 15]. These equations provide an analytical method for relating the vehicle crush to the energy the vehicle absorbed during the impact and then, for relating that absorbed energy to the severity and approach speed for the impact.

These crush analysis methods typically utilize the following concepts and assumptions: (1) *Each of the impacting vehicles is divided into two regions, a deforming region and a non-deforming region.* Based on the testing and observations reported by Severy [1], this is also an appropriate assumption for motorcycle collisions. He noted that "damage was confined almost exclusively to the front wheel and front wheel suspension system…As front tire contact is made with the opposing car sheet metal, initial flattening of the tire occurs, accompanied by some yielding of the car body panel and cycle forks; this is followed by complete deceleration of the front wheel assembly, generally without significant distortion of the wheel. Additional car sheet metal intrusion and bending of the forks above and rearward of the suspension system occurs as the front wheel crushes further into the car side panel. Simultaneously, the principal mass of the motorcycle (all portions to the rear of the front wheel and suspension) continues forward while undergoing moderate deceleration. Contact is finally made by the forward surfaces of the engine with the trailing surfaces of the front wheel… for 30 mph and higher impact speeds…the motorcycle front wheel generally deforms permanently and even completely collapses in some cases." (2) *The vehicle structure is assumed to resist deformation in a spring-like manner, where the impact force is proportional to the magnitude of the crush (constant stiffness).* The validity of this assumption for motorcycles is examined in this chapter. (3) *A common velocity is assumed to be achieved on the contact surface between the impacting vehicles at the time when the maximum crush depth is achieved.* This assumption is valid for the collisions analyzed in this chapter. Application of these methods to the analysis of real-world collisions should, of course, be attentive to possible instances when this condition is not met.

Searle pursued this approach, reporting a method in 2010 that used the underlying physics of traditional crush analysis methods [16]. He observed that "a possible approach to the reconstruction of motorcycle accidents would be to extend the CRASH program, assigning motorcycles into categories such as mopeds, scooters, sports and so on. Each category would have stiffness characteristics, as is done with cars now. A motorcycle to car collision could then be reconstructed, on that basis, as car to car collisions are now. However even without a comprehensive treatment of that kind, reconstruction can still be based upon the physics of the collision, resulting in an analytical formula for the motorcycle closing speed."

Though they used different nomenclature than that used in CRASH and its derivatives, Wood, Glynn, O'Dea, and Walsh [17, 18] also reformulated the wheelbase reduction method along the lines of the CRASH method, utilizing relationships between deformation energy and impact speed rather than between wheelbase reduction and speed as has traditionally been done. As a part of this, they included a means of imposing force balance (the collision force applied to the motorcycle is equal in magnitude to the collision force applied to the passenger car). This approach has potential advantages over equations that simply relate wheelbase reduction to impact speed, without considering the deformation to the struck vehicle or imposing force balance. Specifically, this approach considers the stiffness, deformation, and energy absorption of each vehicle involved in the collision and thus, applies to the analysis of any impact. Speed versus wheelbase reduction equations, on the other hand, are often situation-specific with a different equation having to be used depending on which portion of a passenger car is struck by the motorcycle.

Wood [17, 18, 19] analyzed data from 43 motorcycle and scooter impacts with barriers and proposed the following empirical equation for calculating the energy absorbed by a motorcycle ($E_{A,mc}$) based on its wheelbase reduction. In this equation, the average wheelbase reduction (WBR) is entered in meters, the mass (m_{mc}) is entered in kilograms, and the resulting energy is in units of newton-meters. Wood observed that "the specific energy (E/M) absorption characteristics of motorcycles and scooters in frontal impacts are similar where the primary load path is through the front wheel and fork assembly." He reported an r^2 value for Equation (8.7) of 0.845:

$$E_{A,mc} = 641.7 m_{mc} \left(WBR + 0.1 \right)^{1.89} \qquad (8.7)$$

Wood noted that Equation (8.7) should only be used for wheelbase shortening less than 0.45 m (18 in.) and when the front forks and front wheel remain intact. "Barrier test data show that, when the front wheel rim, etc., breaks away from the wheel hub, the resulting wheelbase shortening underestimates the specific energy." Also, during motorcycle-to-car collisions, "the motorcycle-to-car impact takes place before the rider(s) collide against the car and that the motorcycle-to-car and the rider-to-car collisions can be considered as two discrete separate events. Further, the rider-to-car impact occurs at a higher level on the car. Consequently, the crush damage to the motorcycle or scooter and associated deformation to the car can be considered as being due to the motorcycle or scooter to car collision alone." Among other implications of this statement, it implies that the mass of the motorcycle used for Equation (8.7) would not include the mass of the rider(s).

Equation (8.8) is an English-unit version of Equation (8.7). In this equation, the motorcycle weight should be entered in pounds and the wheelbase reduction in inches:

$$E_{A,mc} = 0.224809 \cdot 3.28084 \cdot \frac{641.7}{2.20462} \cdot W_{mc} \left(0.0254 \cdot WBR + 0.1 \right)^{1.89} \qquad (8.8)$$

Wood also noted that the energy absorbed by the car ($E_{A,car}$) could be estimated with the following equation, which he derived by imposing force balance. In this equation, d_{car} is the maximum crush to the side of the car, measured in the same units used to measure the wheelbase reduction. In the analysis that follows, this method is referred to as the Wood force-balance method:

$$E_{A,car} = E_{A,mc} \frac{d_{car}}{WBR} \qquad (8.9)$$

Wood examined 31 staged tests where motorcycles impacted stationary cars at 90° and derived the following empirical equation for estimating the energy absorbed by the side of the struck vehicle. Equation (8.10) is included here in its English-unit form, such that the maximum crush to the car would be entered in inches and the resulting absorbed energy would be in foot-pounds. Wood reported an r^2 value of 0.845 for this equation. In the analysis that follows, this method is referred to as the Wood Empirical Method:

$$E_{A,car} = 0.224809 \cdot 3.28084 \cdot 65,305 \cdot (0.0254 \cdot d_{car} - 0.0576) \tag{8.10}$$

Once the absorbed energies have been obtained, they can be summed and used with the following equation to calculate the collision speed of the motorcycle:

$$S_{mc,impact} = \sqrt{\frac{\gamma_{mc} m_{mc} + \gamma_{car} m_{car}}{\gamma_{mc} m_{mc} \cdot \gamma_{car} m_{car}} \cdot 2 E_{A,total}} \tag{8.11}$$

In Equation (8.11):
  $E_{A,total}$ is the total absorbed energy for the motorcycle and the car combined
  m_{car} is the mass of the car
  γ_{mc} and γ_{car} are the effective mass multipliers

The effective mass multipliers are defined by the following equation:

$$\gamma_i = \frac{k_i^2}{k_i^2 + h_i^2} \tag{8.12}$$

In this equation,
  k_i is the radius of gyration for either the motorcycle or car
  h_i is the moment arm of the collision force about the center of mass of that vehicle

In many motorcycle-to-vehicle collisions, the moment arm of the collision force for the motorcycle will be zero, and so, the effective mass multiplier for the motorcycles will be equal to 1. When the car involved in a collision is not stationary and some component of the car's velocity is directed into the motorcycle (in other words, when the car is moving and the impact angle is something other than 0, 90, or 180), then Equation (8.11) will yield the closing speed between the motorcycle and the car rather than the impact speed of the motorcycle. To apply Equation (8.12), the reconstructionist will need to calculate the radius of gyration of the struck vehicle about its yaw axis. This value is obtained by taking the square root of the yaw moment of inertia divided by the mass. The yaw moment of inertia characterizes the vehicle's resistance to rotation about its yaw axes. MacInnis [20] and Allen [21] examined methods for estimating the whole vehicle (as opposed to sprung mass) moments of inertia for a passenger vehicle.

Other formulations of crush analysis equations for motorcycle-to-car collisions are possible. For example, consider an alternate method that is more consistent with the way these calculations are typically carried out within the CRASH framework. Within this framework, Equation (8.13) yields the energy absorbed by each vehicle during the collision:

$$E_A = \left(\frac{B}{2} C_R^2 + A C_R + \frac{A^2}{2B} \right) \cdot w_0 \tag{8.13}$$

FIGURE 8.4 Graph illustrating the meaning of the *A* and *B* stiffness coefficients.

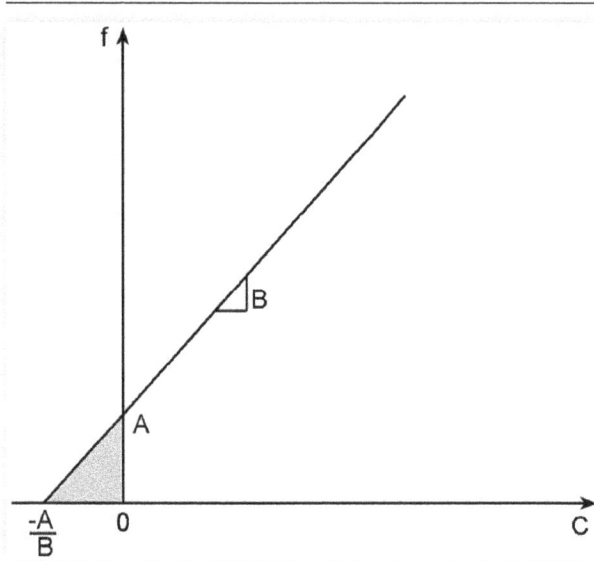

FIGURE 8.4 Graph illustrating the meaning of the *A* and *B* stiffness coefficients.

In this equation,

E_A is the absorbed crush energy

C_R is the average residual crush (or the wheelbase reduction for the motorcycle)

w_0 is the width of the damaged region

A and B are stiffness coefficients describing the resistance of the vehicle structures to deformation

Figure 8.4 illustrates the meaning of the *A* and *B* stiffness coefficients. This figure shows the linear relationship between force and crush. The horizontal axis represents the residual crush depth, and the vertical axis represents the force per unit width of damage. The *B* value is the slope of the linear force-crush relationship, and it governs the proportionality between residual crush and impact force. The *A* value is the force intercept on the force-crush plot, and it represents the force that can be applied to the vehicle structure before the onset of permanent crush.

The force-crush line intersects the crush axis at a value of $-A/B$. This negative intercept on the crush axis has traditionally been interpreted as the elastic recovery of the vehicle structure, which is the difference between the dynamic crush and the residual crush. With this interpretation, the *A* value arises because of the use of residual crush in the model and shifting the force-residual crush line over a distance of A/B would yield the dynamic force-crush line.

A method for obtaining the *A* and *B* stiffness coefficients has been developed by recognizing that Equation (8.13) is quadratic in the residual crush depth, C_R. Application of the quadratic formula to Equation (8.13) yields the following equation:

$$\sqrt{\frac{2E_A}{w_0}} = \sqrt{B}C_R + \frac{A}{\sqrt{B}} \tag{8.14}$$

The left side of Equation (8.14) is a normalized energy term, which has been referred to as the Energy of Approach Factor (EAF) [22]. For a barrier impact crash test, in which the barrier is both non-deforming and immovable, the damage energy in Equation (8.14) would be set equal to the initial kinetic energy of the vehicle. This assumes that all the approach energy is absorbed by the vehicle during the impact. For other impact types, say a vehicle-to-vehicle frontal impact, the damage energy would be set equal to the damage energy absorbed by the vehicle of interest during the impact. Each crash test provides one point for constructing an EAF versus residual crush plot. If multiple tests are available, a best-fit line for the points can be obtained. The slope and the intercept of the EAF versus residual crush plot yield the *A* and *B* coefficients. Such a plot has been referred to as a CRASH plot.

As an illustration of this procedure, consider the barrier impacts reported by Adamson. In these tests, the barrier was not fixed to the ground, and the weight was insufficient to ensure it did not move during the tests. Thus, analysis of these tests needs to consider the motion of the barrier. It is reasonable, however, to assume that the barrier does not absorb any energy through deformation. Thus, Equation (8.15) is an energy balance equation for these tests:

$$\frac{1}{2}m_{mc}v_{mc,i}^2 = E_{A,mc} + \frac{1}{2}m_{mc}v_{mc,f}^2 + \frac{1}{2}m_{barrier}v_{barrier,f}^2 \tag{8.15}$$

In this equation,

m_{mc} is the mass of the motorcycle

$v_{mc,i}$ is the speed of the motorcycle immediately prior to its impact with the barrier

$v_{mc,f}$ is the speed of the motorcycle at the time the maximum wheelbase reduction is achieved

$v_{barrier,f}$ is the speed of the barrier at the same time

$E_{A,mc}$ is the deformation energy absorbed by the motorcycle.

There is no term in this equation for the initial kinetic energy of the barrier because it was initially at rest, and there is no absorbed energy term for the barrier because the barrier would not absorb any significant energy through deformation.

Figure 8.5 is the CRASH plot that results from using Equation (8.15) to calculate the absorbed energy for the motorcycle in each test, using this absorbed energy to calculate an EAF for each test, and then plotting the results. The EAF was obtained by using a 1 ft damage width for the motorcycle. This dimension is arbitrary for these motorcycle collisions and 1 ft was chosen to simplify the math. This same 1 ft dimension would need to be used for the crush zone width when applying the resulting stiffness coefficients to the wheelbase reduction. A best-fit line is included on the graph of Figure 8.5, along with the resulting A and B stiffness coefficients (603 lb/in. and 225 lb/in.^{2}, respectively).*

Equation (8.13) can be applied to calculate the absorbed energy for both the car and the motorcycle in the motorcycle-to-car collisions. The A and B stiffness coefficients are unknown for the car, but they can be estimated by imposing the condition

FIGURE 8.5   CRASH plot for the Adamson barrier impact tests.

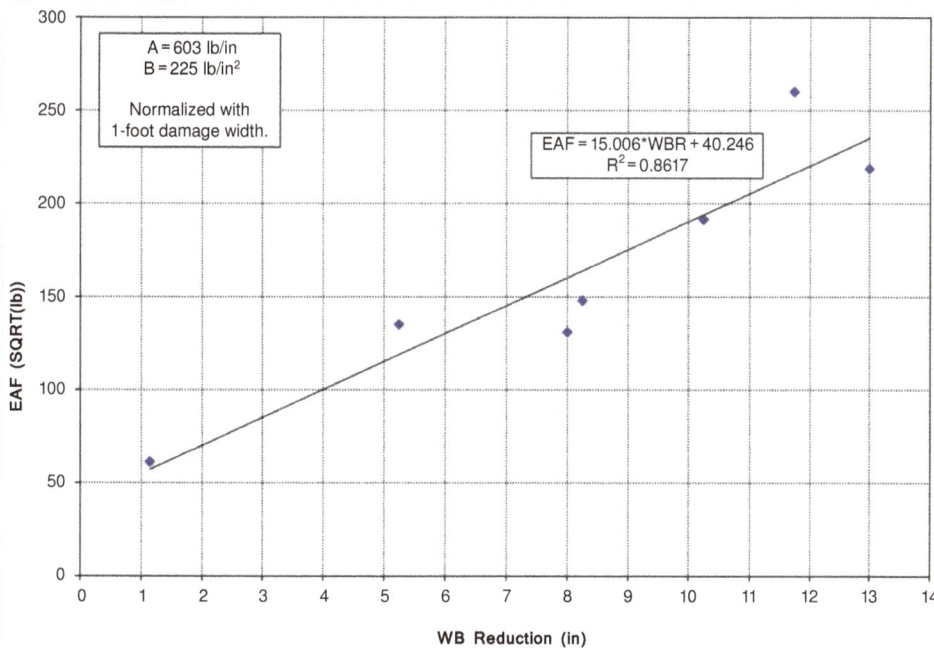

---

* These stiffness values are different than those reported by Deyerl and Cheng [23, 24]. This is because they used a damage width of 18 in., rather than the 12 in. damage width utilized here. For motorcycle collisions, this emphasizes the importance of using the same damage width for stiffness coefficient calculations and calculations with these stiffness coefficients.

that the collision force applied to the car and the motorcycle will be equal. In the calculations performed here, for the side impacts, it was assumed the car's *A* stiffness coefficient would be double the *B* coefficient. For the front or rear impacts, it was assumed the car's *A* stiffness coefficient would be triple the *B* coefficient. These are simply rules of thumb based on the authors' past observations and used here for illustration.

Before applying this approach, it is worth noting that there are few motorcycle-to-barrier collisions available in the literature, and so, applying the CRASH approach on a vehicle-specific basis (as is done with crush analysis for car-to-car collisions) is unlikely to be a practical approach for most instances. The WREX 2000 tests are unique in this sense. For most cases, an approach that lumps all the motorcycles and scooters into one group (such as the Wood approach encapsulated in Equations (8.7) through (8.10)) will typically be necessary. Nonetheless, in introducing and explaining wheelbase reduction methods for analyzing motorcycle-to-car collisions, there is still value in introducing the CRASH approach, so that the reader can see how these methods relate to the methods that are commonly applied for car-to-car collisions.

Bartlett, Focha, and Kauderer [25] reported data from a series of 25 motorcycle to stationary car collisions which were conducted in 2009 by the CA²RS. These tests were conducted on an asphaltic concrete runway, which was smooth, dry, flat, weathered, and traffic-polished. The authors reported a coefficient of friction for the surface of 0.64, a value that was obtained by averaging the results of three skid tests with a 2001 Ford Crown Victoria Police Interceptor. The struck vehicles were passenger cars, and the motorcycles included standard, cruiser, touring, and sport motorcycles. The tests included impacts to the struck vehicle doors, fenders, pillars, wheels, and axles. The authors reported the motorcycle wheelbase reduction and maximum car crush for the struck vehicle in each test. They also reported the yaw rotation of the struck vehicle that occurred as a result of each collision. The authors plotted the total crush for each test (wheelbase reduction plus maximum car crush) against the impact speed, and the data exhibited a generally linear relationship.

Another set of motorcycle-to-car collisions was conducted at the World Reconstruction Exposition in 2016 (WREX 2016). Table 8.3 summarizes the tests in this series that involved Harley-Davidson motorcycles. This table includes the motorcycle and the passenger vehicle utilized in each test, the impact configuration, the motorcycle impact speed, the resulting wheelbase reduction for the motorcycle, and the maximum crush to the vehicle. The passenger vehicles were stationary prior to the collision in these tests. Motorcycle impact speeds varied between 30.3 and 46.3 mph. These tests were conducted on an asphalt roadway near Orlando International Airport. The coefficient of friction for this surface was measured by performing three skid tests with a Chevrolet Silverado, and the average value was reported as 0.7.

Peck et al. [26] analyzed this set of tests with eight different equations and concluded that the modified Eubanks equations presented earlier—Equations (8.4) and (8.6)—yielded the greatest accuracy, with an average error of 0.4 mph and a standard deviation of 4.8 mph. In addition to the WREX2016 tests, Peck also reported results from four motorcycle collision conducted at ARC-CSI 2016. These tests also involved Harley-Davidson motorcycles. In three of the tests, the motorcycles struck passenger cars, and in the fourth the motorcycle struck a concrete barrier. The involved vehicles and resulting deformations for these tests are summarized in Table 8.4.

Peck developed an updated set of Eubanks-style equations by adding additional data published since Bartlett updated them in 2009. Instead of parsing the data into two sets (door/fender and pillar/axle), Peck parsed the data into four sets, with separate equations for axles, pillars and bumpers, doors, and fenders. When applied to analyze

TABLE 8.3 Motorcycle-to-vehicle collisions performed at WREX 2016

Test	Motorcycle	Motorcycle weight (lb)	Struck vehicle	Struck vehicle weight (lb)	Impact location	Motorcycle impact speed (mph)	Motorcycle wheelbase reduction (in.)	Max crush to car (in.)
3	2013 H-D Softail Breakout FXSB	667	2006 Nissan Maxima	3449	Passenger's side front door	43.0	11.3	18.7
5	2013 H-D Dyna Street Bob FXDBA	633	2006 Nissan Maxima	3449	Driver's side rear door	36.9	12.8	8.6
8	2012 H-D Dyna Fat Bob FXDF	678	2005 Dodge Durango	4740	Driver's side rear quarter panel	46.3	3.3	9.1
11	2012 H-D Dyna Low Rider FXDL	649	2005 Dodge Durango	4740	Driver's side front door	42.9	10.7	10.3
22	1997 H-D Sportster 883	498	2006 Hyundai Sonata	3547	Passenger's side rear quarter panel	30.3	4.3	2.1
23	2002 H-D Sportster 883	500	2006 Hyundai Sonata	3547	Passenger's side rear door	42.7	8.8	7.1
24	2003 H-D Sportster 883	483	2006 Hyundai Sonata	3547	Driver's side rear door	35.5	8.9	4.2

TABLE 8.4 Summary of motorcycle collisions from ARC-CSI 2016

Test	Motorcycle	Motorcycle weight (lb)	Struck vehicle	Struck vehicle weight (lb)	Impact location	Motorcycle impact speed (mph)	Motorcycle wheelbase reduction (in.)	Max crush to car (in.)
1	2006 H-D Sportster XL1200C	579	Barrier			25.6	7.2	
3	2011 H-D Road King FLHRC	794	2012 Volkswagen Passat	3360	Wheel	31.9	5.0	6.2
5	2011 H-D Electra Glide FLHTCU	881	2012 Volkswagen Passat	3360	Pillar	29.0	6.5	2.7
9	2011 H-D Softail FLSTC	649	2011 Ford Crown Vic	4057	Fender	32.8	3.8	10.3

the WREX2016 tests, these equations produced an average error of 3.5 mph (standard deviation = 4.3 mph). These equations are as follows:

$$\text{Axle: } S = 2.16\left(L + C\right) + 17.33 \tag{8.17}$$

$$\text{Bumper/pillar: } S = 1.36\left(L + C\right) + 19.50 \tag{8.18}$$

$$\text{Door: } S = 1.50\left(L + C\right) + 9.27 \tag{8.19}$$

$$\text{Fender: } S = 1.26\left(L + C\right) + 22.95 \tag{8.20}$$

Peck also included a table of the available crash tests that were used for developing Equations (8.17) through (8.20). This data is plotted, along with Equations (8.17) through (8.20), in the graphs that follow. Figure 8.6 contains a point for each of the motorcycle-to-axle collisions. The horizontal axis is the motorcycle wheelbase reduction plus the maximum car crush in inches. The vertical axis is the motorcycle collision speed in miles per hour. The dark black line represents Equation (8.17). Figure 8.7 contains a point for each of the motorcycle-to-bumper (squares) and motorcycle-to-pillar collisions (triangles). The dark black line represents Equation (8.18). Figure 8.8 contains a point for each

FIGURE 8.6   Equation (8.17) plotted with the crash test points.

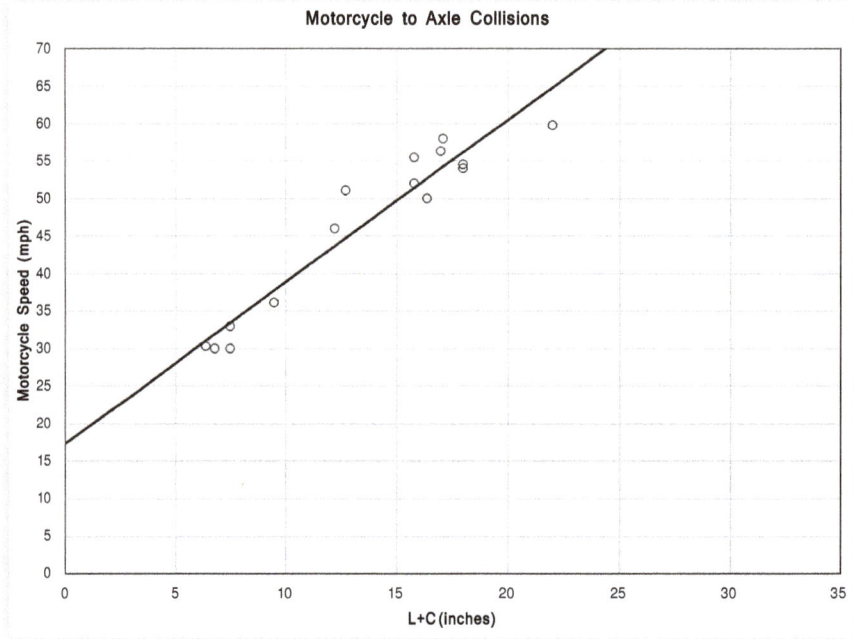

FIGURE 8.7   Equation (8.18) plotted with the crash test points.

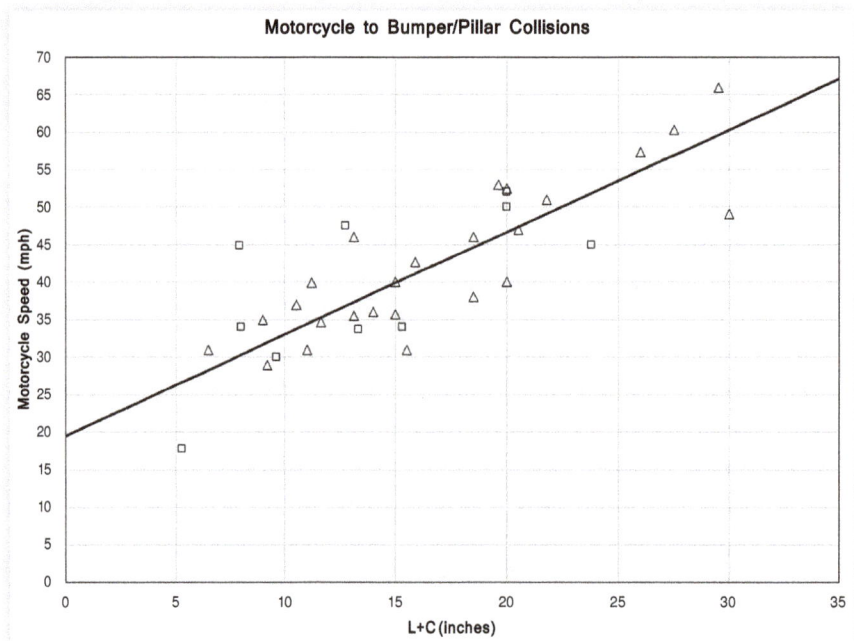

FIGURE 8.8 Equation (8.19) plotted with the crash test points.

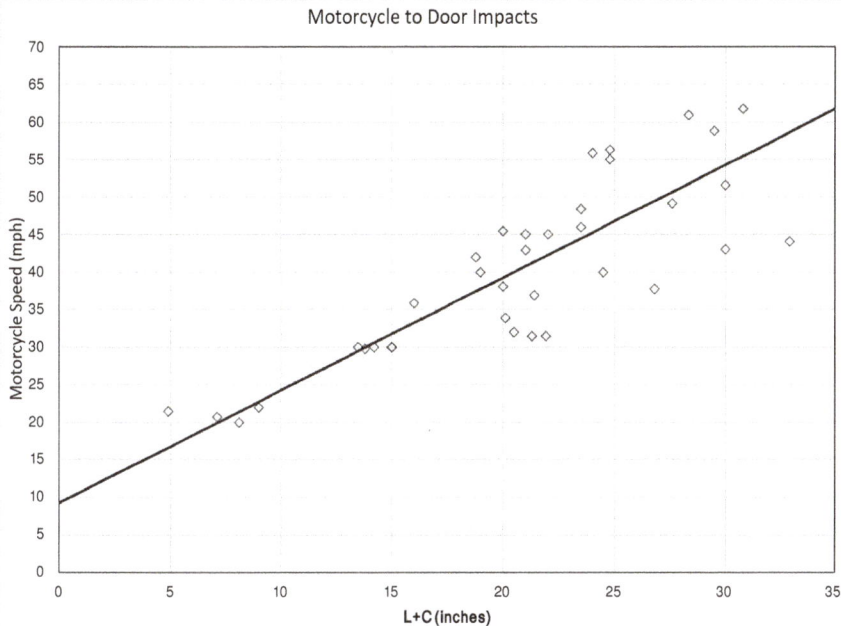

Motorcycle to Door Impacts

FIGURE 8.9 Equation (8.20) plotted with the crash test points.

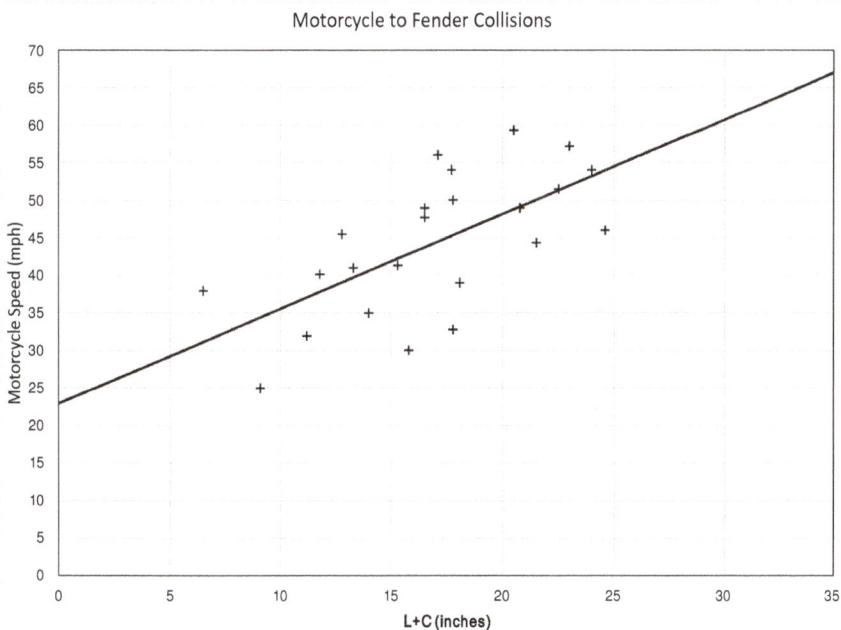

Motorcycle to Fender Collisions

of the motorcycle-to-door collisions. The dark black line represents Equation (8.19). Finally, Figure 8.9 contains a point for each of the motorcycle-to-fender collisions. The dark black line represents Equation (8.20).

It is worth mentioning the following observation that Peck made in his article: "the vast majority of data feeding current equations" are from motorcycles with traditional forks rather than upside down (USD) forks. He noted that "only four documented tests involving motorcycles equipped with USD forks are available at this time…three of those are included in the source data used to create the [above] equations…For these three USD fork tests, the data fit well with that of the traditional fork, with an average error of –2.5 mph. However, additional testing and analysis is desired to determine how confident an analyst can be when establishing impact speed for motorcycles equipped with USD forks, which are so stiff that they commonly fracture in a manner that traditional forks do not."

In the collisions reported by Adamson, the motorcycle struck the car at an angle of either 0°, 90°, or 180°. Clearly, this will not always be the case in the real world. Wood [19] noted that, when the collision is angled, the damage energy for the car should be adjusted with the following equation:

$$E_{A,car} = \frac{E_{car,90}}{\cos \alpha} \tag{8.21}$$

In this equation,

$E_{car,90}$ is the calculated energy absorption for the car assuming a 90° impact angle to the side of the vehicle

α is the angle of the collision to the side of the vehicle

The same concept could be applied for front and rear collisions to the vehicle. To apply this calculation, the deformation would be measured perpendicular to the car.

8.2 Determining Motorcycle Speed from the Struck Vehicle Translation and Rotation

One indicator of a motorcycle's impact speed with a passenger vehicle is the magnitude of the translation and rotation experienced by the passenger vehicle following the impact. Simulation can be an effective means to determine the motorcycle impact speed necessary to cause a documented magnitude of translation and rotation of the struck vehicle. Deyerl and Cheng [23, 24] illustrated this type of analysis using EDSMAC4 simulation. In their study, Deyerl and Cheng simulated the WREX2000 motorcycle-car collisions and assessed the degree to which the simulations accurately predicted the vehicle rest positions. They concluded that "the use of EDSMAC4 in the simulation of motorcycle-into-vehicle collisions provides a valid means for analyzing collisions with configurations similar to these crash tests…The simulation effort described resulted in good to excellent correlation of post-impact translations and heading angle changes of the vehicles struck by the motorcycles."

Other software packages commonly used by accident reconstructionists can be used for similar analysis. As an example, this section describes analysis with PC-Crash of four of the WREX2016 collisions. Numerous studies conducted over the last two decades have demonstrated that the impact and trajectory models of PC-Crash can accurately model vehicular crashes [27]. Thus, the simulations described here are not a validation but rather a calibration in which reasonable inputs for this type of simulation are determined and described. For example, to simulate a motorcycle-car collision in PC-Crash, a reasonable coefficient of restitution will need to be selected. This section gives recommendations on this input and others for conducting this type of simulation.

Two additional issues are worth mentioning. First, some collisions induce steering of the struck vehicle's front wheels during the post-impact motion [28]. These steering angles develop, in part, because the frictional forces between the tires and ground cause the yaw rotation of the tires to lag the yaw rotation of the vehicle. The development of these steering angles also depends, in part, on moments generated due to the caster angle, which would cause some steering to occur even for a crash test where a significant yaw velocity did not develop. Rose demonstrated that simulations can be improved by including this steering. Such steering did occur in some of the WREX collisions and can also occur in real-world crashes. Including this steering in the simulation can improve the match with the known evidence.

Second, Deyerl and Cheng noted that "EDSMAC4 is a planar analysis which does not explicitly model a two-wheeled vehicle, and so does not simulate the tipover regime of motorcycle motion…a two-wheeled vehicle was modeled in EDSMAC4 by generating a four-wheeled vehicle in which the left side and right side tire-ground contact points are a very short distance apart." This same method can be employed in PC-Crash. In practice, Deyerl and Cheng's observation means that simulation of motorcycle-to-vehicle collisions with PC-Crash or EDSMAC4 will usually focus on modeling the post-collision motion of the struck vehicle, not the post-collision motion of the motorcycle. It may be possible to match the post-impact travel direction of the motorcycle but likely not the exact rest position and orientation of the motorcycle.

8.2.1 Case Study: WREX2016, Test #3

WREX2016, Test #3 involved a 2013 Harley-Davidson FXSB 103B Softail Breakout motorcycle impacting the passenger's side front door of a stationary 2006 Nissan Maxima near its center, at an approximate 90° angle and at a speed of 43.0 mph. Figure 8.10 shows the damage to these vehicles, their rest positions, tire marks, and chalk marks identifying the passenger's side wheel positions both pre- and post-collision. As these photographs show, the front wheels of the Nissan were steered to the left at rest. Review of the video for this test confirmed that these wheels were oriented straight ahead prior to the collision and that they steered to the left during the post-impact motion of the Nissan. The motorcycle in this test weighed 667 lb, and the Nissan weighed 3449 lb. The motorcycle experienced a wheelbase reduction of 11.3 in. and the car a maximum crush of 18.7 in.

In the simulation for this test, the roadway coefficient of friction was set at 0.7, and the TM-Easy tire model was used with default values for both vehicles. The impact height was set at 1.0 ft. A leftward steering input of 15°, occurring over 250 ms, was used in modeling the post-impact motion of the Nissan. Brake factors of 100% were used for the front drive wheels of the Nissan and 1% for the rear wheels. Brake factors of 100% were applied to the front wheel of the motorcycle, though the simulation was not sensitive to this input. An integration time step of 1 ms was used. The actual impact speed was entered, and the simulation was optimized using the coefficient of restitution. A high-quality match with the actual rest position of the Nissan was obtained with the actual motorcycle impact speed and a coefficient of restitution of 0.17 (Figure 8.11).

FIGURE 8.10   Impact damage and rest positions for WREX2016, Test #3.

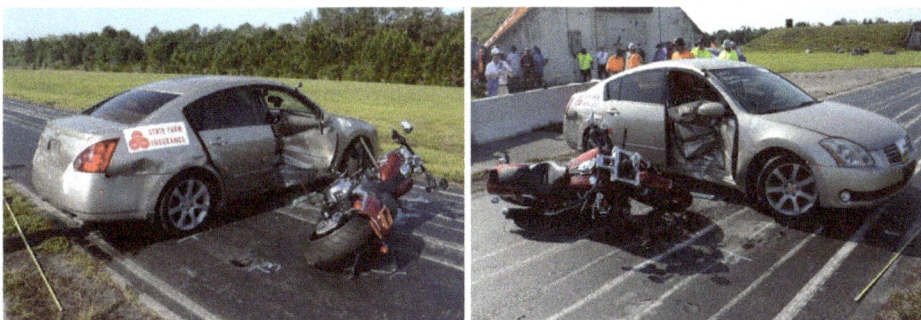

FIGURE 8.11 Optimized PC-Crash simulation for WREX2016, Test #3.

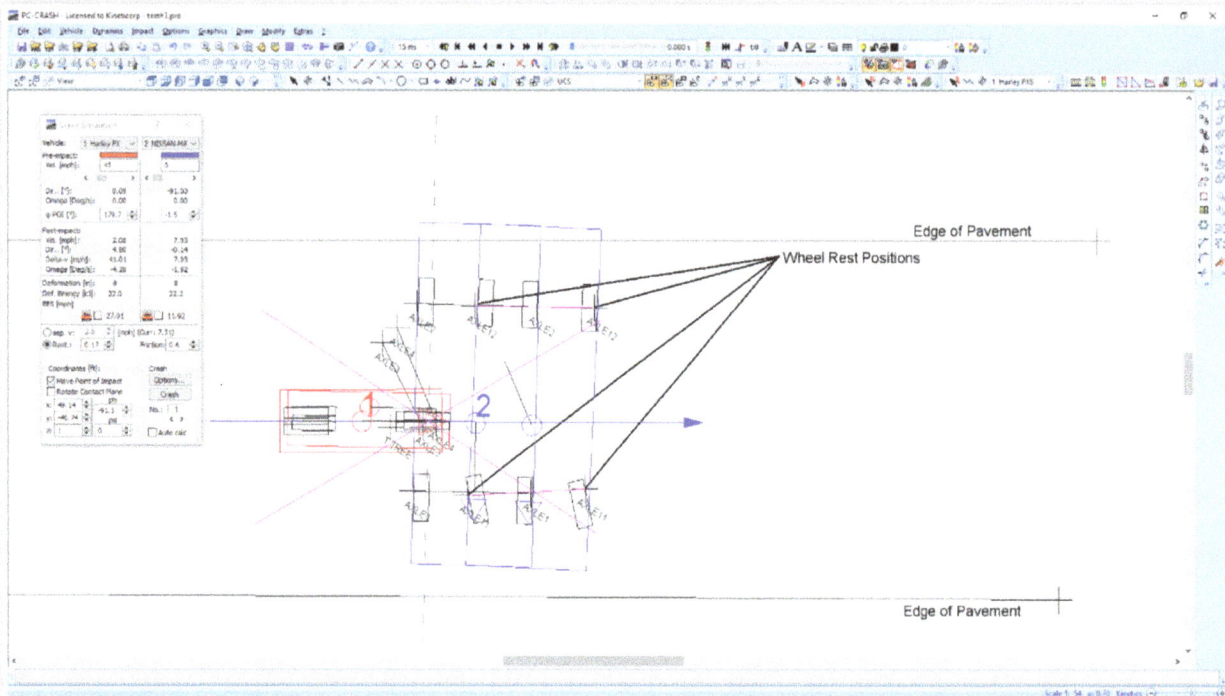

8.2.2 Case Study: WREX2016, Test #5

Test #5 involved a 2013 Harley-Davidson Dyna Street Bob FXDBA motorcycle impacting the driver's side rear door of stationary 2006 Nissan Maxima at a 90° angle and at a speed of 36.9 mph. Figure 8.12 shows the damage to these vehicles, their rest positions, tire marks, and chalk marks identifying the driver's side wheel positions both pre- and post-collision. As these photographs show, the front wheels of the Nissan were steered to the right at rest. Review of the video for this test confirmed that these wheels were oriented straight ahead prior to the collision and that they steered to the right during the post-impact motion of the Nissan. The motorcycle in this test weighed 633 lb, and the Nissan weighed 3449 lb. The motorcycle in this test experienced a wheelbase reduction of 12.8 in. and the car a maximum crush of 8.6 in.

In the simulation for this test, the roadway coefficient of friction was set at 0.7, and the TM-Easy tire model was used with default values for both vehicles. The impact height

FIGURE 8.12 Impact damage and rest positions for WREX2016 Test #5.

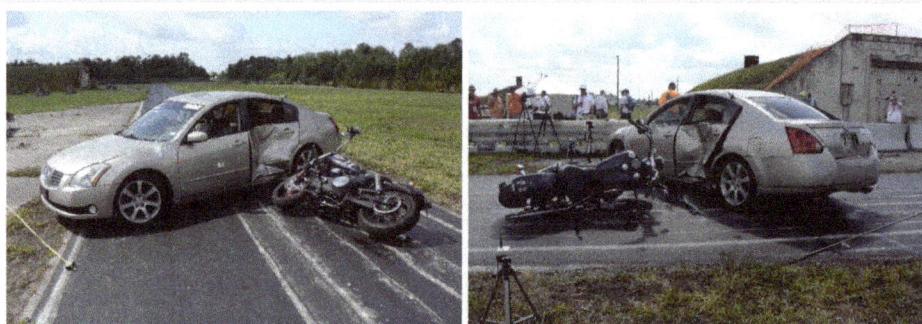

FIGURE 8.13 Optimized PC-Crash simulation for WREX2016, Test #5.

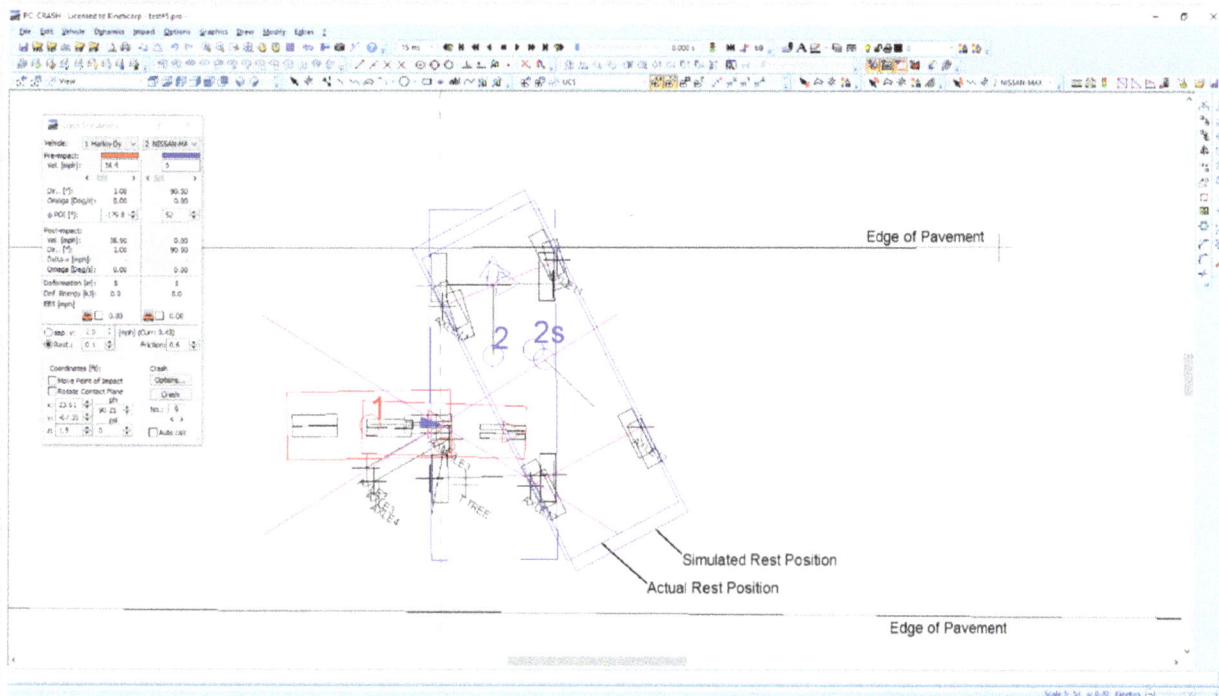

was set at 1.5 ft. A rightward steering input of 10° occurring over 250 ms was used for the post-impact motion of the Nissan. Brake factors of 100% were used for the front drive wheels of the Nissan and 1% for the rear wheels. Brake factors of 100% were applied to the front wheel of the motorcycle, though the simulation was not sensitive to this input. An integration time step of 1 ms was used. The actual impact speed was entered for the motorcycle, and the simulation was optimized using the coefficient of restitution. Figure 8.13 shows the optimized simulation for this test. The post-impact rotational motion of the Nissan was well matched with a coefficient of restitution of 0.1. There was a small translational discrepancy between the simulated and actual rest positions of the vehicle.

8.2.3 Case Study: WREX2016, Test #8

WREX2016, Test #8 involved a 2012 Harley-Davidson FXDF Dyna Fat Boy motorcycle impacting the driver's side rear of a stationary 2005 Dodge Durango at a 90° angle and at a speed of 46.3 mph. Figure 8.14 contains two photographs showing the damage to these vehicles, their rest positions, tire marks, and chalk marks identifying the driver's side wheel positions both pre- and post-collision. The motorcycle in this test weighed 678 lb, and the Dodge weighed 4740 lb.

In the simulation for this test, the impact height was set at 2.0 ft. Brake factors of 1% were used for the front wheels of the Nissan and 100% for the rear drive wheels. An integration time step of 1 ms was used. The simulation was optimized using the coefficient of restitution. Figure 8.15 shows the optimized simulation for this test. The post-impact rotational motion of the Nissan was well matched with a coefficient of restitution of 0.09. There was a small translational discrepancy between the simulated and actual rest positions of the vehicle.

| **FIGURE 8.14** | Impact damage and rest positions for WREX2016, Test #8. |

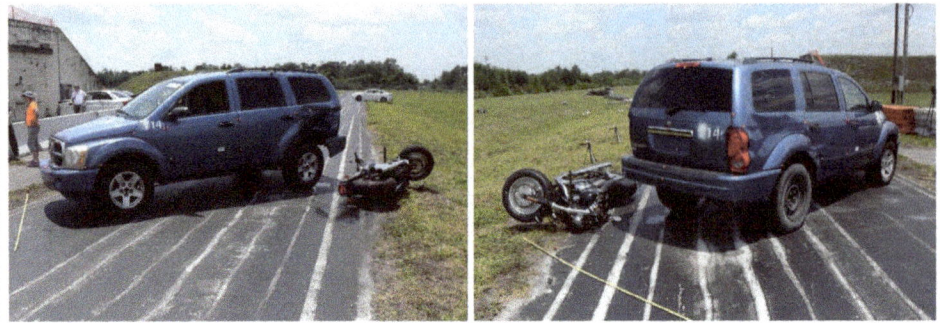

| **FIGURE 8.15** | Optimized PC-Crash simulation for WREX2016, Test #8. |

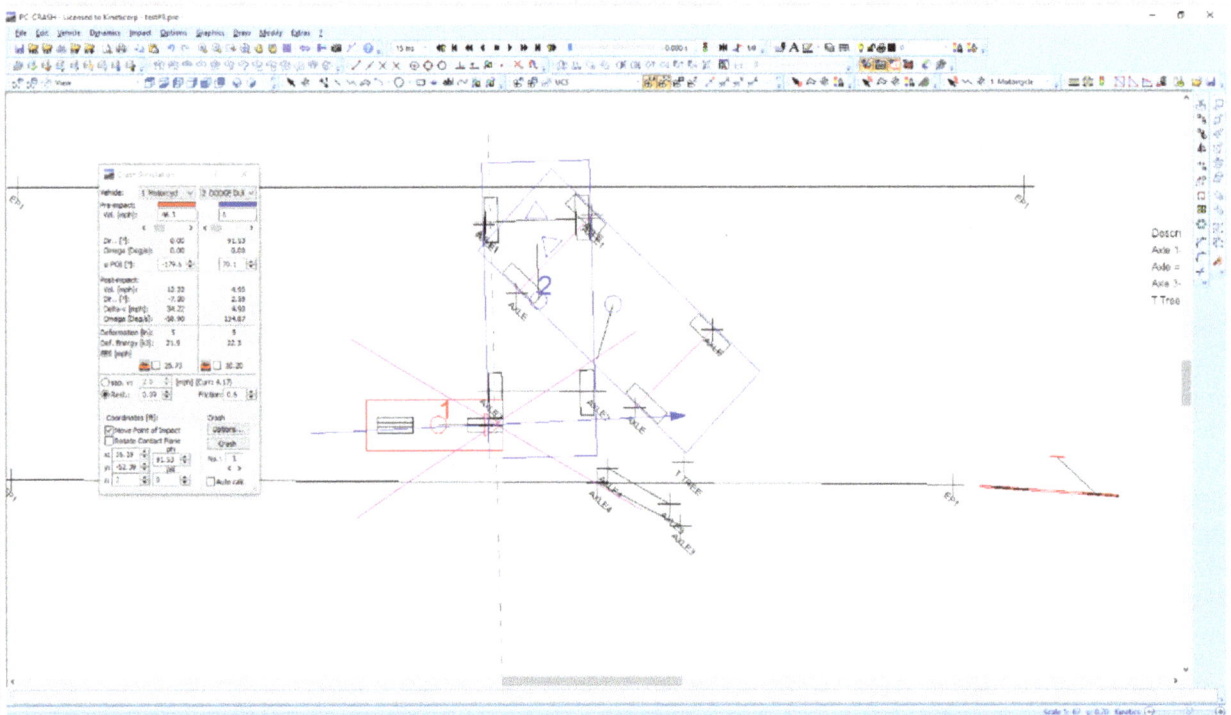

8.2.4 Case Study: WREX2016, Test #11

WREX2016, Test #11 involved a 2012 H-D Dyna Low Rider FXDL motorcycle impacting the passenger's side front door of a stationary 2005 Dodge Durango at a 90° angle and at a speed of 42.9 mph. The rear tires of the Dodge Durango were initially positioned on moist dirt and grass, and the front tires were positioned on asphalt. Figure 8.16 shows the damage to these vehicles, their rest positions, tire marks, and chalk marks identifying the passenger's side wheel positions both pre- and post-collision. The motorcycle in this test weighed 649 lb. and the Dodge weighed 4740 lb.

In the simulation for this test, a coefficient of friction of 0.6 was used for the dirt and grass surface. The impact height was set at 2.0 ft. A leftward steering input of 5°, occurring over 250 ms, was used for the post-impact motion of the Dodge. Brake factors of 1% were used for the front wheels of the Dodge and 100% for the rear drive wheels.

FIGURE 8.16 Impact damage and rest positions for WREX2016, Test #11.

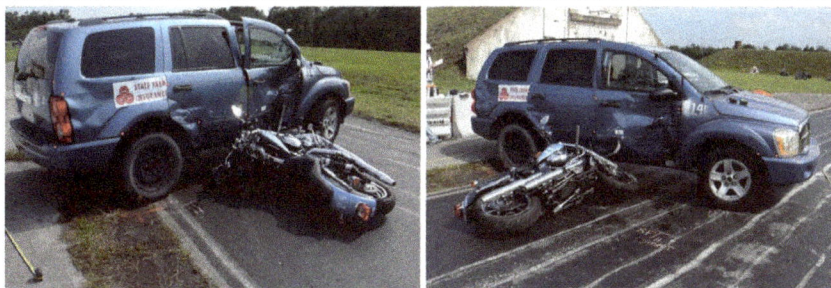

FIGURE 8.17 Optimized PC-Crash simulation for WREX2016, Test #11.

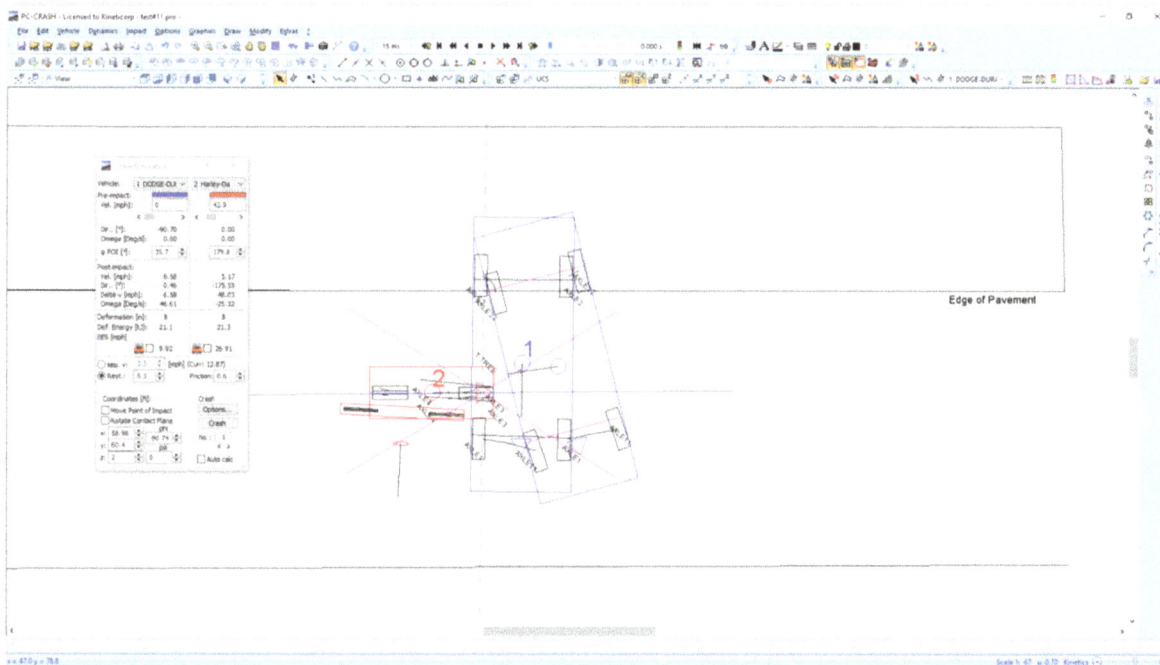

Brake factors of 100% were applied to the front wheel of the motorcycle, though the simulation was not sensitive to this input. An integration time step of 1 ms was used. The simulation was optimized using the coefficient of restitution (Figure 8.17). The post-impact motion of the Dodge was well matched with a coefficient of restitution of 0.3.

8.2.5 Case Study: WREX2016, Test #22

Test #22 involved a 1997 Harley-Davidson Sportster 883 motorcycle impacting the passenger's side rear wheel of a stationary 2006 Hyundai Sonata at a 90° angle and at a speed of 30.3 mph. Figure 8.18 shows the damage to these vehicles and their rest positions. The motorcycle in this test weighed 498 lb, and the Hyundai weighed 3547 lb.

In the simulation for this test, the impact center height was set at 2.0 ft. Brake factors of 100% were used for the front drive wheels of the Hyundai and 1% for the rear wheels. An integration time step of 1 ms was used. Attempts were made to optimize the simulation using the coefficient of restitution. However, with the reported motorcycle impact

FIGURE 8.18 Impact damage and rest positions for WREX2016, Test #22.

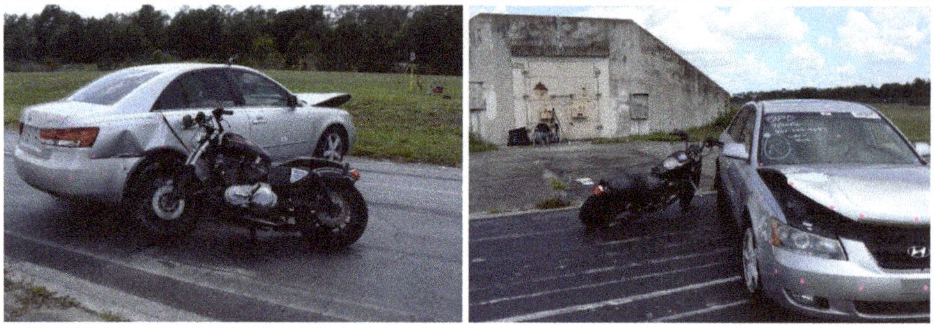

FIGURE 8.19 PC-Crash simulation for WREX2016, Test #22.

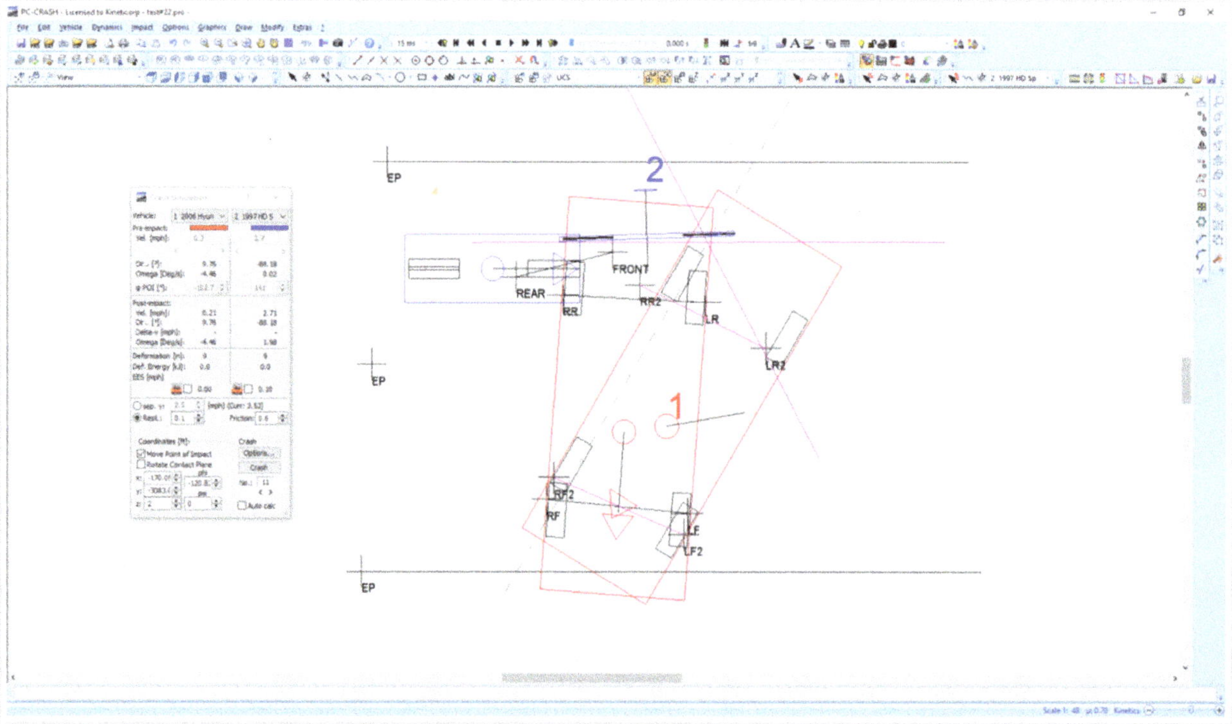

speed of 30.3 mph, the Hyundai translated and rotated too much, even with a coefficient of restitution of 0.0. For the sake of illustration, Figure 8.19 shows a simulation for this scenario with a coefficient of restitution of 0.1.

8.2.6 Case Study: WREX2016, Test #23

Test #23 involved a 2002 Harley-Davidson Sportster 883 motorcycle impacting the passenger's side rear door of a stationary 2006 Hyundai Sonata, just in front of the rear wheel, at a 90° angle and at a speed of 42.7 mph. Figure 8.20 shows the vehicles at rest after the test, along with the damage that the collision caused. The motorcycle in this test weighed 500 lb, and the Hyundai weighed 3547 lb.

In the simulation for this test, the impact center height was set at 1.5 ft. Brake factors of 100% were used for the front wheels of the Hyundai and 1% for the rear wheels. An integration time step of 1 ms was used. The simulation was optimized using the

FIGURE 8.20   Impact damage and rest positions for WREX2016, Test #23.

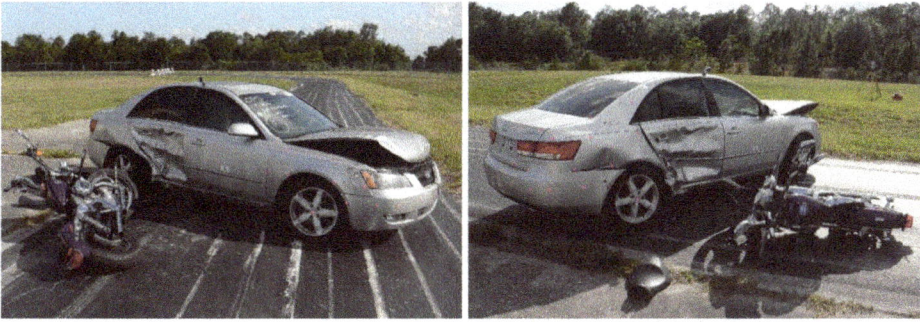

FIGURE 8.21   Optimized PC-Crash simulation for WREX2016, Test #23.

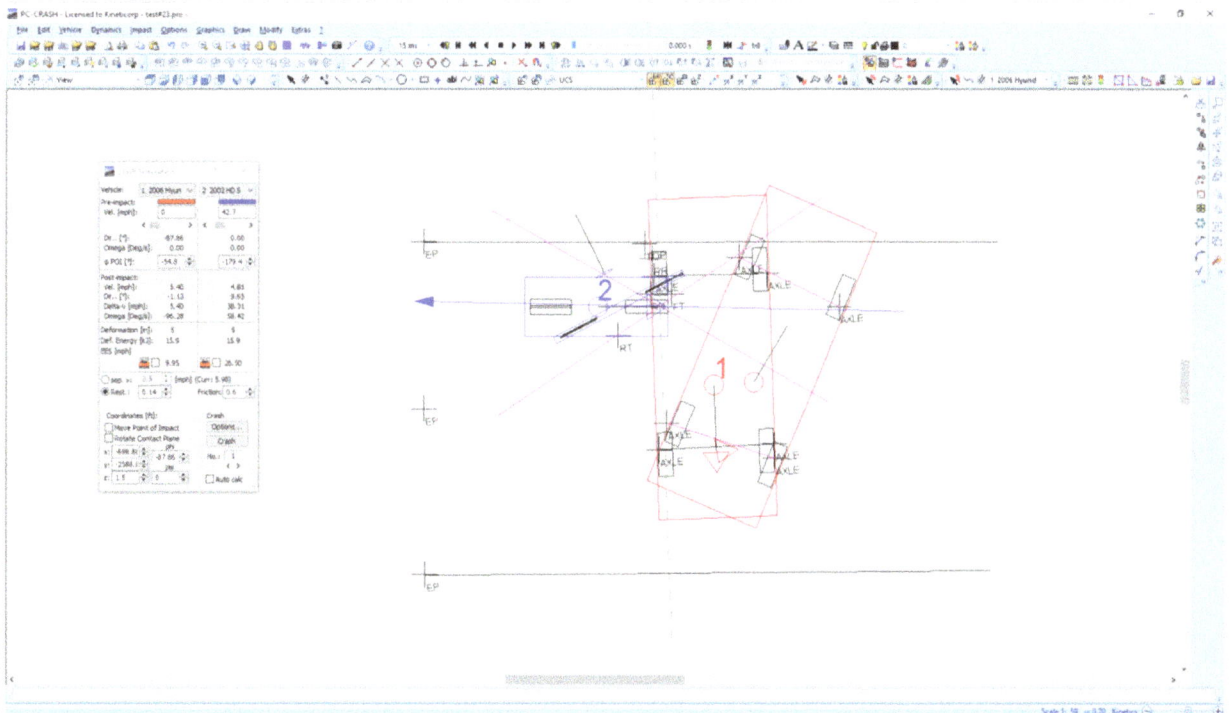

coefficient of restitution. Figure 8.21 shows the optimized simulation for this test. The post-impact translation and rotation of the Dodge were well matched with a coefficient of restitution of 0.14.

8.2.7 Case Study: WREX2016, Test #24

Test #24 involved a 2003 Harley-Davidson Sportster 883 motorcycle impacting the driver's side rear door of a stationary 2006 Hyundai Sonata at a 90° angle and at a speed of 35.5 mph. Figure 8.22 shows the damage to the vehicles along with their rest positions. The motorcycle in this test weighed 483 lb, and the Hyundai weighed 3547 lb.

In the simulation for this test, the impact center height was set at 1.5 ft. Brake factors of 100% were used for the front wheels of the Hyundai and 1% for the rear wheels. An integration time step of 1 ms was used. The simulation was optimized using the

FIGURE 8.22 Impact damage and rest positions for WREX2016, Test #24.

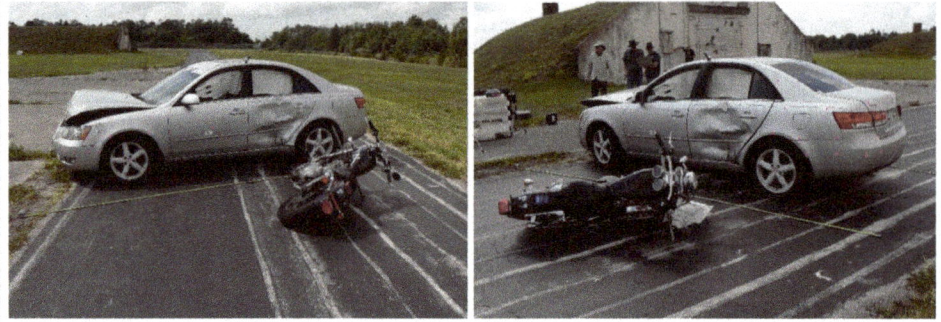

FIGURE 8.23 Optimized PC-Crash simulation for WREX2016, Test #24.

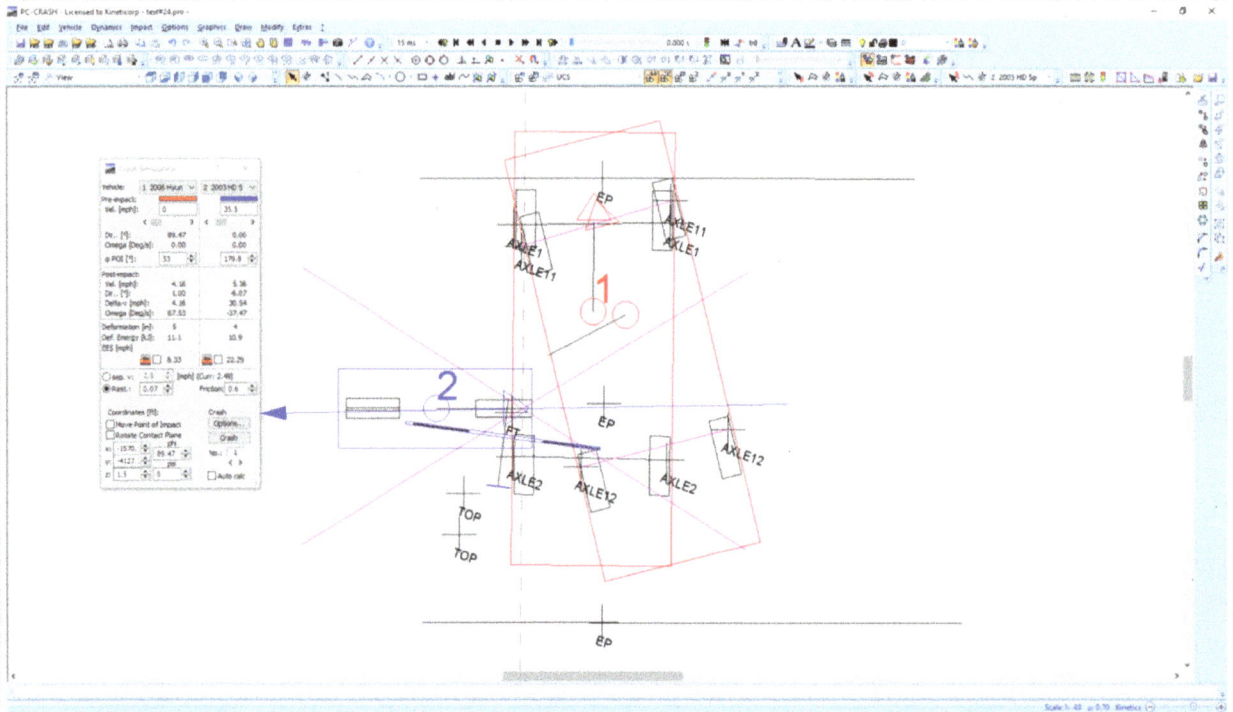

TABLE 8.5 Coefficients of restitution for the WREX2000 tests

Test #	Impact speed (mph)	Struck surface	Coefficient of restitution
8	46	Fender	0.12
9	39	Wheel	0.26
10	34	Bumper	0.19
12	30	Wheel	0.25
13	42	Door	0.10
14	30	Bumper	0.17
16	41	Wheel	0.26
18	45	Bumper	0.17
19	49	Fender	0.22

coefficient of restitution. Figure 8.23 shows the optimized simulation for this test. The post-impact translation and rotation of the Dodge were well matched with a coefficient of restitution of 0.07.

8.2.8 Discussion of WREX Tests

The authors have utilized PC-Crash to simulate both the WREX2000 collisions and the remaining 2016 collisions. Table 8.5 lists the coefficients of restitution that resulted from optimizing the WREX2000 simulations. In each simulation, the actual motorcycle impact speed was entered, and the simulation was optimized using the coefficient of restitution.

Similar data is reported for the WREX2016 tests in Table 8.6. The struck vehicle in the simulation of Test #22 rotated too much even with a coefficient of restitution of zero; therefore the coefficient of restitution for this test is reported as unknown. In practice, this could have been resolved by lowering the impact speed in the simulation. That would have led to a slight underestimation of the speed but a good match with the evidence. This was not done because the intention was to explore reasonable inputs for the simulations with the actual impact speeds. The coefficients of restitution in Tables 8.5 and 8.6 can be used as reference values and a general guideline for simulations of real-world motorcycle-to-vehicle collisions.

TABLE 8.6 Coefficients of restitution for the WREX2016 tests

Test #	Impact speed (mph)	Struck surface	Coefficient of restitution
3	43.0	Door	0.17
5	36.9	Door	0.10
8	46.3	Fender	0.09
11	42.9	Pillar	0.30
22	30.3	Wheel	Unknown
23	42.7	Door	0.14
24	35.5	Door	0.07

8.2.9 Should the Rider's Weight Be Included?

The WREX2000 and WREX2016 motorcycle-to-vehicle collisions did not utilize anthropomorphic test devices (ATDs) to represent riders of the motorcycles. Therefore, the discussion so far leaves an important issue unaddressed. When analyzing real-world collisions, the rider will need to be considered. As Niederer [29] has observed: "A major difficulty in the reconstruction of motorcycle-vehicle collisions derives from the fact that the motorcycle-rider and the motorcycle itself execute in general different trajectories after a collision with another vehicle." The previous section noted that, when using damage-based methods to analyze the energy dissipation during the collision, the weight of the rider should generally not be included in the motorcycle weight. This is because the rider will typically continue moving forward as the motorcycle is decelerated out from under them. Any collision between the rider and the passenger vehicle will typically occur later, after the collision between the motorcycle and the car is complete. When using simulation to model the collision, this situation is different. Even though there is a time delay between the motorcycle and rider collisions with the vehicle, the rider collision to the vehicle could influence the amount of translation and rotation the passenger vehicle experiences following the collision.

In PC-Crash and HVE, there is really no way to simulate the collisions of the motorcycle and rider to the vehicle as separate events. These collisions will have to be collapsed into one, with the option to either include or not include the weight of the rider. This is an issue that will have to be dealt with on a case-by-case basis, and the reconstructionist will need to determine the degree to which the rider's body engages with the vehicle. In some instances, there will be significant engagement, and, in others, there will be little engagement. In the former case, the weight of the rider would be included, and, in the later, it would not. There might also be some warrant for including part, but not all, of the rider weight. Describing the damage to the motorcycle fuel tank damage observed in a crash test, Smith [30] observed: "As the rider moved forward on the motorcycle and engaged the fuel tank, the loading to the fuel tank created by the rider's legs and pelvis was symmetric and produced a balanced damage pattern. This damage is consistent with fuel tank damage observed by the authors in similar 'real world' accidents." Such loading of the motorcycle by the rider would indicate that at least part of the rider's weight is participating with the motorcycle in the collision with the car.

Frank [31] applied such an approach in the EDSMAC4 and SIMON simulations he reported, noting that "the initial weight used was the as-tested weight of the [motorcycle], ignoring the weight of the [anthropomorphic test device]. However, after performing some initial simulations it was determined that the ATD was a factor in the impact. Review of the test video showed interaction between the ATD and the [car] during the impact; however, it appeared that the interaction involved only a portion of the ATD's mass. Currently, EDSMAC4 and SIMON are not capable of simulating the free body movement of the ATD traveling forward off of a motorcycle and impacting the side of a car. So, after some experimentation, it was determined that adding half of the ATD's weight to the motorcycle improved the results of the simulations significantly."

Simulation software does exist that can simulate the motion of the motorcycle and rider independently, along with their interaction with the vehicle. For example, Nieboer [32] presented simulation of motorcycle collisions using MADYMO. Nieboer noted that "computer simulation of motorcycle rider behavior during a collision event is far more difficult than the simulation of passenger car occupants. This is due to the complex way in which motorcycles and their riders behave after impact and the numerous contact interactions required in a mathematical model associated with this...The motorcycle rider interacts with the motorcycle, the motorcycle interacts with the passenger car (or another collision partner), but the rider interacts with the car directly as well. Considering these complex interactions, a step-by-step approach to specify more complete mechanical properties for each model component is often needed to improve the accuracy of the simulation." This type of simulation is often used in safety system research and development. However, because of the detailed component-level knowledge necessary for the application of this type of modeling, it is not customarily used in a collision reconstruction context.

8.3 Impacts into Moving Vehicles

In the crash tests discussed so far, the motorcycle struck a stationary barrier or vehicle. In real-world crashes, a struck vehicle could be moving, and this will influence the collision forces and the resulting motion of the vehicles. As Smith [30] has observed, "For two-moving-vehicle accidents, the rotation of the motorcycle front wheel and the resulting asymmetric compression and deformation of the front forks affects the post-impact motion of the motorcycle rider and the deformation of both the motorcycle and the other vehicle." Smith reported four crash tests where both the motorcycle and the car were moving. These tests are summarized in Table 8.7. The motorcycles in the first two tests were ridden by Hybrid III, 50th-percentile male adult ATDs with a full-face helmet. The motorcycles in the third and fourth tests, were ridden by Hybrid II, 5th-percentile female adult ATDs.

For these tests, Smith observed that "the post-impact motion of the motorcycle and the rider...was significantly influenced by the velocity of the car...the area of direct contact is typically wider on the side of the car than the comparable direct contact area for a stationary car crash test. The direct contact is not symmetric around the first point of contact and there is typically no direct contact damage from the motorcycle on the car forward of the initial point of contact...After contact, the front tire and wheel assembly of the motorcycle turns to align with the travel direction of the moving car...As a result of this rotation, the wheel and tire do not become trapped between the forward-most components of the motorcycle body and the car. Therefore, symmetric damage to the wheel is typically not evident...As a result of the impact, the motorcycle develops rotational motion primarily in yaw...Fork tube damage was also related to the speed of the moving car..." These observations imply that the extent of the damage on the struck car will be one indicator of the direction and magnitude of that car's motion at the time of the collision. They also imply

TABLE 8.7 Summary of the crash tests reported by Smith [30]

Test	Bullet vehicle	Bullet vehicle speed (mph)	Target vehicle	Target vehicle speed (mph)	Test description
1	1981 Kawasaki KX750E	30.0	1986 Ford Mustang	14.0	The Kawasaki (449 lb + 172 lb ATD) impacted the driver's side of the Mustang (2771 lb), near the rear of the driver's door; 90° impact angle
2	1981 Kawasaki KZ750E	29.9	1986 Ford Mustang	30.1	The Kawasaki (456 lb + 172 lb ATD) impacted the passenger's side of the Mustang (2771 lb), near the rear of the passenger's door; 90° impact angle
3	2007 Kawasaki Ninja ZX-10R	63.2	1986 Jaguar XJ6	41.9	The Kawasaki (407 lb + 103 lb ATD) impacted the passenger's side of the Mustang (4360 lb), near the rear of the passenger's door; 60° impact angle
4	2006 Kawasaki Ninja ZX-10R	68.1	1986 Jaguar XJ6	46.6	The Kawasaki (409 lb + 103 lb ATD) impacted the passenger's side of the Mustang (4362 lb), near the rear of the passenger's door; 60° impact angle

that, as the speed of the struck vehicle increases, wheelbase reduction methods for determining the motorcycle impact speed become less and less applicable. Smith observes that for the lowest car speed (14.0 mph), the fork tubes "bent in a manner similar to an impact into a stationary car." This was not the case for the higher car impact speeds.

Frank [31] presented the analysis of Smith's tests using EDSMAC4 and SIMON. He concluded that "the results demonstrate that it is indeed possible to simulate a motorcycle in these packages and that both packages can simulate two-moving motorcycle-to-car crashes reasonably well." There are a several details of these simulations that will be useful to a reconstructionist carrying out simulation analysis of a motorcycle-to-vehicle collision. First, "in both EDSMAC4 and SIMON a two-wheeled motorcycle must be modeled as a narrow-track four-wheeled vehicle. In all of the simulations discussed in this article the rear track width was set to 2 inches and the front track width was set to 4 inches. This configuration kept the contact patches of the front and rear tires sufficiently close to the simulate a single tire, while also providing the capacity to input front wheel steering without generating a software error code." Second, Frank shortened the distance from the motorcycle CG to the front of the motorcycle by 6 in. in each simulation. He stated that "a thorough review of the crash test footage and data traces revealed that the motorcycles did not experience any substantial deceleration until they had traveled some distance beyond initial contact. On closer examination it was determined that immediately after the initial contact steering inputs produced by the relative motion across the engagement interface, coupled with bending of the front forks, allowed the motorcycle to move approximately six inches forward before sustaining significant deceleration." Third, Frank noted that "it was expected that the post-impact motion of the motorcycle would be difficult to match. This expectation was borne out by the results of the simulations. In reality the simulation packages cannot be held accountable for this because they do not claim the ability to model a motorcycle."

Frank also observed that "initially there was some difficulty achieving the [car's] measured rest position in the simulation. A review of the test photos and video showed that the front tires of the [car] experienced caster steer post-impact. This was due to the fact that the steering gear was free to respond to tire forces once the vehicle was released from tow. To mimic the steering response observed in this test a fixed post-impact clockwise steering wheel input of 270° was added. With this simulated caster steer applied it became possible to produce a rest position for the [car] that closely approximated the measured rest position."

8.4 Summary of Motorcycle-to-Car Collision Analysis Methods

8.4.1 Speed Analysis Based on Wheelbase Reduction

Following is the progression of steps that a reconstructionist could use to analyze the motorcycle impact speed based on the motorcycle's wheelbase reduction:

- Determine the original wheelbase of the motorcycle.
- Document the postcrash wheelbase of the motorcycle and quantify the shortening.
- Determine which portion of the struck vehicle was engaged by the motorcycle.
- Quantify the maximum crush to the struck vehicle.
- Add the motorcycle wheelbase shortening to the maximum car crush.
- Apply either Equation (8.17), (8.18), (8.19), or (8.20).

8.4.2 Speed Analysis Based on a Known Translation and Rotation of the Struck Vehicle

Following is the progression of steps that a reconstructionist could use to analyze the motorcycle impact speed based on the translation and rotation of the struck vehicle. This progression assumes that the analyst will utilize a simulation software, such as EDSMAC4, SIMON, or PC-Crash. A reconstructionist that chooses to carry out this analysis in a spreadsheet can adapt this progression to fit that approach. In some instances, not all of these steps will be necessary:

- Obtain geometric specifications and the weight of the motorcycle and the struck vehicle.
- Estimate the longitudinal position of the centers of mass of the motorcycle and the struck vehicle. If a three-dimensional simulation will be used, the vertical positions of the center of mass will also be needed.
- Use the physical evidence to determine the impact and rest positions of the motorcycle and struck vehicle.

- Create an evidence diagram that can be used in the simulation. Ideally, this diagram would include the impact positions, the rest positions, and any physical evidence that was deposited on the roadway (tire marks, scrapes, and gouges).

- Import the evidence diagram and create the vehicles in the simulation software.

- Estimate the roadway coefficient of friction between the tires and the roadway for the simulation. Depending on the software package utilized, suitable tire model parameters may also be necessary.

- Estimate the degree to which the wheels of the motorcycle and struck vehicle are impinged or impeded following the collision and enter appropriate inputs into the software.

- Set up the collision. The procedure for carrying this out will vary from software package to software package but may involve inputting stiffness coefficients, establishing the impact location, establishing the contact surface, and inputting a coefficient of restitution.

- Vary the impact speed of the motorcycle until the translation and rotation of the struck vehicle match the rest position on the evidence diagram. In instances where the struck vehicle is moving at the time of the collision, this speed may need to be varied as well.

8.5 Motorcycle Collisions with Roadside Barriers

In 2007, Gabler examined U.S. accident statistics related to fatal motorcycle collisions with guardrails [33]. He observed that "in 2005 for the first time, motorcycle riders suffered more fatalities (224) than the passengers of cars (171) …involved in a guardrail collision. In terms of fatalities per registered vehicle, motorcycle riders are dramatically overrepresented in number of fatalities resulting from guardrail impacts… Motorcycle-guardrail crash fatalities are a growing problem. From 2000-2005, the number of car occupants who were fatally injured in guardrail collisions declined by 31% from 251 to 171 deaths. In contrast, the number of motorcyclists fatally-injured in guardrail crashes increased by 73% from 129 to 224 fatalities during the same period. Over two-thirds of motorcycle riders who were fatally injured in a guardrail crash were wearing a helmet."

Also in 2007, Ibitoye et al. reported MADYMO simulations of upright motorcyclists colliding with w-beam guardrails adjacent to lanes designated exclusively for motorcycles [34]. They also reported a crash test that they used to validate the MADYMO finite element modeling of the guardrail system and the multi-body model of the motorcycle and rider. This study was focused on improving the safety of motorcyclists in Malaysia where motorcycles constitute 49% of registered vehicles and "about 68% of all road accident injuries involved motorcyclists with overall relative risks of about 20 times higher than that of passenger cars." The simulations utilized a 110 kg motorcycle impacting the guardrail at speeds of 32, 48, and 60 kph at angles of 15°, 30°, and 45°. Ibitoye reported that "the kinematics of [the] rider for all impact conditions are similar during the initial stage with the dummy having leg contact with the guardrail surface and projecting with head forward. But, the dynamics of [the] rider towards the landing depend on the impact speeds and angles." Further, the w-beam guardrail "causes the rider to slide and tumble along the top of [the] guardrail before landing on the ground with [their] head."

In 2010, Bambach reported a study of 78 crashes in which motorcyclists were fatally injured in Australia and New Zealand following a collision with a roadside barrier [35]. The study period was 2001 to 2006. "Of particular note were the findings that 97% of the motorcyclists were wearing a helmet prior to the crash, 86% of the crashes were single vehicle run-off crashes, 80% occurred on a corner, 92% of motorcyclists were male with a mean age of 34.2 years, 72% were less than 40 years and 81% of motorcyclists died at the crash scene. Motorcyclist behavior such as speeding and alcohol/drug use were identified as common causal factors...In Australia and New Zealand the main barrier types installed are steel W beam barriers...followed by concrete and wire rope (steel cable) barriers. Amongst motorcyclists fatally injured in barrier crashes, 77% involved W beams, 10% involved concrete barriers, 8% involved wire rope barriers and 5% involved other barriers...In the 78 cases the majority of motorcycles were sports motorcycles (n = 51), followed by touring motorcycles (n = 17) and off-road motorcycles (n = 3), with insufficient information to classify the motorcycle in seven cases."

Bambach found that in 37 cases the motorcyclist was upright at impact with the barrier and in 34 cases the motorcycle and rider were sliding on the ground into the barrier. He noted that in the upright crashes, "the motorcycle is typically redirected along the barrier. Due to the impact trajectory angle of the motorcycle relative to the barrier, momentum causes the upper body of the motorcyclist to want to continue over the barrier. In nine cases the motorcyclist was ejected over the barrier upon impact. In 20 cases this momentum and the redirection of the motorcycle along the barrier resulted in the motorcyclists scraping/tumbling/skidding along the top of the barrier. After scraping along the top of the barrier for some distance the motorcyclist was then ejected from the barrier, and in 15 of the 20 cases this occurred as a result of the motorcyclist impacting a barrier post."

Rizzi et al. [36] examined the influence of the barrier type and the motorcycle's orientation (upright or capsized) at the time of the collision on the injury outcome for the riders. They utilized police-reported crashes in Sweden from between 2003 and 2010. They also conducted in-depth interviews with 55 Swedish motorcyclists who had been involved in collisions with roadside barriers. Rizzi et al. found no statistically significant difference in the injury outcomes between wire rope barriers, Kohlswa-beam (similar to W-beam) barriers, and W-beam barriers. They noted that "the small number of in-depth case findings, however, showed that injury severity was lower in crashes in which the motorcyclists were in an upright position during the collision."

Maza et al. [37] noted that "a particularly severe type of motorcycle collision is the crash into road barriers due to losing control of the motorcycle." Noting the past research efforts that have examined this issue, these researchers state that "some of these efforts resulted in the adoption of the European Technical Specification CEN/TS 1317-8 in which a modified Hybrid III test dummy with a helmet is launched sliding on the ground in a head-on impact at 30° and 60 km/h against different locations of [a] Motorcycle Protective Systems (MPS). [An] MPS consist[s] of a lower continuous rail that is installed in existing W-beam barriers to prevent the sliding motorcyclist from passing under the upper W-beam and impact into other rigid roadside obstacles. However, there is evidence that a significant share of motorcyclist impacts against roadside barriers happen in upright position with the rider still attached to the motorcycle." Maza et al. also observed that "the International Federation of Motorcycles (FIM) proposed an internal regulation of roadside protection used in the racing tracks during competition. This regulation requires barriers to provide a certain level of deceleration of a body-block in vertical position, impacting the barrier at different speeds in free flight." These researchers sought to determine the most common orientations of riders impacting roadside barriers on normal roads and on racing tracks. Ultimately, they sought to assess the realism of the test standards.

In conducting their research, Maza et al. examined 110 motorcycle collisions with roadside barriers that were captured on video and posted to YouTube. These researchers concluded that "For race track crashes, the pilot spine – ground angle distribution found in the video analysis shows mostly low angles, which is not well represented in the barrier test procedure applied, consisting of a body-block vertically impacting the barrier at different speeds in free flight. For normal road crashes, the motorcyclist spine-ground angle distribution found is consistent with the barrier test procedure defined by CEN/TS 1317-8, consisting of a full dummy sliding and impacting the barrier in supine position."

8.5.1 Case Study: Motorcycle-to-Roadside Barrier Crash Tests

Berg and Rücker reported crash tests of motorcycles (Kawasaki ER 5 Twisters) and rider dummies colliding with three different barrier systems-a conventional steel barrier, a concrete barrier, and a modified steel guardrail design [38, 39]. Tests were conducted with the motorcycle and rider initially upright and with the motorcycle and rider capsized prior to colliding with the barrier. The nominal collision speed for each test was 60 kph (37.3 mph). For the upright tests, the impact angle was approximately 12°, and for the capsized tests, the impact angle was approximately 25°. The motorcycles in these tests had a mass of approximately 180 kg (397 lb), and the rider dummies had a mass of approximately 92 kg (198 lb).

8.5.1.1 STEEL GUARDRAIL: UPRIGHT

In the upright test into the steel guardrail, the motorcycle exited the sled at 60 kph (37.3 mph) and collided with the steel barrier at a speed of approximately 58 kph (36.0 mph). From first contact to rest, the motorcycle traveled 28 m (91.9 ft). The dummy traveled 21 m (68.8 ft). Thus, from first contact to rest, the motorcycle decelerated at an average rate of 0.47 g, and the rider decelerated at an average rate of 0.63 g. Figure 8.24 is a series of frames from the video of this test showing the motion of the motorcycle and rider from the time of contact with barrier until the motorcycle is nearly capsized. As these images show, the motorcycle collided with the barrier with its right side leading. The motorcycle quickly began rebounding, leaning, and steering to the left. The upper body of the rider continued to the right and folded over the barrier. Eventually, the front tire of the motorcycle steered back to the right as the motorcycle continued to be in contact with the lower extremities of the rider. The motorcycle began leaning right and eventually capsized onto its right side.

Figure 8.25 is another series of frames from the test video showing the motion of the motorcycle and rider following capsize of the motorcycle. As these images show, the motorcycle capsized onto its right side and remained on its right side as it slid and spun to rest. The upper body of the rider dummy continued interacting with and sliding along the barrier, while the dummy's lower body began sliding on the pavement.

FIGURE 8.24 Upright, steel barrier, frames from the test video showing the motion of the motorcycle and rider from the time of contact with barrier until the motorcycle is nearly capsized.

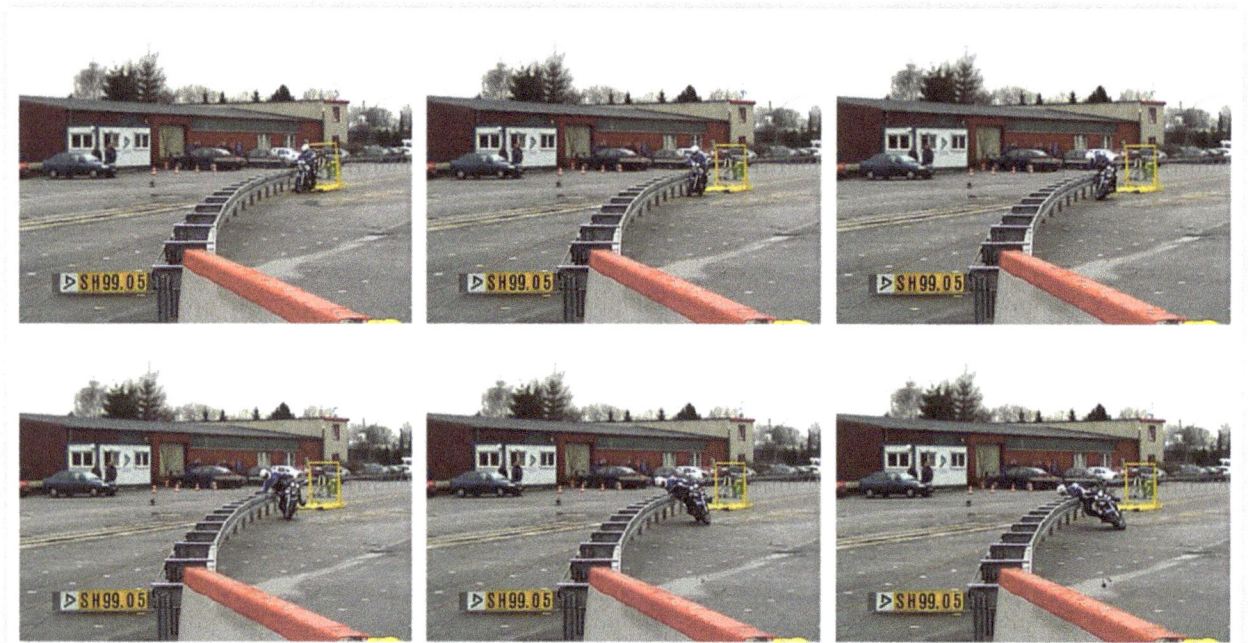

FIGURE 8.25 Upright, steel barrier, frames from the test video showing the motion of the motorcycle and rider after capsize.

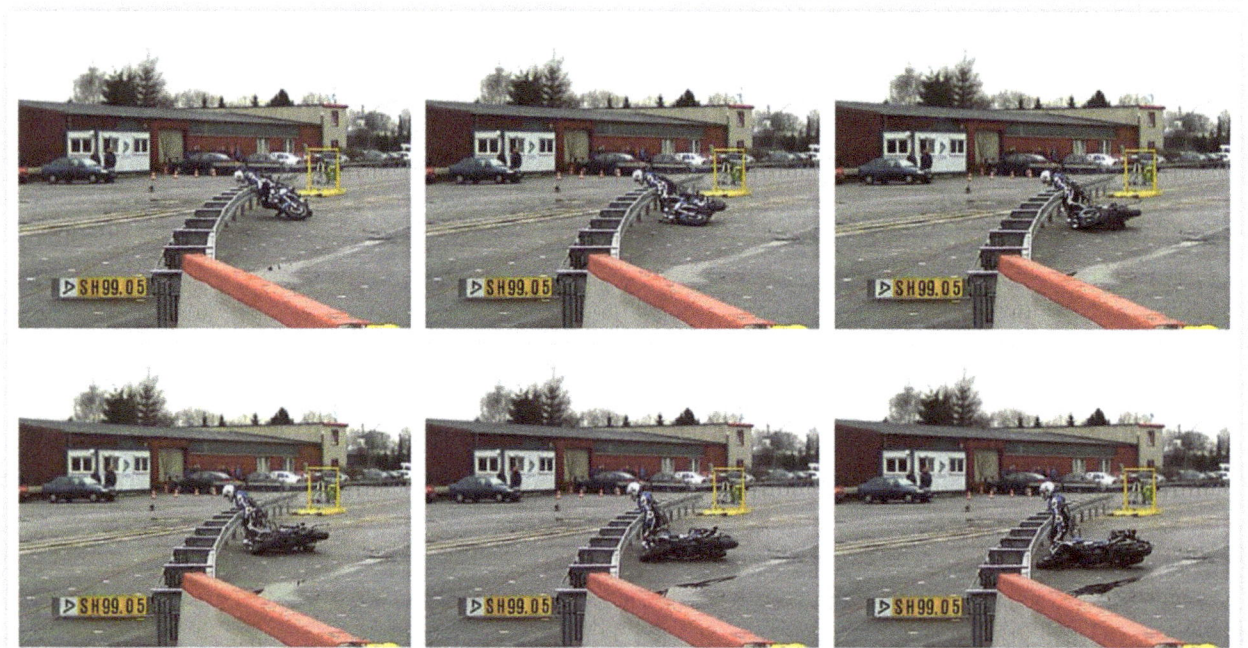

8.5.1.2 CONCRETE BARRIER: UPRIGHT

In the upright test into the concrete barrier, the motorcycle again exited the sled at 60 kph (37.3 mph) in an upright position. After the motorcycle collided with the barrier, the dummy separated from the motorcycle and traveled over the barrier, coming to rest on the opposite side of the barrier. The motorcycle traveled 38 m (124.7 ft) from first contact with the barrier to rest. The dummy traveled 26 m (85.3 ft) from first contact to rest. Thus, from first contact to rest, the motorcycle decelerated at an average rate of 0.37 g, and the rider decelerated at an average rate of 0.54 g. Figure 8.26 is a series of frames from the test video showing the motion of the motorcycle and rider as it contacts the barrier. The motorcycle begins sliding along the barrier, and the rider is thrown over the barrier.

8.5.1.3 MODIFIED STEEL GUARDRAIL: UPRIGHT

Berg, Rücker, and their colleagues designed a modification to the steel guardrail system in which "an additional underrun protection board was mounted near to the ground to prevent both the direct impact onto a post and movement of the motorcyclist underneath the barrier protection system." In relationship to the upright motorcycle collision into this modified barrier, again at a speed of 60 kph (37.3 mph), Berg and Rücker observed that "after first contact into the barrier the motorcycle was redirected away from the barrier. The dummy separated from the motorcycle and fell onto the protection system. After sliding for a short distance on the guard rail the dummy fell to the ground on the opposite side. Because of the closed shape of the box-type profile, snagging did not occur and injury risk from impact was low as observed from the analysis of the film." Figure 8.27 is a series of frames from the video of this test. The motorcycle traveled 23 m (75.5 ft) from first contact to rest, and the dummy traveled 22 m (72.2 ft). Thus, from first contact to rest, the motorcycle decelerated at an average rate of 0.61 g, and the rider decelerated at an average rate of 0.64 g.

FIGURE 8.26 Upright, concrete barrier, frames from the test video showing the motion of the motorcycle and rider.

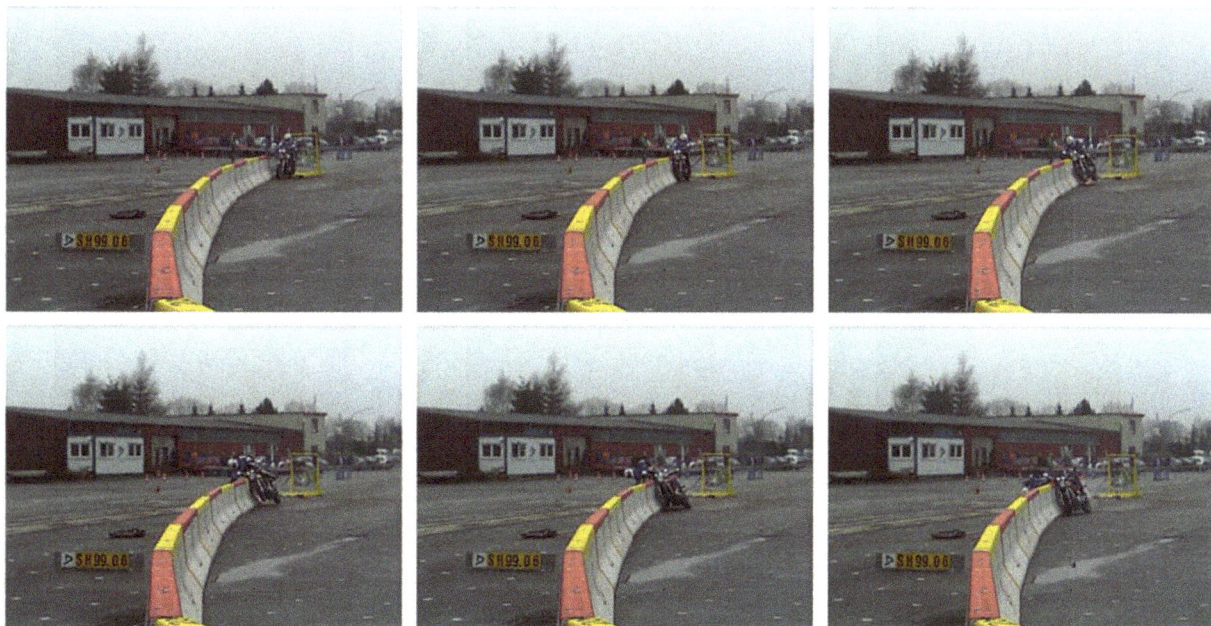

FIGURE 8.27 Upright, modified steel guardrail, frames from the test video showing the motion of the motorcycle and rider.

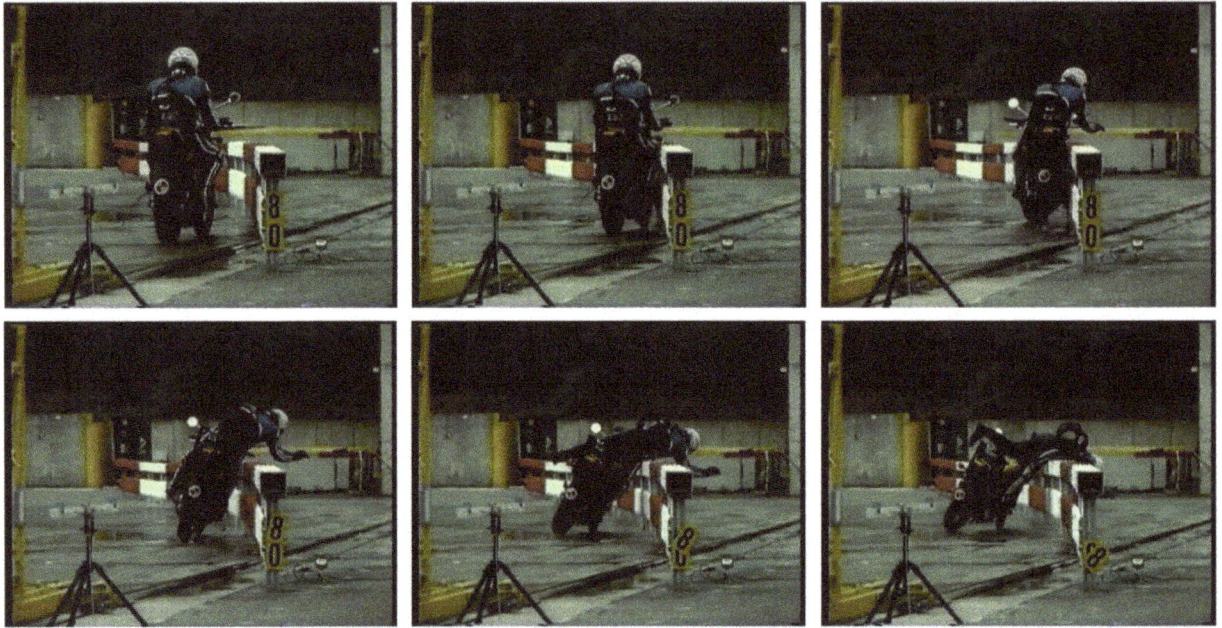

8.5.1.4 STEEL GUARDRAIL: CAPSIZED

In this test, the motorcycle exited the sled at 60 kph (37.3 mph). As it slid on its side, the motorcycle decelerated, and, at the time it collided with the barrier, it was traveling a speed of 47 kph (29.2 mph). Because it was on its side, the motorcycle bypassed the metal rail and directly impacted one of the posts of the barrier system. This impact brought the motorcycle to a stop quickly, and the motorcycle came to rest underneath the guardrail. The dummy slid toward the barrier behind the motorcycle. When the motorcycle struck the barrier, the dummy separated from the motorcycle and struck a post of the barrier system. The motorcycle traveled 2 m during its interaction with the barrier, and the dummy traveled 5 m. Figure 8.28 is a series of frames from the video of this test.

8.5.1.5 CONCRETE BARRIER: CAPSIZED

In this test, the motorcycle exited the sled at 59 kph (36.7 mph). At the time it collided with the barrier, it was traveling 46 kph (28.6 mph). The collision with the barrier system redirected the motorcycle and the rider along the barrier, and they both slid to rest traveling parallel with the barrier. Figure 8.29 is a series of frames from the video of this test. In relationship to this test, the authors observed that the "deceleration of the motorcycle and dummy were not as rapid as during the impact where the motorcycle slid into the guard rail made from steel. Nevertheless, the measured dummy decelerations for the primary impact were high, indicating a risks of severe and life-threatening injuries."

8.5.1.6 MODIFIED STEEL GUARDRAIL: CAPSIZED

In this test, the motorcycle exited the sled at a speed of 60 kph and impacted the barrier at a speed of 54 kph. The authors observed that "due to the impact the underrun

FIGURE 8.28 Capsized, steel barrier, frames from the test video showing the motion of the motorcycle and rider.

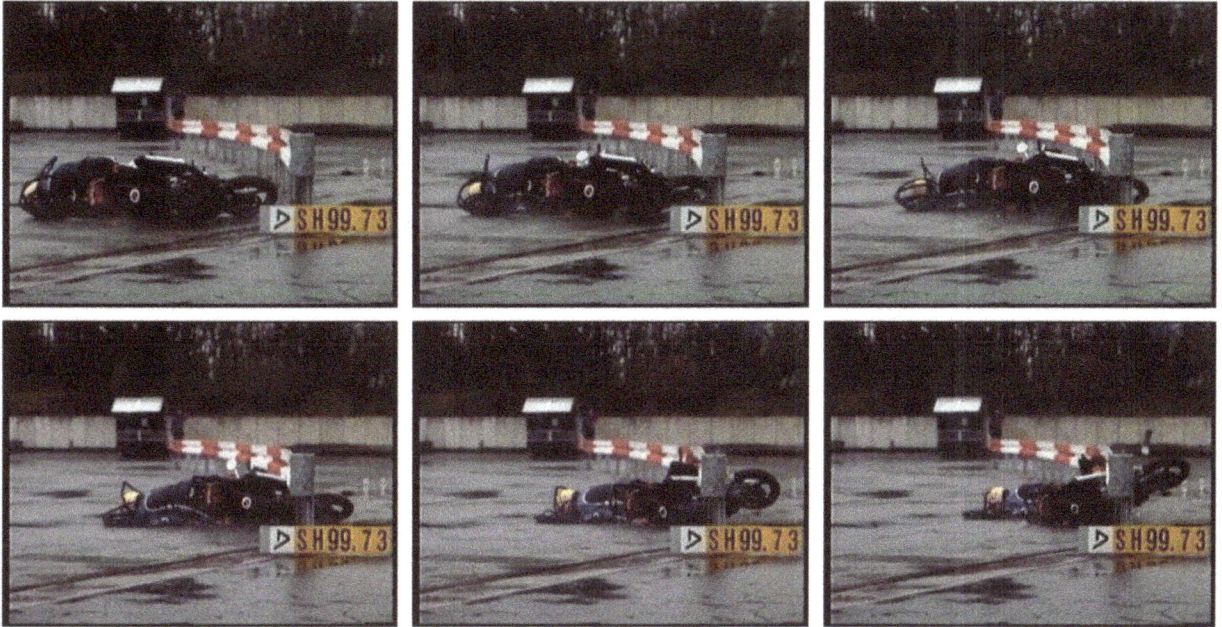

FIGURE 8.29 Capsized, concrete barrier, frames from the test video showing the motion of the motorcycle and rider.

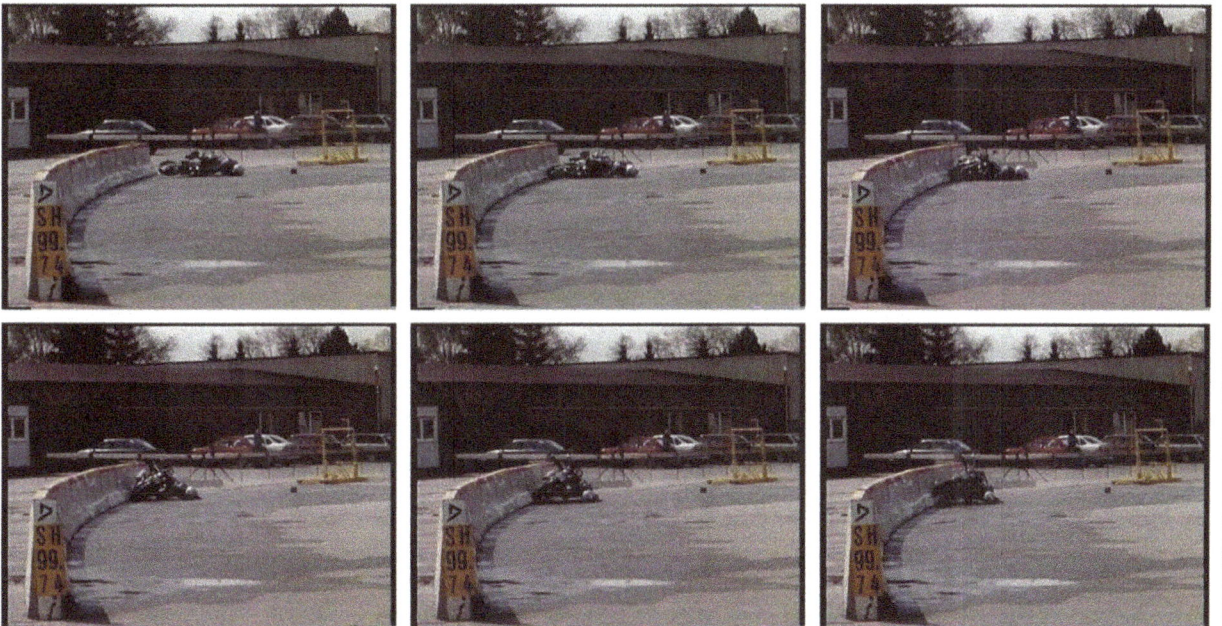

protection board broke and the motorcycle struck a Sigma post. The dummy separated from the motorcycle immediately after the initial primary impact and then the helmeted head struck the underrun protection board." Following first contact with the barrier, the motorcycle traveled 1 m, and the dummy traveled 7 m.

References

1. Severy, D., Brink, H., and Blaisdell, D., "Motorcycle Collision Experiments," SAE Technical Paper 700897, 1970, doi:10.4271/700897.

2. Adamson, K.S., "Seventeen Motorcycle Crash Tests into Vehicles and a Barrier," SAE Technical Paper 2002-01-0551, 2002, doi:10.4271/2002-01-0551.

3. Baxter, A.T., *Motorcycle Crash Investigation*, (Jacksonville, FL: Institute of Police Technology and Management, 2017), ISBN:978-1-934807-18-7.

4. Bartlett, W., "Motorcycle Crush Analysis," *Accident Reconstruction Journal* (March/April 2009): 25-29, ISSN:1057-8153.

5. Eubanks, J., "Motorcycle Speed-from-Damage Estimates Update," *Society of Accident Reconstruction* (October 1991): 22.

6. Campbell, K., "Energy Basis for Collision Severity," SAE Technical Paper 740565, 1974, doi:10.4271/740565.

7. McHenry, R.R., "A Comparison of Results Obtained with Different Analytical Techniques for Reconstruction of Highway Accidents," SAE Technical Paper 750893, 1975, doi:10.4271/750893.

8. McHenry, R.R., "Extensions and Refinements of the CRASH Computer Program Part II," DOT HS-801 838, February 1976.

9. McHenry, R.R. and Jones, I.S., "Extensions and Refinements of the CRASH Computer Program Part III, Evaluation of the Accuracy Reconstruction Techniques for Highway Accidents," DOT HS-801 839, February 1976.

10. McHenry, R.R., "Computer Aids for Accident Investigation," SAE Technical Paper 760776, 1976, doi:10.4271/760776.

11. McHenry, R.R. and McHenry, B.G., "A Revised Damage Analysis Procedure for the CRASH Computer Program," SAE Technical Paper 861894, 1986, doi:10.4271/861894.

12. Rose, N., Fenton, S., and Ziernicki, R., "An Examination of the CRASH3 Effective Mass Concept," SAE Technical Paper 2004-01-1181, 2004, doi:10.4271/2004-01-1181.

13. Rose, N., Fenton, S., and Ziernicki, R., "Crush and Conservation of Energy Analysis: Toward a Consistent Methodology," SAE Technical Paper 2005-01-1200, 2005, doi:10.4271/2005-01-1200.

14. Rose, N., Fenton, S., and Beauchamp, G., "Restitution Modeling for Crush Analysis: Theory and Validation," SAE Technical Paper 2006-01-0908, 2006, doi:10.4271/2006-01-0908.

15. Rose, N. and Carter, N., "Further Assessment of the Uncertainty of CRASH3 ΔV and Energy Loss Calculations," SAE Technical Paper 2014-01-0477, 2014, doi:10.4271/2014-01-0477.

16. Searle, J., "The Reconstruction of Speed in Motorcycle Collisions from the Extent of Damage," *IMPACT: Journal of the ITAI* 18, no. 1 (Spring 2010).

17. Wood, D.P., Glynn, C., and Walsh, D., "Estimation of the Collision Speed in a Collision of a Motorcycle or Scooter with a Car from Individual Vehicle Deformation," *Proc IMechE Part D: J Automobile Engineering* 228, no. 3 (2014): 295-309, doi:10.1177/0954407012471272.

18. Wood, D.P., Glynn, C., O'Dea, C., and Walsh, D., "Physical and Empirical Models for Motorcycle Speed Estimation from Crush," *International Journal of Crashworthiness* 19, no. 5 (2014): 540-554, doi:10.1080/13588265.2014.918300.

19. Wood, D.P., Glynn, C., and Walsh, D., "Motorcycle-to-Car and Scooter-to-Car Collisions: Speed Estimation from Permanent Deformation," *Proc IMechE Part D: J Automobile Engineering* (2009), doi:10.1243/09544070JAUTO1069.

20. MacInnis, D., Cliff, W., and Ising, K., "A Comparison of Moment of Inertia Estimation Techniques for Vehicle Dynamics Simulation," SAE Technical Paper 970951, 1997, doi:10.4271/970951.

21. Allen, R., Klyde, D., Rosenthal, T., and Smith, D., "Estimation of Passenger Vehicle Inertial Properties and Their Effect on Stability and Handling," SAE Technical Paper 2003-01-0966, 2003, doi:10.4271/2003-01-0966.

22. Varat, M.S., Husher, S.E., and Kerkhoff, J.F., "An Analysis of Trends of Vehicle Frontal Impact Stiffness," SAE Technical Paper 940914, 1994, doi:10.4271/940914.

23. Deyerl, E. and Cheng, L., "Computer Simulation of Staged Motorcycle-Vehicle Collisions Using EDSMAC4," white paper presented at *the 2008 HVE Forum*, HVE-WP2008-3, http://www.edccorp.com/library/whitepaper.html.

24. Deyerl, E. and Cheng, L., "Computer Simulation of Staged Motorcycle-Vehicle Collisions Using EDSMAC4," *Accident Reconstruction Journal* (July/August 2007).

25. Bartlett, W., Focha, B., and Kauderer, C., "25 Moving Motorcycle into Stationary Car Tests: CA²RS 2009 Data," *Accident Reconstruction Journal* (July/August 2013): 23-27, 64, ISSN:1057-8153.

26. Peck, L., Bartlett, W., Joseph, M., Dickerson, C. et al., "Eleven Instrumented Motorcycle Crash Tests and Development of Updated Motorcycle Impact-Speed Equations," SAE Technical Paper 2018-01-0517, 2018, doi:10.4271/2018-01-0517.

27. Rose, N. and Carter, N., "An Analytical Review and Extension of Two Decades of Research Related to PC-Crash Simulation Software," SAE Technical Paper 2018-01-0523, 2018, doi:10.4271/2018-01-0523.

28. Rose, N.A., Carter, N., and Beauchamp, G., "Post-Impact Dynamics for Vehicles with a High Yaw Velocity," SAE Technical Paper 2016-01-1470, 2016, doi:10.4271/2016-10-1470.

29. Niederer, P., "Some Aspects of Motorcycle-Vehicle Collision Reconstruction," SAE Technical Paper 900750, 1990, doi:10.4271/900750.

30. Smith, J., Frank, T., Bosch, K., Fowler, G. et al., "Full-Scale Moving Motorcycle into Moving Car Crash Testing for Use in Safety Design and Accident Reconstruction," SAE Technical Paper 2012-01-0103, 2012, doi:10.4271/2012-01-0103.

31. Frank, T., Smith, J., Fowler, G., Carter, J. et al., "Simulating Moving Motorcycle to Moving Car Crashes," SAE Technical Paper 2012-01-0621, 2012, doi:10.4271/2012-01-0621.

32. Nieboer, J., Wismans, J., Versmissen, A., van Slagmaat, M. et al., "Motorcycle Crash Test Modelling," SAE Technical Paper 933133, 1993, doi:10.4271/933133.

33. Gabler, H.C., "The Emerging Risk of Fatal Motorcycle Crashes with Guardrails," January 2007, https://www.sbes.vt.edu/gabler/publications/TRB-07-3456-Motorcycles-Final.pdf.

34. Ibitoye, A.B., Radin, R.S., and Hamouda, A.M.S., "Roadside Barrier and Passive Safety of Motorcyclists Along Exclusive Motorcycle Lanes," *Journal of Engineering Science and Technology* 2, no. 1 (2007): 1-20.

35. Bambach, M.R., Grzebieta, R.H., and McIntosh, A.S., "Crash Characteristics of Motorcyclists Impacting Road Side Barriers," *2010 Australasian Road Safety Research, Policing and Education Conference*, Canberra, Australian Capital Territory, August 31-September 3, 2010.

36. Rizzi, M., Strandroth, J., Sternlund, S., Tingvall, C. et al., "Motorcycle Crashes into Road Barriers: The Role of Stability and Different Types of Barriers for Injury Outcome," *IRCOBI Conference 2012*, Dublin, Ireland, IRC-12-41.

37. Maza, M., Larriba, J., Juste-Lorente, O., and Lopez-Valdes, F.J., "Motorcyclists Crashes into Race Tracks and Normal Road Barriers: Kinematic Analysis and Correlation with Test Procedures," *IRCOBI Conference 2016*, Seoul, South Korea, IRC-16-103.

38. Berg, F.A. et al., "Motorcycle Impacts into Roadside Barriers – Real World Accident Studies, Crash Tests and Simulations Carried Out in Germany and Australia," *International Technical Conference on the Enhanced Safety of Vehicles*, Washington, DC, June 2005, Paper Number 05-0095.

39. Berg, F.A., Rücker, P., and König, J., "Motorcycle Crash Tests – An Overview," *International Journal of Crashworthiness* 10, no. 4 (2005): 327-339, doi:10.1533/ijcr.2005.0349.

Event Data Recorders in Motorcycle Accidents

9.1 Data from the Struck Vehicle

Crash data from passenger cars and heavy truck event data recorders (EDRs) are now well established and widely used in the industry. Currently, the EDR data most likely to aid a reconstructionist in analyzing a motorcycle crash will be data from the vehicle the motorcycle struck, since most motorcycles are not equipped with crash data recorders. Bortles [1] presented a comprehensive review of the literature related to the accuracy of the velocity change (ΔV) and pre-crash speed reported by original equipment (OEM) EDRs installed in passenger vehicles. Bortles reported that "event data recorders accurately measure and record the vehicle wheel (or transmission output) speed and integrated accelerations of the module. Reported values of vehicle velocity change (ΔV) and Pre-Crash vehicle speed tend to be less than the actual values…Analysts should consider event recorder data within the context of an accident reconstruction and account for factors that cause discrepancies between the reported and actual values."

In reaching these conclusions, Bortles and his colleagues compiled 187 sources of information, including peer-reviewed studies, textbooks, legal opinions, governmental rulemaking policies, industry publications, and presentations pertaining to EDRs. Sixty-four of those studies contained physical test data related to the accuracy of the EDR data. Of those 64 studies, 27 of them "contained paired data points from EDR and independent instrumentation suitable to validate the accuracy of ΔV and Pre-Crash vehicle speed… Of these 27 papers, there were nine that contained Pre-Crash data, nine that contained ΔV data and nine that contained both data types."

As Bortles noted, the speeds reported by passenger vehicle EDRs are typically measured by sensors monitoring the output of the transmission or an average of the speed of the drive wheels. While these sensors accurately report the speed they are measuring, during a crash, this speed does not necessarily correspond to the actual over-the-ground speed of the vehicle. For example, during a loss of control, the vehicle may develop a sideslip angle, where there is a discrepancy between the heading of the vehicle and the velocity direction. When this occurs, the EDR-reported speed will be the longitudinal component of the speed but not the total over-the-ground speed. Also, if the driver applies the brakes or the accelerator, longitudinal wheel slip may be induced that will cause there to be a difference between the wheel speed and the actual over-the-ground speed of the vehicle. Other possibilities include differences between the rolling radius of the OEM tires for a vehicle and the tires that are installed on the vehicle at the time of the crash and changes to the final drive ratio compared to the vehicle's original equipment. In addition to these causes, differences can also exist due to rounding, truncation, or unit conversion.

Bortles and his colleagues produced the graph of Figure 9.1 based on the studies they reviewed. In this graph, the actual pre-crash speed is plotted on the horizontal axis, and the vertical axis plots the difference between the EDR-measured pre-crash speed and the actual pre-crash speed based on other instrumentation. Positive values on the vertical axis represent the EDR overestimating the actual speed and negative values represent the EDR underestimating the actual speed. The data in the graph has been sorted by vehicle operational condition. Steady-state driving (designated with green circles) was found to be associated with minor speed differences and a tendency to underreport vehicle speed. Active braking was associated with greater underreporting and more variance in reported vehicle speed.

Heavy braking causes a discrepancy between the actual speed of the vehicle and the speed reported by the CDR, as shown in Figure 9.1. More broadly, anything that affects the rotational speed of the wheels can affect the speed reported by the CDR.

FIGURE 9.1 Differences between EDR-reported and actual pre-crash speeds in the studies reviewed by Bortles [1].

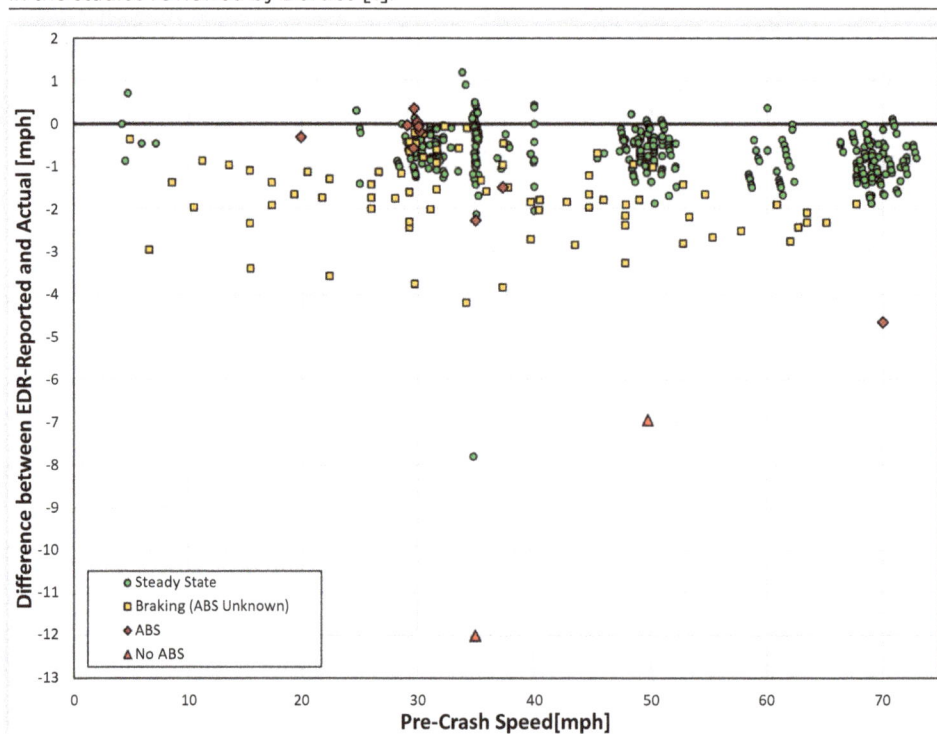

FIGURE 9.2 Differences between EDR-reported and actual ΔVs in the studies reviewed by Bortles [1].

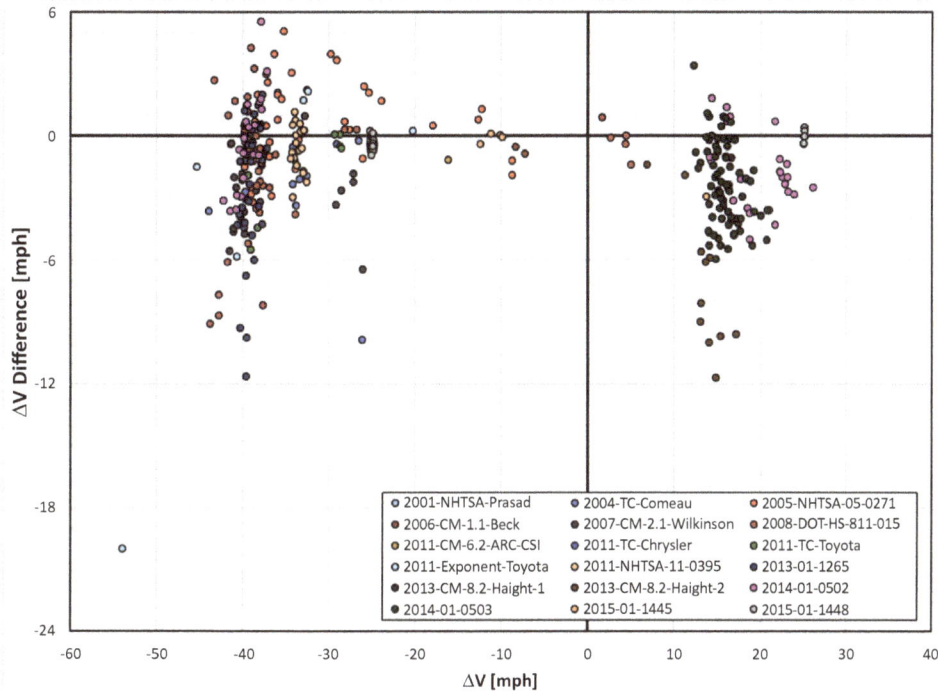

When a vehicle yaws and the tires generate a sideslip angle, the wheel speed will not be consistent with the over-the-ground speed of the vehicle. As an extreme example, if a vehicle is sliding perpendicular to its heading (a slip angle of 90°), the wheels will stop rotating. In this case, the CDR could report zero mph when the actual speed could be anything greater than zero. By measuring the wheel speeds or output speed of the transmission, the CDR is measuring the longitudinal speed of the vehicle.

Bortles and his colleagues also produced Figure 9.2, which contains data from 401 tests from 18 studies cited on the graph (refer to the Bortles article for these citations). The plot shows the difference between the EDR-reported ΔV values and the independently measured values for all tests and impact modes. The ΔVs are plotted in accordance with the SAE J1733 sign convention (frontal- and right-side impacts, negative, rear- and left-side impacts, positive).

As Bortles noted, much of the data in this graph was from tests conducted as a part of the National Highway Traffic Safety Administration's (NHTSA) New Car Assessment Program (NCAP)—35 mph frontal barrier crash tests, side moving barrier tests, and lateral pole tests. While informative, only 12 of the 401 tests plotted in this graph fall in the band of ΔVs between –10 and 10 mph. Given the large weight discrepancies that often exist between the motorcycle and the struck vehicle in motorcycle crashes, this is the region where the struck vehicle's ΔV would be likely to fall. The crash reconstruction literature would benefit from EDR studies specifically related to motorcycle crashes.

One such study was reported in 2006 by Beck [2]. He conducted three collinear impact tests in which a 2002 Chevrolet Cavalier was driven, braked, and then impacted a stationary, upright 1989 Kawasaki EX500 and 160 lb dummy. The weight ratio between the Chevrolet and Kawasaki was approximately 4.6:1. In the first test, the Chevrolet was driven and braked to an impact speed of approximately 12 mph. No event was recorded by the EDR in this impact. A second test was conducted at an impact speed of 27 mph and a non-deployment event was recovered by the EDR. In a third test, the speed of the Chevrolet at impact was approximately 37 mph and resulted in the recovery of a deployment event. Comparing the ΔV from the EDR to independent instrumentation, Beck found that the EDR underreported the actual ΔV by 0.53 mph (~6%) and 0.86 mph (~12%) for the second and third test.

EDR data from a vehicle struck by a motorcycle will clearly be useful in the investigation of a motorcycle crash, as was demonstrated in the previous chapter's analysis of the WREX2016 motorcycle-to-vehicle collisions. Still, there are issues that arise in the use of this data for analyzing motorcycle collisions that should be considered. For instance, as the tests reported by Severy, Brink, and Blaisdell in 1970 demonstrated, in a motorcycle-to-vehicle collision, there is a time delay between when the motorcycle strikes the vehicle and when the rider strikes the vehicle. In these tests, this delay ranged from 80 to 195 ms [3]. Depending on the recording interval of a particular EDR system, the system could fail to record the collision between the rider and the vehicle. In addition to that, the full weight of the rider may not participate in the collision. This will influence the analysis when the analyst uses the ΔV measured by the EDR to estimate the motorcycle impact speed. In such a case, the analyst will have to estimate the percentage of the rider weight that participates in the collision to accurately assess the motorcycle impact speed necessary to cause the reported ΔV of the struck vehicle. This assessment can be aided by consideration of other evidence—what gear the motorcycle was in or the magnitude of the translation and rotation experienced by the struck vehicle—since the calculated speed of the motorcycle would also need to be consistent with these other pieces of evidence.

9.1.1 Case Study: Utilizing EDR Data from the Struck Vehicle

This section describes the reconstruction of an intersection collision involving a motorcycle. EDR data from the sport utility vehicle that was struck by the motorcycle is incorporated into the reconstruction. This collision involved a motorcyclist riding eastbound through the subject intersection. The driver of a westbound SUV attempted to turn left to go southbound and the motorcycle struck the passenger's side rear of the SUV. The driver of the SUV stated that she did not see the motorcycle prior to initiating her turn on a yellow traffic signal. A witness who observed the motorcycle prior to the collision stated that the motorcyclist accelerated into the intersection to make it through on the yellow light. The speed limit for east-west traffic through the intersection was 60 mph. An investigating officer noted that sun glare could have been a factor contributing to the SUV driver not seeing the motorcyclist.

The photograph in Figure 9.3 depicts the motorcycle and the SUV at rest in the intersection following the collision. The photograph in Figure 9.4 also depicts the SUV at rest and shows the damage to the vehicle from the collision. The motorcycle struck and damaged the passenger's side rear of the SUV, directly contacting the rear wheel behind the axle. This caused the wheel to deform and rotate clockwise relative to the vehicle and the tire to go flat. The collision caused significant clockwise yaw rotation of the SUV, on the order of 180°, and the SUV deposited prominent tire marks between impact and rest. Figure 9.4 also shows that the front tires of the Ford are steered to the left following the collision.

The subject intersection was inspected, and its geometry mapped with a Faro Focus3D X 330 scanner. Some of the resulting scan data is depicted in Figure 9.5. The SUV was also inspected, and its post-collision geometry documented with the same scanner.

FIGURE 9.3 Motorcycle and SUV at rest in the intersection.

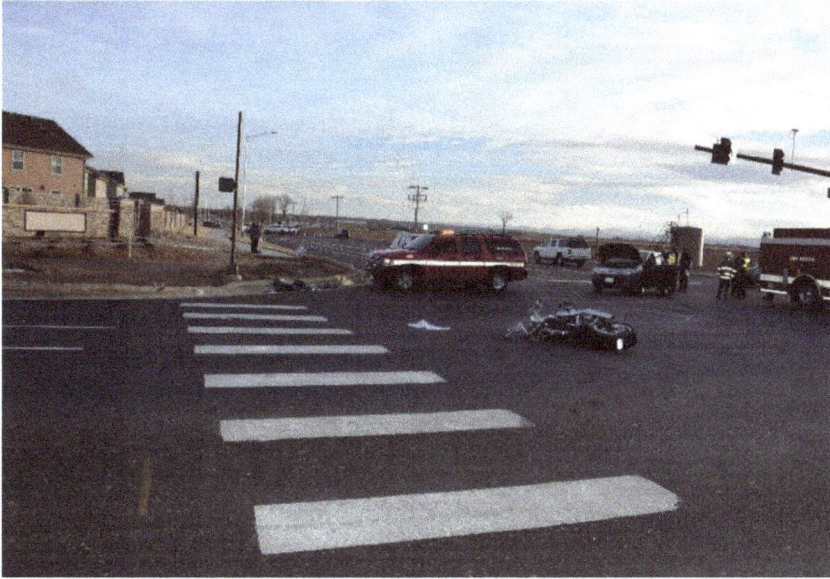

FIGURE 9.4 EDR-equipped SUV involved in the subject collision.

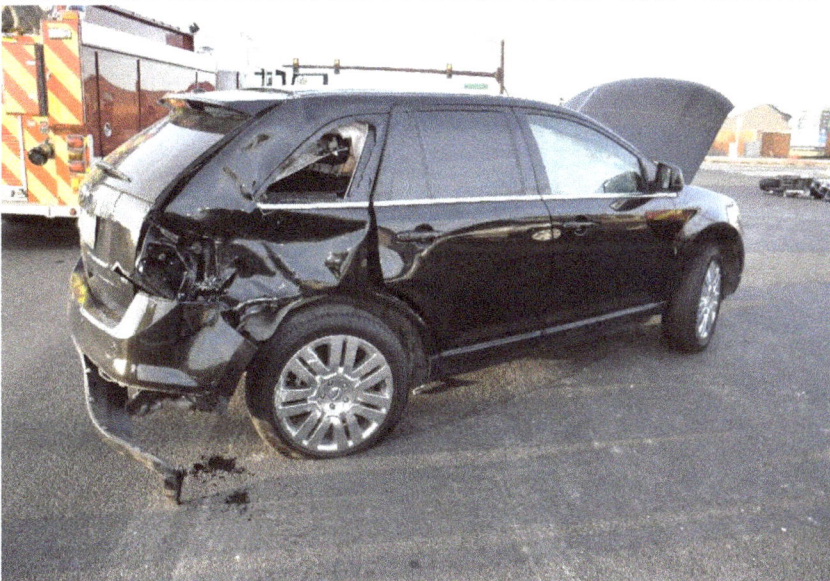

The resulting scan data for this vehicle is depicted in Figure 9.6. The clockwise rotation of the passenger's side rear wheel due to deformation was measured from this scan data at 17° relative to the vehicle. In the photographs of the SUV at rest in the intersection, the leftward steer angle of the right front wheel appears to be of greater magnitude than the 17° the right rear wheel was angled.

The Bosch Crash Data Retrieval system was used to image data from both the restraint control module (RCM) and the powertrain control module (PCM) on the SUV. Data from one event was recovered from the RCM-a side deployment event. The data indicated that the driver pretensioner and both the driver and passenger curtain airbags deployed 28 ms after the system began sensing the collision. The data also indicated that

FIGURE 9.5 Faro laser scan data for the accident site.

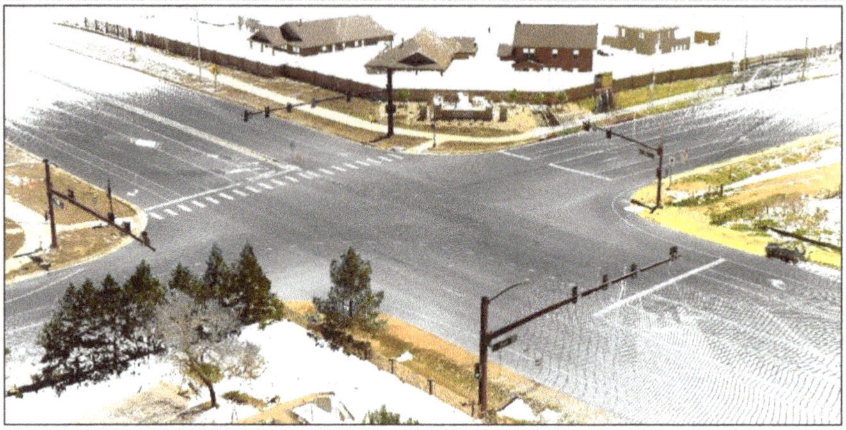

FIGURE 9.6 Faro laser scan data for the SUV.

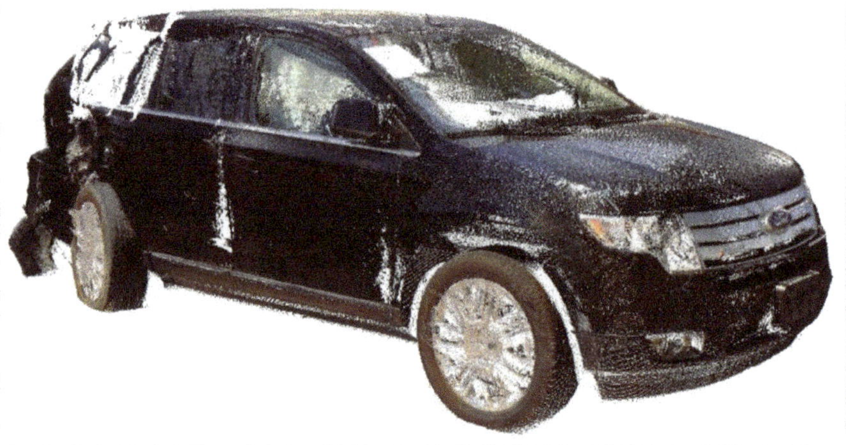

the driver, who was the sole occupant of the vehicle, was buckled at the time of the collision. The RCM data included pre-crash data at five indicated time intervals (−4 s, −3 s, −2 s, −1 s, and 0 s). This data is included in Table 9.1. Finally, the RCM data reported a lateral change in velocity of 2.49 mph. However, the reporting window for the lateral change in velocity was only 50 ms. Based on the timing reported in Table 8.2 for the crash tests reported by Severy, this recording window would be too short to capture the entire collision between the SUV and the motorcycle and certainly too short to capture the collision between the rider and the SUV. The graphical data for this lateral change in velocity is depicted in Figure 9.7. As this figure shows, the horizontal axis of the graph starts at −49 ms and goes to 0 ms. The first non-zero acceleration reading is at −28 ms. Given that the system reports that the curtain airbags deployed 28 ms after the collision began being sensed, it seems likely that, in this case, the EDR only reported the timeframe from the start of the collision until the deployment of these airbags.

Data was also recovered from the PCM on the SUV. The graphical data, which is depicted in Figure 9.8, included the vehicle indicated speed, the accelerator pedal percentage, brake switch status, antilock brake status, and engine rpms for 20 s prior to and 5 s after time zero. Tabular data was also reported for each of the variables included in the graph. In addition, the tabular data added transmission status (reverse or not reverse),

TABLE 9.1 Pre-crash data from the SUV's RCM

Pre-crash data (first record)					
Time (s)	-4	-3	-2	-1	0
Accelerator pedal position (%)	0	0	22	40	99
Vehicle speed (MPH [km/h])	6.0 [9.7]	3.2 [5.1]	4.1 [6.6]	10.8 [17.4]	17.3 [27.9]
ABS event in progress	No	No	No	No	No
ESP event in progress	No	No	No	No	No
TCS event in progress	No	No	No	No	No
Brake lamp switch depressed (from PCM)	Yes	Yes	No	No	No
RCM serial number received by OCS	No	No	No	No	No
OCS sensor status	Empty	Empty	Empty	Empty	Empty
OCS system level 1 fault	No	No	No	No	No
OCS system level 2 fault	No	No	No	No	No
Vehicle calibration ID	56	56	56	56	56
Vehicle model year calibration ID	07	07	07	07	07

FIGURE 9.7 Lateral velocity change data from the SUV's RCM.

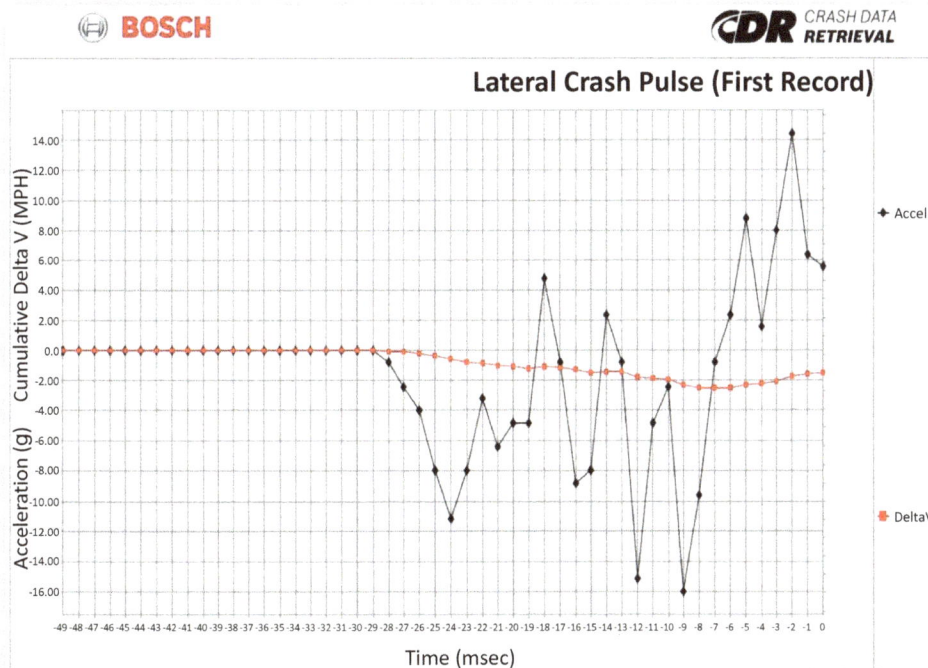

speed control status (on or off), traction control status (active or inactive), and stability control status (active or inactive). According to the data limitations in the CDR report, time zero corresponds to the time at which the PCM received a restraint deployment signal from the RCM. However, "The Restraint Deployment Signal (RDS) may not be recorded on the PCM immediately at impact. Time lags within the system may result in the Restraint Deployment Signal being recorded a few data samples after impact has occurred." The SUV was equipped with electronic stability control, and the tabular data from the PCM indicates that it was activated from +0.2 through +1.4 s. After that, it was inactive. The AdvanceTrac system utilizes the ABS system, and the data also reports the ABS system was active during the same timeframe.

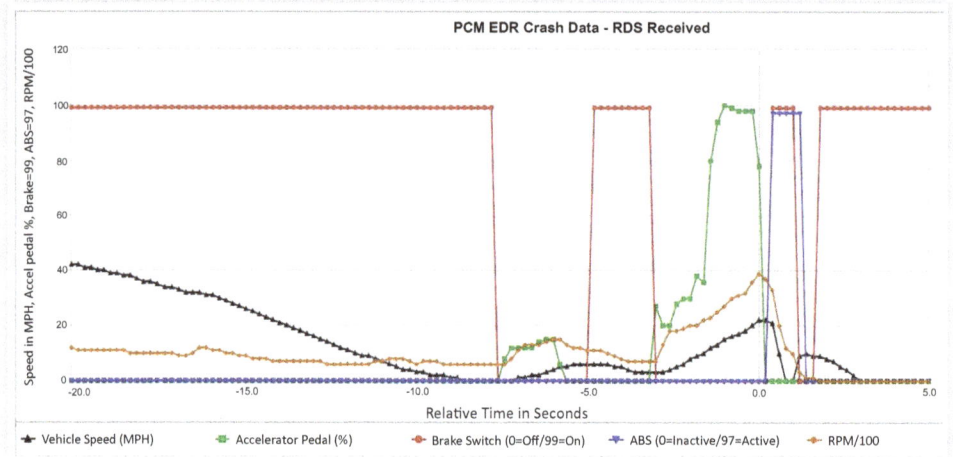

Arndt et al. [4] reported a study of the accuracy of the speeds reported by the PCM on a 2005 Ford Explorer during high slip angle maneuvers and during acceleration and braking. This test vehicle was equipped with electronic stability control (ESC) system. Tests were conducted with and without the ESC active. Arndt noted that "in testing with ESC enabled, speed error was associated with ESC intervention…A Ford PCM download which provides recorded speed every 0.2 seconds appears to provide enough data that an accurate speed trend can be discriminated." For the subject collision, ESC intervention *did* occur, but not until after the collision. The tabular data identifying this ESC intervention is included in Table 9.2. The second to last column states that the ESC was intervening from +0.2 to +1.4 s. Based on Arndt's results, there would likely be intervention-related error in the reported speeds during this timeframe. In addition to that error source, the significant yaw rate of the SUV following the collision would be expected to result in errors in the reported speeds because of the discrepancy between the heading and velocity directions of the vehicle.

That said, the speeds reported by the PCM prior to the collision are likely to be accurate. These speeds were recorded when the vehicle would have a low slip angle and when there was no ESC intervention. Ruth et al. [5] reported testing to evaluate the accuracy of PCM-reported speeds under steady-state conditions. They compared PCM-reported speeds to speeds measured with a 100 Hz VBOX and with a speed trap and found a maximum difference of 0.61 kph (0.38 mph).

The tabular data indicated that the speed of the SUV at time zero (the time of the restraint deployment signal) was 35 kph (21.7 mph). This data also indicated that the vehicle was accelerating in the seconds leading up to the collision. The data from the RCM, on the other hand, reported a speed at time zero of 27.9 kph (17.3 mph). This is 4.4 mph lower than the speed reported by the PCM for time 0. The RCM and the PCM are obtaining their speeds from the same sensor—a speed sensor on the transmission output shaft. However, they are sampling from this sensor at different rates. The PCM obtains a speed reading every 0.2 s, whereas the RCM obtains a reading every 1 s. The speed reported by the RCM for time 0 would simply be the last speed reading obtained by the RCM prior to the collision. Thus, the RCM did not capture the actual speed at the time of the collision; rather it captured a speed sometime in the 1 s time window preceding the collision. Looking at the tabular data from the PCM, the 17.3 mph speed reported by the RCM would have been measured sometime between −0.6 and −0.4 s in the PCM data. For the analysis reported here, the collision speed was estimated from the PCM data.

TABLE 9.2 Tabular data from the PCM showing ESC intervention

Buffer address (Hex)	Relative time (calc. seconds)	Transmission – reverse (reverse/ not reverse)	Speed control (on/off)	Engine RPM (RPM)	Engine output torque calculated (N-m)	Driveline output torque calculated (N-m)	Traction control (active/ inactive)	Stability control (active/ inactive)	Key on timer 63.75 max (s)
EA000290	−7.2	Not reverse	OFF	768	51	300	Not active	Not active	63.75
EA0002A0	−7.0	Not reverse	OFF	1113	71	434	Not active	Not active	63.75
EA0002B0	−6.8	Not reverse	OFF	1287	69	401	Not active	Not active	63.75
EA0002C0	−6.6	Not reverse	OFF	1301	58	316	Not active	Not active	63.75
EA0002D0	−6.4	Not reverse	OFF	1289	64	342	Not active	Not active	63.75
EA0002E0	−6.2	Not reverse	OFF	1385	84	448	Not active	Not active	63.75
EA0002F0	−6.0	Not reverse	OFF	1507	90	476	Not active	Not active	63.75
EA000300	−5.8	Not reverse	OFF	1485	81	386	Not active	Not active	63.75
EA000310	−5.6	Not reverse	OFF	1330	42	156	Not active	Not active	63.75
EA000320	−5.4	Not reverse	OFF	1205	36	124	Not active	Not active	63.75
EA000330	−5.2	Not reverse	OFF	1152	25	69	Not active	Not active	63.75
EA000340	−5.0	Not reverse	OFF	1138	25	69	Not active	Not active	63.75
EA000350	−4.8	Not reverse	OFF	1120	1	−31	Not active	Not active	63.75
EA000360	−4.6	Not reverse	OFF	1061	−5	−63	Not active	Not active	63.75
EA000370	−4.4	Not reverse	OFF	970	−8	−77	Not active	Not active	63.75
EA000380	−4.2	Not reverse	OFF	872	−2	−56	Not active	Not active	63.75
EA000390	−4.0	Not reverse	OFF	818	2	−33	Not active	Not active	63.75
EA0003A0	−3.8	Not reverse	OFF	728	5	−25	Not active	Not active	63.75
EA0003B0	−3.6	Not reverse	OFF	662	20	37	Not active	Not active	63.75
EA0003C0	−3.4	Not reverse	OFF	729	28	89	Not active	Not active	63.75
EA0003D0	−3.2	Not reverse	OFF	714	13	14	Not active	Not active	63.75
EA0003E0	−3.0	Not reverse	OFF	728	5	−37	Not active	Not active	63.75
EA0003F0	−2.8	Not reverse	OFF	1256	121	626	Not active	Not active	63.75
EA000400	−2.6	Not reverse	OFF	1755	133	752	Not active	Not active	63.75
EA000410	−2.4	Not reverse	OFF	1772	122	637	Not active	Not active	63.75
EA000420	−2.2	Not reverse	OFF	1946	173	893	Not active	Not active	63.75
EA000430	−2.0	Not reverse	OFF	1967	158	748	Not active	Not active	63.75
EA000440	−1.8	Not reverse	OFF	2015	166	751	Not active	Not active	63.75
EA000450	−1.6	Not reverse	OFF	2206	187	817	Not active	Not active	63.75
EA000460	−1.4	Not reverse	OFF	2348	191	801	Not active	Not active	63.75
EA000470	−1.2	Not reverse	OFF	2535	214	878	Not active	Not active	63.75

TABLE 9.2 (*Continued*) Tabular data from the PCM showing ESC intervention

Buffer address (Hex)	Relative time (calc. seconds)	Transmission - reverse (reverse/not reverse)	Speed control (on/off)	Engine RPM (RPM)	Engine output torque calculated (N-m)	Driveline output torque calculated (N-m)	Traction control (active/inactive)	Stability control (active/inactive)	Key on timer 63.75 max (s)
EA000480	−1.0	Not reverse	OFF	2744	216	884	Not active	Not active	63.75
EA000490	−0.8	Not reverse	OFF	2958	225	920	Not active	Not active	63.75
EA0004A0	−0.6	Not reverse	OFF	3086	226	927	Not active	Not active	63.75
EA0004B0	−0.4	Not reverse	OFF	3212	228	933	Not active	Not active	63.75
EA0004C0	−0.2	Not reverse	OFF	3629	234	961	Not active	Not active	63.75
EA0004D0	0.0	Not reverse	OFF	3858	242	991	Not active	Not active	63.75
EA0004E0	0.2	Not reverse	OFF	3725	218	889	Not active	Active	63.75
EA0004F0	0.4	Not reverse	OFF	3301	49	159	Not active	Active	63.75
EA000500	0.6	Not reverse	OFF	2039	92	241	Not active	Active	63.75
EA000510	0.8	Not reverse	OFF	1232	61	355	Not active	Active	63.75
EA000520	1.0	Not reverse	OFF	955	60	348	Not active	Active	63.75
EA000530	1.2	Not reverse	OFF	304	55	254	Not active	Active	63.75
EA000540	1.4	Not reverse	OFF	105	89	135	Not active	Active	63.75
EA000550	1.6	Not reverse	OFF	105	114	448	Not active	Not active	63.75
EA000560	1.8	Not reverse	OFF	0	142	1030	Not active	Not active	63.75
EA000570	2.0	Not reverse	OFF	0	117	828	Not active	Not active	63.75
EA000580	2.2	Not reverse	OFF	0	117	825	Not active	Not active	63.75
EA000590	2.4	Not reverse	OFF	0	117	841	Not active	Not active	63.75
EA0005A0	2.6	Not reverse	OFF	0	117	833	Not active	Not active	63.75
EA0005B0	2.8	Not reverse	OFF	0	117	824	Not active	Not active	63.75
EA0005C0	3.0	Not reverse	OFF	0	117	813	Not active	Not active	63.75
EA0005D0	3.2	Not reverse	OFF	0	117	813	Not active	Not active	63.75
EA0005E0	3.4	Not reverse	OFF	0	117	813	Not active	Not active	63.75
EA0005F0	3.6	Not reverse	OFF	0	117	813	Not active	Not active	63.75
EA000600	3.8	Not reverse	OFF	0	117	813	Not active	Not active	63.75
EA000610	4.0	Not reverse	OFF	0	117	813	Not active	Not active	63.75
EA000620	4.2	Not reverse	OFF	0	117	813	Not active	Not active	63.75
EA000630	4.4	Not reverse	OFF	0	117	813	Not active	Not active	63.75
EA000640	4.6	Not reverse	OFF	0	117	813	Not active	Not active	63.75
EA000650	4.8	Not reverse	OFF	0	117	813	Not active	Not active	63.75
EA000660	5.0	Not reverse	OFF	0	117	813	Not active	Not active	75

Camera-matching photogrammetry was utilized to locate the vehicle rest positions, tire marks from the SUV, and scrapes and gouges on the asphalt from the motorcycle. As was described in Chapter 5, camera matching involves reconstructing the location and characteristics of the camera that took the photograph being analyzed. Once the camera location and characteristics are obtained, physical evidence within the photograph can be located. This technique involves the following steps:

1. A photograph is selected for analysis.

2. The scene geometry depicted in the photograph is mapped.

3. The mapping data is imported into a computer modeling software package and viewed using a virtual camera with a vantage point similar to that shown in the photograph.

4. Lens distortion is removed from the photograph.

5. The corrected photograph is then imported into the modeling software and is designated as a background image for the virtual camera.

6. Adjustments are then made to the location, focal length, and viewing plane of the virtual camera until an overlay is achieved between the mapping data and the scene geometry shown in the photograph. Once a match is obtained, then the camera has been reconstructed.

7. Once the camera location and characteristics have been obtained, the evidence visible in the photograph can be located.

This process was carried out for several police photographs that depicted evidence related to the subject collision. A sample of these photogrammetry results is included in the following figures. Figure 9.9 is one of the police photographs that depicts the tire marks deposited by the SUV following the collision. Figure 9.10 shows the scan data from the accident site overlaid on this photograph, indicating that the camera location and characteristics have been reconstructed. Figure 9.11 shows the tire marks located and traced with dark blue outlines. A set of scrapes and gouges on the asphalt are also shown in this image (with light blue lines) that were traced from another police photograph that was also analyzed.

FIGURE 9.9 Police photograph selected for analysis.

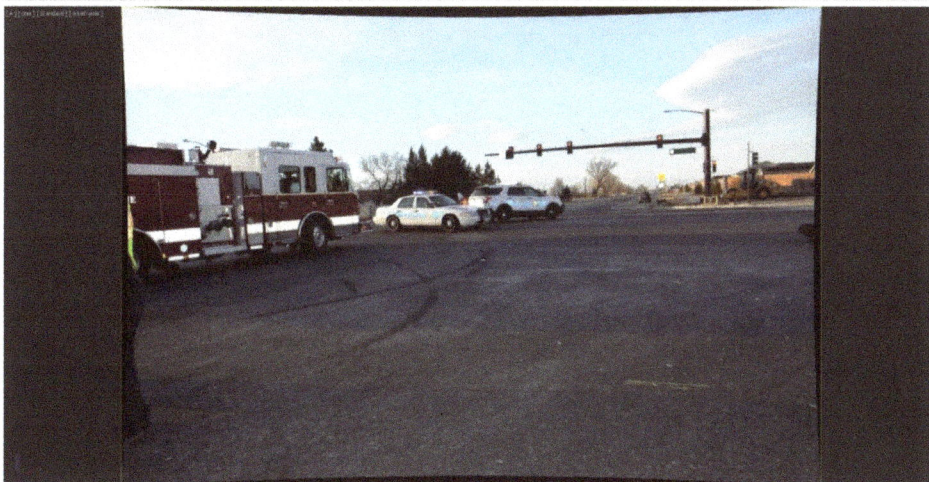

FIGURE 9.10   Scan data overlaid onto the police photograph via camera matching.

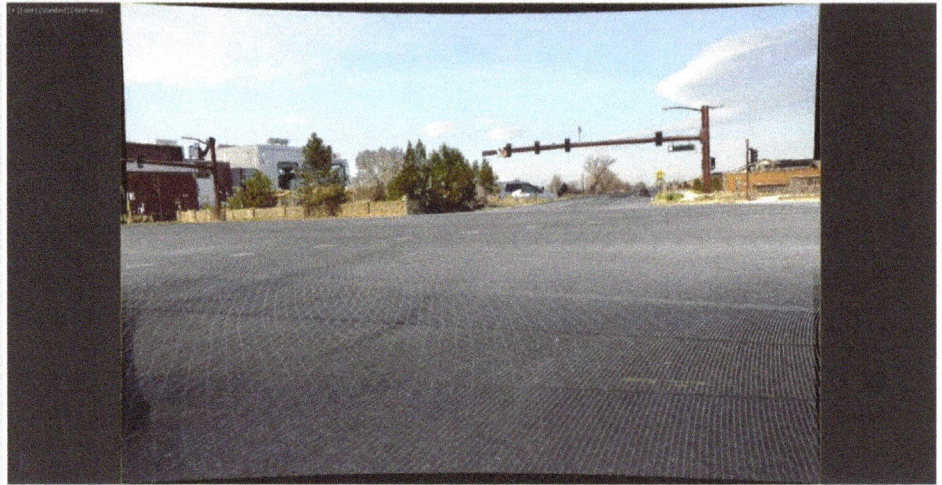

FIGURE 9.11   Physical evidence located in the photograph.

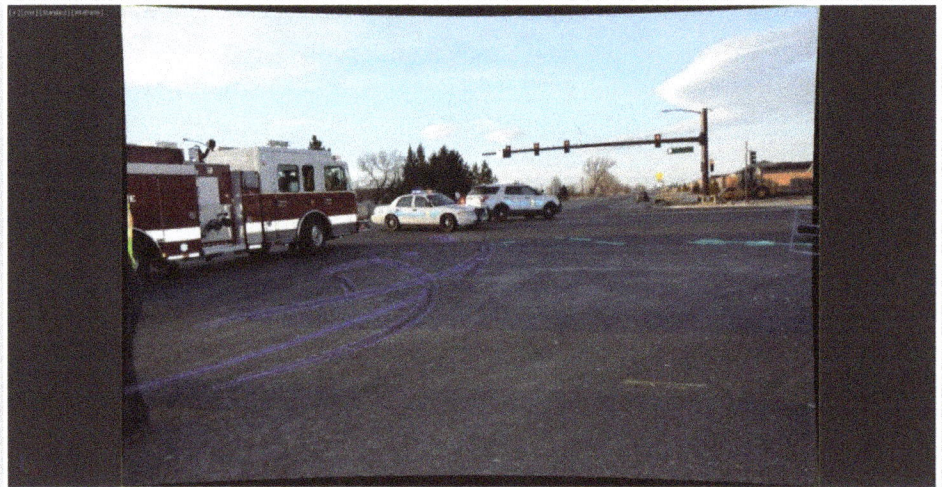

As Chapter 8 described, one indicator of a motorcycle's impact speed with a passenger vehicle is the magnitude of the translation and rotation experienced by the struck vehicle following the impact. PC-Crash simulation software was used to simulate the subject collision, specifically to determine the motorcycle impact speed necessary to cause the documented post-collision rotation of the SUV. In setting up this simulation, manufacturer specifications were obtained for each of the vehicles to obtain the geometric dimensions and weights. The SUV was equipped with a 3.5 L, V6 gasoline engine, an automatic transmission, all-wheel drive, antilock brakes, and ESC. Based on the manufacturer specifications for this vehicle, the weight at the time of the collision was estimated at 4385 lb, including the weight of the driver. The motorcycle was equipped with a 1584 cc V-Twin engine, a manual transmission, and a conventional braking system. The weight of the motorcycle at the time of the collision was approximately 714 lb, and the weight of the rider was approximately 170 lb. The rider's weight was included in the motorcycle's weight within the simulation.

In the simulation of this collision, the roadway coefficient of friction was set at 0.76, and the TM-Easy tire model was used with default values for both vehicles.

The integration time step was set at 5 ms. Because the motorcycle struck the passenger's side rear wheel of the SUV, the coefficient of restitution was set at 0.25, consistent with the coefficients of restitution for other wheel impacts reported in Chapter 8. Based on the EDR data, the impact speed of the SUV was initially set at 21.7 mph. Sequences in PC-Crash were used to steer the passenger's side rear wheel of the Ford 17° to the right immediately following the collision. The simulation was optimized using the impact speed of the motorcycle, the precise location of the collision on the roadway, the inter-vehicular friction, the impact center height, the steering angles of the front wheels, and the brake factors for each wheel. Small changes in the impact speed of the Ford were also utilized for the final step in the optimization. Consistent with the discussion in Chapter 8 and with the orientation of the front wheels of the Ford when it was at rest in the intersection, leftward steering inputs of 23° at the left front wheel and 19° at the right front wheel were ultimately utilized, developing over 2.3 s. The SUV was an all-wheel drive vehicle, and brake factors of 5% were used for the front wheels and the left rear wheel. A brake factor of 100% was used for the wheel that was struck and deformed by the motorcycle—the right rear wheel. The exception to these brake factors was during the interval of ESC intervention, during which a 100% brake factor was assigned to the left front wheel, and when the system indicated that the driver applied the brakes near the rest position. Brake factors were not applied to the wheels of the motorcycle because it fell on its side shortly after the collision. The coefficient of friction between the body of the motorcycle and the ground was set ultimately at 0.4, though this parameter was also iterated in optimizing the simulation.

Figure 9.12 is a screen capture from PC-Crash showing the final impact parameters and the motion of the vehicles following the collision. A high-quality match was obtained with the rest positions for both vehicles and the SUV's post-collision motion matched very well with the documented tire marks. The optimization process led to the conclusion that the motorcycle was traveling 69 mph at the time of the collision, 9 mph greater

FIGURE 9.12   Motion from optimized simulation.

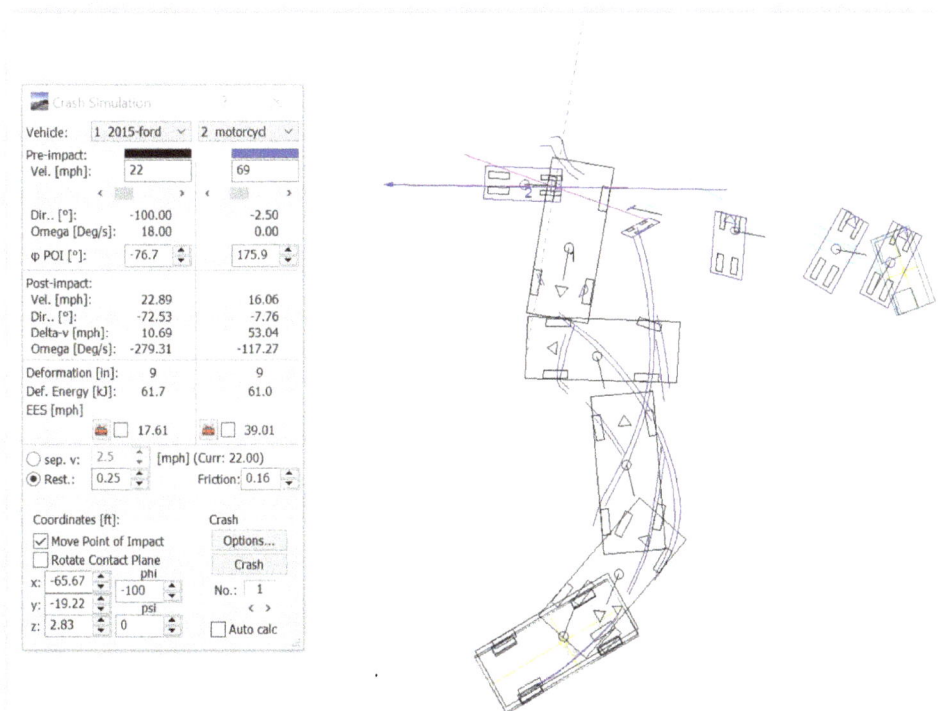

than the speed limit and consistent with the statement by a witness that the motorcyclist accelerated into the intersection in response to the yellow traffic signal. During the optimization process, it was recognized that the overall rotation of the Ford could be matched with a wide range of motorcycle impact speeds. However, the rate of rotation, as represented by the tire marks that were deposited, could only be matched with a narrow band of motorcycle impact speeds. In this case, a high-quality match was obtained with the motorcycle rest position, though the trajectory of the motorcycle was slightly below the documented scrapes and gouges. Such a quality match of the motorcycle's rest position would not be expected in every case, but often matching at least the postimpact velocity direction of the motorcycle will help with the simulation optimization.

The change in velocity calculated for the SUV in this simulation was 10.7 mph with a principal direction of force of 81°. Thus, the total lateral velocity change for the SUV was approximately 10.6 mph, 8.1 mph more than what was reported by the RCM. The simulation calculated a change in yaw rotational speed of the SUV of approximately 280° per second.

9.2 **Data from the Motorcycle**

For now, it is much less common to have EDR data from the motorcycle than from the struck vehicle, since most motorcycles do not have EDRs. Fatzinger [6] categorized the motorcycle EDRs that do exist into three groups: (1) those that give diagnostic codes, (2) those that log data for measuring performance, and (3) those that record crash-related data. The second and third categories have the greatest potential for use in crash reconstruction. That said, data from such systems is rarely available for now in a reconstruction context. As Fatzinger noted, performance data loggers have the limitation that they are typically only present and turned on in instances where the motorcycle operator has chosen this. EDRs that record crash-related data are currently installed on few motorcycles. As of 2017, Kawasaki was the only manufacturer including crash-sensing EDRs on their motorcycles and (at times) making the data available to crash reconstructionists. The owner's manual will typically specify whether a motorcycle is equipped with an EDR.

Fatzinger examined the EDR data on 2013-2016 Kawasaki Ninja 300 motorcycles. He noted that "a thorough research effort was conducted in order to establish methods for downloading EDR data, determining which data was recorded in collision events, validating its accuracy, and determining the triggering conditions." For the physical testing that Fatzinger conducted, he utilized a 2013 Ninja EX300A equipped with a Denso ECU. He was able to trigger EDR events by positioning the motorcycle in a rear wheel stand, idling the engine in sixth gear so that the rear wheel was spinning at approximately 16 mph, then "applying a hard brake application to stop the rear wheel and motor [and] then manually tilting the tip-over sensor…After learning how to trigger events, it was quickly discovered that the three EDR event locations in the ECU memory were all 'locked' events, or events that could not be overwritten. Once all three EDR event memory locations were full, no new EDR events could be recorded. The events were populated in chronological order 1-3, with Event 3 being the most recent." Fatzinger also discovered that "if the rear wheel speed gradually came to a stop, followed by an immediate tip-over, an EDR event was not recorded. It was apparent that a rear wheel deceleration rate threshold had to be exceeded in order to trigger an EDR event if the rear wheel stopped rotating before time zero (emergency engine shut-down)." He discovered that the braking deceleration threshold to trigger an event was approximately 0.6 g. Finally, "if the rear wheel was still moving at the time of emergency shut-down, an EDR event would always be triggered… at an indicated speed of approximately 2 mph or higher…Anything below this value would not trigger an EDR event." After generating events, Fatzinger accessed the following data for EDR events at a rate of 2 Hz: vehicle speed, gear position, inlet air temperature, coolant temperature, battery voltage, and diagnostic trouble codes. He accessed the following data at a rate of 10 Hz: throttle position, engine RPM, clutch in/out, fuel injector pulse, timing BTDC, and fuel cutout.

In another study, Fatzinger tested the EDR capabilities and behavior on Kawasaki Ninja ZX-6R and ZX-10R motorcycles [7]. Like the prior study, he reported that EDR recording would be triggered by activation of the tip-over sensor. Activation of this sensor also triggered the engine to shut off. Fatzinger reported that "an EDR event was only recorded if the motorcycle was commanded to shut-down by the tip-over sensor, and either had rear wheel movement at the time of shut-down or the rear wheel experienced a certain amount of deceleration in the several seconds prior to shut-down. The 'time zero' data element was synchronous with the tip-over commanded shut-down signal."

Peck [8] described several data loggers that fall in the category of those that log data for measuring performance. For instance, the Woolich Racing Log Box, installation of which requires some modification of the motorcycle's wiring system. This data logger can access a plethora of data from the motorcycle's ECU. The data available depends on the specific motorcycle but could include wheel speed, throttle position, brake switch status, transmission gear position, engine speed, and other potentially useful parameters. Captured data is stored on a micro SD card, allowing for straightforward retrieval.

The HP Race Datalogger is a similar device manufactured by BMW. This data logger can also record GPS data. This system can be plugged directly into the original wiring harness of certain BMWs, but the owner must choose to install the device. Some more technologically advanced motorcycles, such as Yamaha's 2015+ YZF-R1M, are equipped with GPS-enabled onboard data acquisition systems and can pair with smartphones and tablets. Peck recommended that reconstructionists be aware of the potential presence of such data and preserve any devices where it might be stored.

Peck reported testing focused on Ducati's data logger, the Ducati Data Analyzer (DDA). First introduced in 2007, the initial system was comprised of a single component resembling a USB drive, with the ability to log vehicle speed, engine speed (RPM), engine temperature, throttle aperture, gear position (calculated value), engine temperature, and total distance traveled. Ducati introduced a GPS-enabled version of the device in June 2012, which adds a GPS sensor (usually mounted behind the windscreen) to record vehicle position data. Peck reported testing of a 2008 Ducati 848 equipped with an early version of the DDA. He rode this motorcycle while collecting data with the DDA and with a VBOX Sport, a GPS data acquisition device with a sampling rate of 20 Hz (Racelogic, Farmington Hills, MI). He compared the data from these two devices.

After the test runs, the DDA was removed from the motorcycle and plugged into a laptop running a 32-bit version of Windows XP (required for this version of the DDA) for data download. To perform this operation, the *DDA Graphic Analyzer* application had to be installed. Peck noted that this software can be downloaded for free at dda. prosa.com. After retrieval, the data can be viewed using the same software. Once the DDA file is opened, there is a small icon beside each channel that gives the user the ability to examine several parameters of the data including the min, max, and average values. The sampling frequency is also reported. The frequency for each parameter is listed in Table 9.3. The DDA software package does not have the ability to export the recorded data into a text format, as would be convenient for analysis in a spreadsheet program like Microsoft's Excel. As such, an application called *DDA Converter* (Version 1.5.0), designed for use with Droid devices, was utilized for conversion. Data acquired using the VBOX Sport was exported to text format using the manufacturer's PerformanceBox Tools software package (Version 1.8.2, Build 012). Upon exportation,

TABLE 9.3 Sampling frequency and precision for each parameter captured by the DDA system

Parameter	Frequency (Hz)	Precision
Speed	10	0.25 kph
Engine speed	50	1 RPM
Throttle aperture	20	1%
Gear position	10	1
Engine temp.	1	0.2°F
Tot. distance trav.	1	1 km

the DDA data was then compared to the VBOX data in Excel. Five runs were performed on relatively urban streets with traffic signals, stop signs, and elevation changes.

Peck concluded that the vehicle speeds reported by the DDA were accurate and aligned well to those reported by the VBOX Sport. When the rear wheel of the Ducati was locked by applying the rear brake, there was a notable discontinuity in the speed trace reported by the DDA, as was expected. When such a discontinuity is observed, the analyst should be alerted to the possibility that the front or rear brake of the motorcycle was locked during the collision sequence. Of course, physical evidence should be analyzed to corroborate any suspicion of a locked wheel. When the rear tire was locked via braking, there was a sudden, noticeable drop in the reported vehicle speed. However, the speed did not drop to zero as might be expected if the system was simply monitoring the rear wheel speed. Nor did the speed drop to half of the actual speed, as might be expected if the system was monitoring both front and rear wheel speeds.

9.2.1 Case Study: Video as a Source of Data from the Motorcycle

Video from a camera on a motorcyclist's helmet or chest, or surveillance footage from a security camera on a nearby business, can be another source of data about the events leading to a collision. For example, the images included in Figure 9.13 are several frames of footage from a GoPro camera attached to a motorcyclist's helmet. These frames depict a straight truck turning left in front of the motorcyclist. This resulted in a collision with the motorcyclist. The frames from this GoPro camera could be used, in conjunction with measurements from the accident site and vehicle dimensions to determine the speeds of the motorcycle and the straight truck and the timing of the straight truck's turn.

Following are a series of observations related to the analysis of videos like this one. These observations may assist a reconstructionist as they incorporate such video evidence into a reconstruction:

- The view of a camera will have a limit. Keep in mind that there will always be what the camera does show and what it does not. A complete reconstruction may require knowledge of more than what is captured within the viewing area of the camera, and so, additional information may need to be obtained from physical evidence, principles of physics, or electronic data. In the example covered here, the camera shows the motion of the straight truck from the vantage point of the motorcyclist but not the motion of the motorcyclist from the vantage point of the truck driver.

- A camera captures a finite number of frames in any given second. Just as there is motion that occurs outside the view of the camera, there is also motion that can occur between frames and during the time an image is being captured. There can also be uncertainty about the precise time between frames.

- Each of the images contained within a video is likely to have lens distortion that may need to be removed for analysis. This distortion will be the same across a series of frames captured with a single camera, lens, and focal length.

- Video analysis will often need to determine the position and motion (translation, rotation, and zooming) of the camera before the motion of objects within the video can be quantified. For a static camera, this process is simplified.

FIGURE 9.13   Video frames from GoPro camera on motorcyclist's helmet.

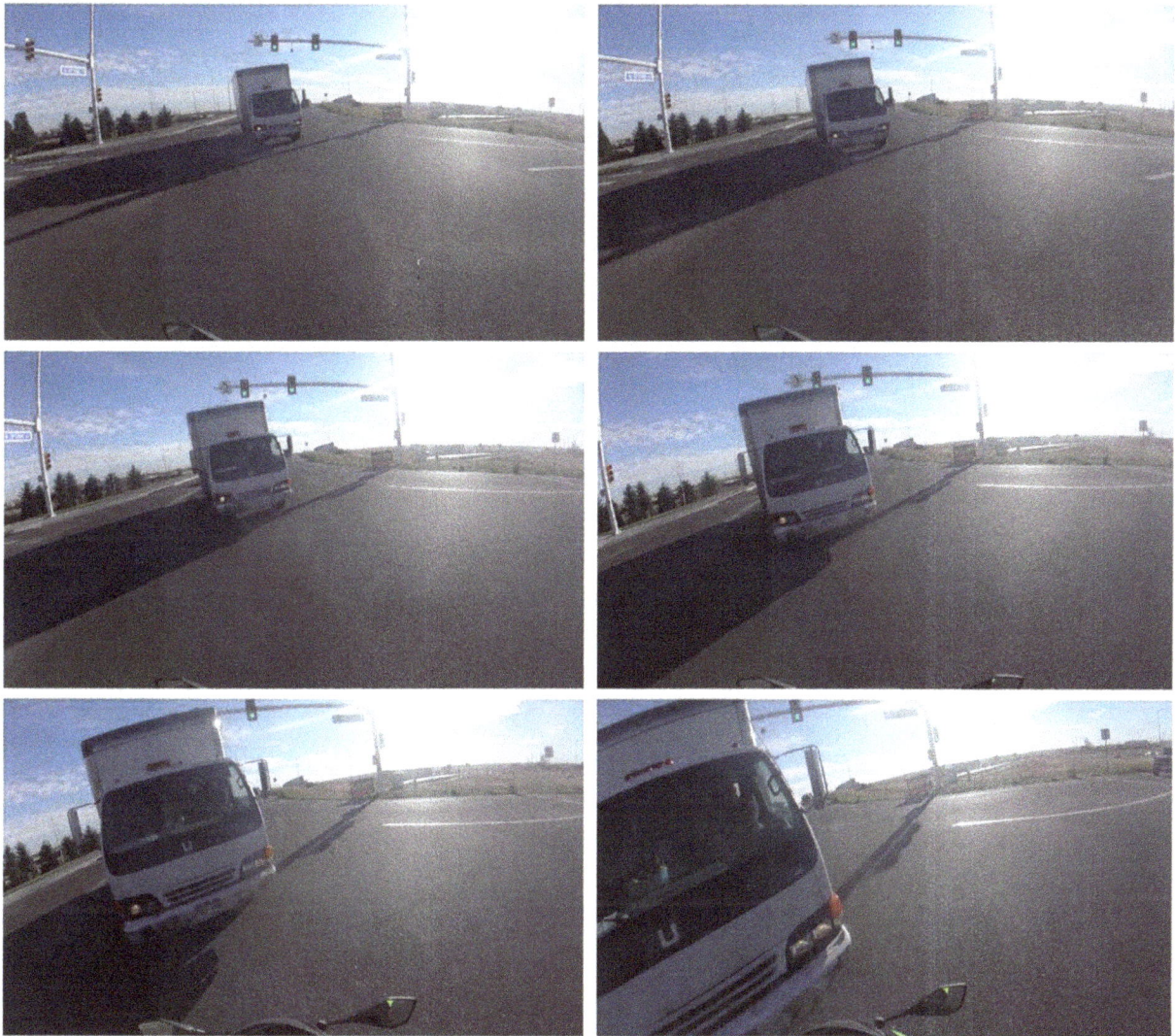

- There will be uncertainty in the reconstructed translation, rotation, and zooming of a camera. There will also be uncertainty in the reconstructed position and orientation of objects within a video frame.

- Some objects depicted by a video frame may be out of focus (blurry). Post-processing of the images cannot bring out-of-focus objects into focus. Blurriness can lead to uncertainty in determining the position of the camera, determining the position and orientation of objects depicted in a frame, and tracking the motion of objects across a series of frames.

- Post-processing can alter the brightness, contrast, and color balance of a video image. That may make the position and orientation of objects within the image more distinct.

- Video analysis results should be consistent with the physical limitations on the motion of objects in the real world. For example, there are limits on the rate at which vehicles can accelerate or decelerate in the real world. If video analysis produces unrealistic results, the source will be an inaccuracy in the calculated position of the tracked object, the frame rate of the video, or both.

References

1. Bortles, W., Biever, W., Carter, N., and Smith, C., "A Compendium of Passenger Vehicle Event Data Recorder Literature and Analysis of Validation Studies," SAE Technical Paper 2016-01-1497, 2016, doi:10.4271/2016-01-1497.

2. Beck, R., Casteel, D., Phillips, E. et al., "Motorcycle Collinear Collisions Involving Motor Vehicles Equipped with Event Data Recorders," *Collision* 1, no. 1 (2006): 82-96, ISSN: 1934-8681.

3. Severy, D., Brink, H., and Blaisdell, D., "Motorcycle Collision Experiments," SAE Technical Paper 700897, 1970, doi:10.4271/700897.

4. Arndt, M.W., Rosenfield, M., Stevens, D., and Arndt, S., "Test Results: Ford PCM Downloads Compared to Instrumented Vehicle Response in High Slip Angle Turning and Other Dynamic Maneuvers," SAE Technical Paper 2009-01-0882, 2009, doi:10.4271/2009-01-0882.

5. Ruth, R.R., West, O., Engle, J., and Reust, T.J., "Accuracy of Powertrain Control Module (PCM) Event Data Recorders," SAE Technical Paper 2008-01-0162, 2008, doi:10.4271/2008-01-0162.

6. Fatzinger, E. and Landerville, J., "An Analysis of EDR Data in Kawasaki Ninja 300 (EX300) Motorcycles," SAE Technical Paper 2017-01-1436, 2017, doi:10.4271/2017-01-1436.

7. Fatzinger, E., "An Analysis of EDR Data in Kawasaki Ninja ZX-6R and ZX-10R Motorcycles Equipped with ABS (KIBS) and Traction Control (KTRC)," SAE Technical Paper 2018-01-1443, 2018, doi:10.4271/2018-01-1443.

8. Peck, L.R., "Exploration and Validation of the Ducati Data Analyzer (DDA)," *Accident Reconstruction Journal* 28, no. 1 (January/February 2018), ISSN: 1057-8153.

10

Motorcycle Visibility and Conspicuity

This chapter describes and illustrates physical factors related to the motorcycle, rider, and the roadway environment that can influence motorcycle visibility and conspicuity. Some of these factors are a consequence of the motorcycle's unique shape, size, design, and operation and can result in visibility issues that differ from passenger cars. For instance, the motorcycle is narrower than other vehicles and has a significantly different headlamp and signal lighting design and configuration. Other physical factors are related to the roadway and its environment. For instance, foliage, signage, power poles, bridge columns, or other structures can influence the visibility and conspicuity of a motorcycle. The geometry of the roadway may also play a role in visibility, particularly when there are curves and hill crests present. Curves and hill crests can create geometrical obstructions to line of sight between a rider and other vehicles.

In addition to these physical properties, there are also operator decisions that can affect visibility. For instance, a motorcycle can occupy different positions within a lane that can affect both the operator's visibility of other traffic, as well as the ability for other traffic to see the motorcyclist. Additionally, movement of the motorcycle and brake lamp actuation are other techniques used in motorcycle riding that are unique and can impact sight lines, conspicuity, and visibility. Motorcycle visibility and conspicuity are presented here from both the perspective of the motorcycle operator as well as from the perspective of other drivers on the roadway. The role any of these factors play in a crash would need to be examined on a case-by-case basis. Whether a motorcycle is visible or conspicuous may be determined by decisions, or lack thereof, by either the motorcyclist, the vehicle that the motorcyclist encounters, or a combination of both. The factors in this chapter point to a line of inquiry for a reconstructionist that can be examined to help determine the role of visibility in a crash.

10.1 **Physical Factors Affecting Visibility**

10.1.1 **The Shape and Size of the Motorcycle**

Motorcycles are thin and small compared to passenger vehicles (Figure 10.1), making motorcycles potentially harder to see than larger vehicles, day or night. Unlike passenger cars, which feature strong outlines in its shape and large painted surfaces, a motorcycle, when viewed from the front, has small surfaces and small parts, often not of high contrast in color or material. A passenger car has contrasting enclosures such as the grill and headlamps that further make the car easier to see as these elements provide contrasting surfaces to the remaining painted panels. A motorcycle has little surface area to provide similar contrast beyond the clothing worn by the operator. However, there is not a specific clothing color that provides contrast in all conditions, since the ability for the clothing to be contrasting depends on the background environment, the lighting in the foreground and background, and the material properties of the clothing. Black clothing may have high contrast during the day against some backgrounds but low contrast at night in the same environment. The size, shape, color, and contrast of the motorcycle and rider can affect the driver's ability to detect a motorcycle. Even if the motorcycle and rider are visible, its relative size and shape may affect the driver's perception of the speed and position of the approaching motorcycle. Larger objects appear to expand in one's field of view from a farther distance away than smaller objects. This phenomenon, referred to as looming (subtended angular velocity), creates a disadvantage to the motorcyclist since the motorcyclist must be closer to the viewer before the viewer can judge its approach speed.

10.1.2 **Foliage, Signage, and Other Environmental Elements**

At intersections, roadside geometry such as power poles, signs, and foliage may exist that can play a role in the visibility of a motorcycle. As an example, consider the three photographs of Figure 10.2. Each of these photographs shows the view to the left from a different vantage point at an intersection. Each of these views represents a possible stopping position and vantage point for a passenger car driver intending to make a left turn at this intersection across the path of an approaching motorcycle. Depending on

FIGURE 10.1 Relative size of a typical motorcycle to a typical passenger vehicle.

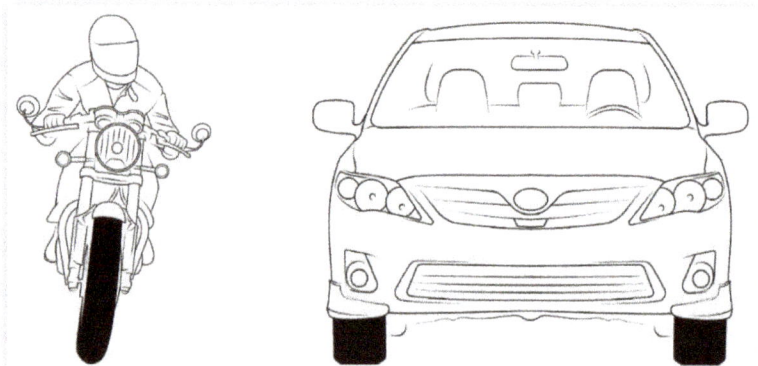

FIGURE 10.2 View of the oncoming traffic lane from three different vantage points at an intersection.

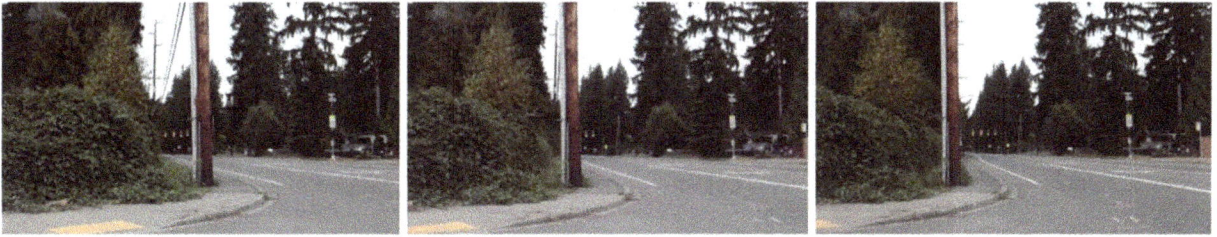

where the driver chooses to stop, the bushes and utility pole would have varying influences on what the driver is able to see. If the driver chose to initiate their turn from the first position, they would be doing so with a much more restricted view of the approaching traffic than the view afforded them by the third position.

Another example of the occlusion that power poles and trees can cause with motorcycles is shown in Figure 10.3. The first three images of this figure show a white passenger vehicle traveling behind the power pole. Because of the size of the vehicle, the pole only partially occludes the view of the car. The next three images show a motorcycle passing behind the same pole. Because the motorcycle is smaller than the passenger car, there is a timeframe during which the motorcycle becomes entirely occluded by the pole. How long the motorcycle is occluded and the degree to which this occlusion may play a role in a crash will depend on several factors, including the speed of the motorcycle, the relative position between the pole, the viewer and the motorcycle, and when and for how long the driver is looking in the direction of the approaching motorcycle. Some of these factors can be assessed during reconstruction of the crash. Other factors, like how long a driver may be looking in a particular direction, may require testimonial support or an assumption of ranges and values for glance times based on research of typical drivers.

When reconstructing a crash where a geometric obstruction may have influenced the visibility of a motorcyclist, on-site photography and testing can be performed. Scaled diagrams can also be used to analyze and illustrate the influence that various objects have on the view available to the driver. Figure 10.4 shows an example of such diagrams. In these graphics, visibility cones have been created to show the influence of the utility

FIGURE 10.3 Occlusion of a passenger car and a motorcycle by a power pole.

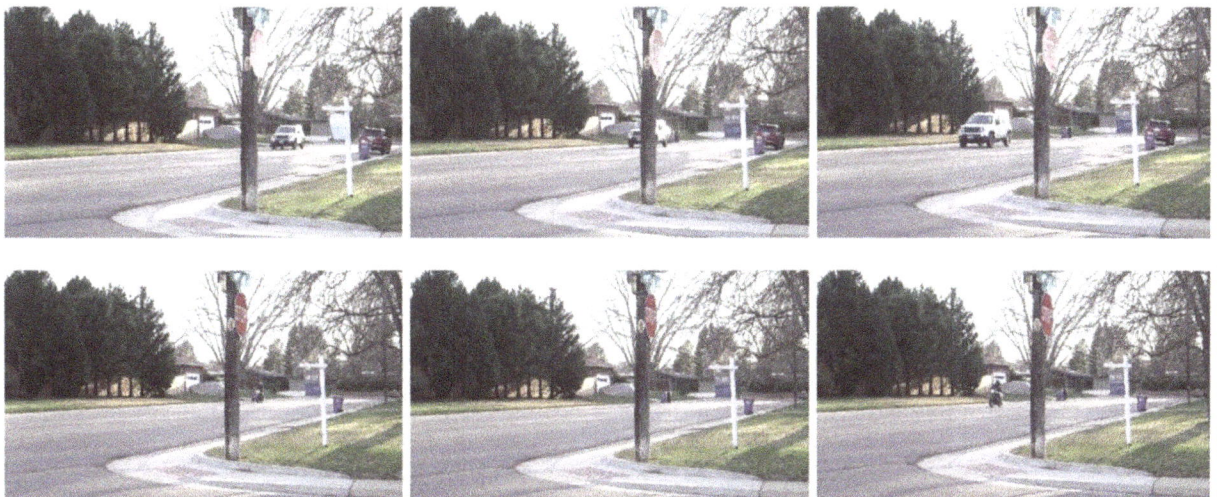

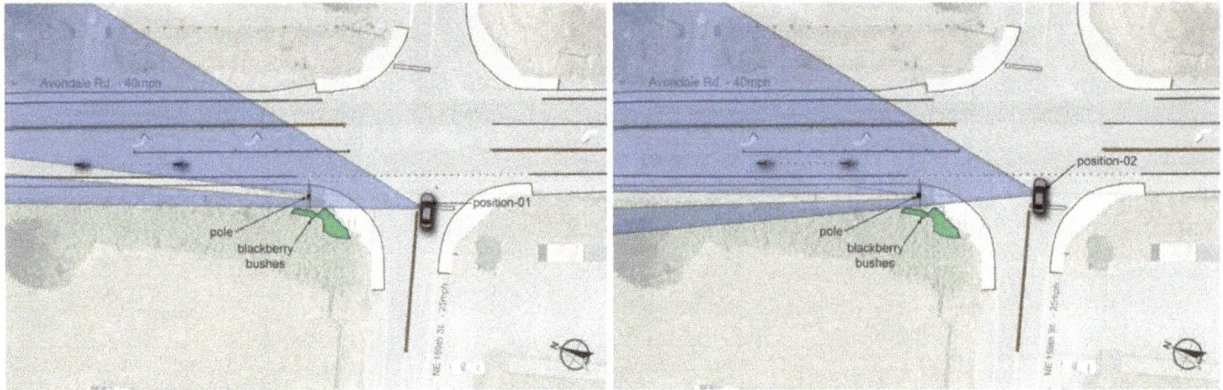

pole and bushes on the driver's view from two different vantage points at the same intersection. This type of graphical demonstrative can be helpful since positions and distances can easily be measured and used in further reconstruction analysis.

Roadway geometry can also affect the ability of car drivers and motorcycle riders to see other traffic and objects. The shape of the roadway and its crests, curvatures, and elevations can create visual obstruction contributing to a motorcycle being fully or partially occluded. In some instances, the motorcycle may be out of view during the moment when a driver is deciding whether or not to change lanes or cross the path of oncoming traffic. Often, the influence of a particular roadway or environmental issue will depend on the speeds of the vehicles and on their relative positions, and therefore, assessment of the role any roadway or environmental factor plays in a crash would depend on the specific time and space relationships of the vehicles relevant in the reconstruction. A geometrical obstruction that prevents one driver from seeing another may provide a physical explanation, but does not necessarily excuse a driver's responsibility to see the vehicle, as this will depend on many other factors, and would need to be assessed on a case-by-case basis.

10.1.3 Visibility over Hill Crests

The geometry of a hillcrest can create visual occlusions, limiting visibility for drivers on either side of the crest. During the day, for passenger cars and trucks, it is typically their roof line and windshield that first emerges over the hillcrest. Due to a lack of contrast at night, this part of the vehicle may not be visible, and it may not be until the headlamps emerge that the vehicle is visible and conspicuous. For a motorcycle, it is the head or helmet of the operator that is typically the first object to emerge over the crest of the hill. Due to its size, shape, color, and relationship to the background, a motorcycle may be less conspicuous than a passenger car. Since most motorcycles have headlamps that are on during both the day and night, when the headlamp emerges over the hill crest, it may increase the conspicuity of the motorcycle. The images in Figure 10.5 demonstrate the effect that a hillcrest has on visibility for both a passenger car and a motorcycle.

At night, the relationship between vehicles and their background may create a low-contrast situation. In this condition, the color and darkness of the vehicle and the color and darkness of the background may create a situation where the vehicles are difficult to see. This lack of contrast is compounded by the brightness of the headlamp and potential glare that it can cause. In addition, at night, motorcycles and passenger cars would likely have their headlamps on. For the car, this means that the two front headlamps may be the first objects visible cresting the hill, and for motorcycles with a single

FIGURE 10.5 Passenger car and motorcycle cresting a hill—daytime.

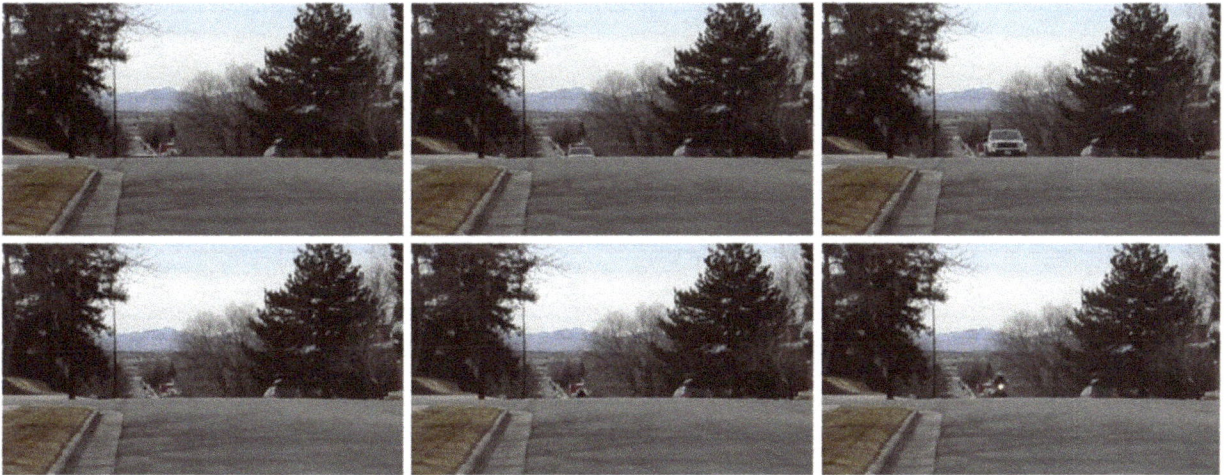

FIGURE 10.6 Passenger car and motorcycle cresting a hill—nighttime.

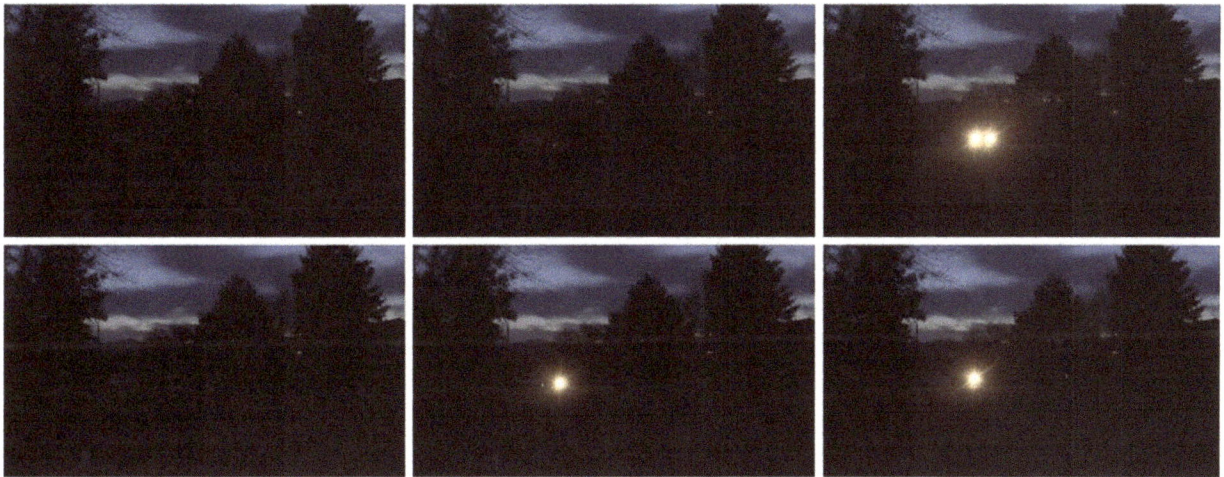

front headlamp, this too would be the first visible object over the crest. This is illustrated in the images of Figure 10.6.

For a nighttime situation, testing can be performed at a site (as shown in the images of Figure 10.6), and the point at which the headlamp becomes visible can be measured from the point of observation. Another method involves geometrically measuring the effect of the hillcrest with a diagram or computer model. This will often involve conducting a site inspection to measure the geometry of the hillcrest. For this analysis, the measurement should be taken from the eye height of the point of observation to the top portion of the headlamp assembly, as this constitutes the first area of the headlamps that would become visible.

As the vehicle crests the hill, it is unlikely that the headlamps will create a visible beam pattern on the roadway or illuminate the surrounding environment from the perspective of the viewer. Headlamps are designed primarily to illuminate the roadway for the driver, and so for observers facing the oncoming vehicle, it is the headlamps themselves that will be visible to the observer, not the illumination of the roadway or environment by the headlamps. This is illustrated in the photographs of Figure 10.7.

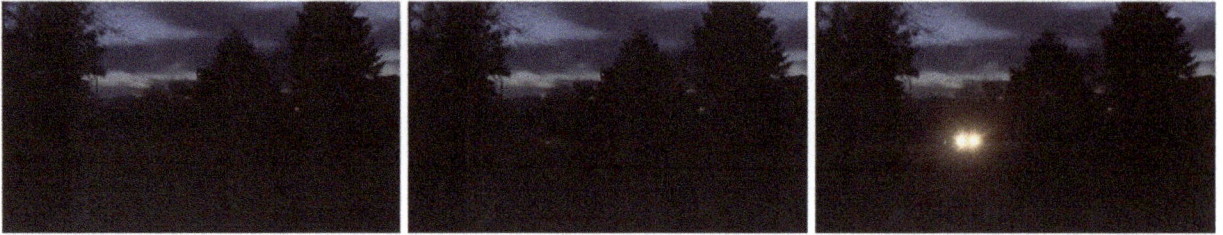

10.1.4 Visibility around a Corner

Curves or corners in the roadway may affect the visibility between a motorcycle and other traffic or of objects in the roadway ahead. The effect of a curve on visibility depends on the radius of curve, the position of the motorcycle as it traverses the corner, and the environment on either side of the shoulder. Environmental conditions such as boulders, trees, shrubbery, and roadway signage can influence the visibility. In the *MSF's Basic RiderCourse Handbook* (Edition 1), two different techniques for negotiating a curve are discussed:

> *...you could use a general strategy of middle-middle-middle: middle on entry, middle at the apex, and middle at the exit, as this provides space on both sides within your lane throughout the curve. Or you could use a performance-type strategy of outside-inside-outside that reduces the lean required and allows you to see farther through the curve, but gets you closer to the center line and the shoulder. For any strategy you use, having a good entry speed is crucial so you do not have to make any major speed or lane position adjustments in the curve.*

Figure 10.8 demonstrates this general concept of how different lane positions influence visibility. In this example, the position of the motorcycle to the left in the lane has a different line of sight than when positioned on the right side of the lane.

FIGURE 10.8   Influence of motorcycle lane position on visibility around a curve.

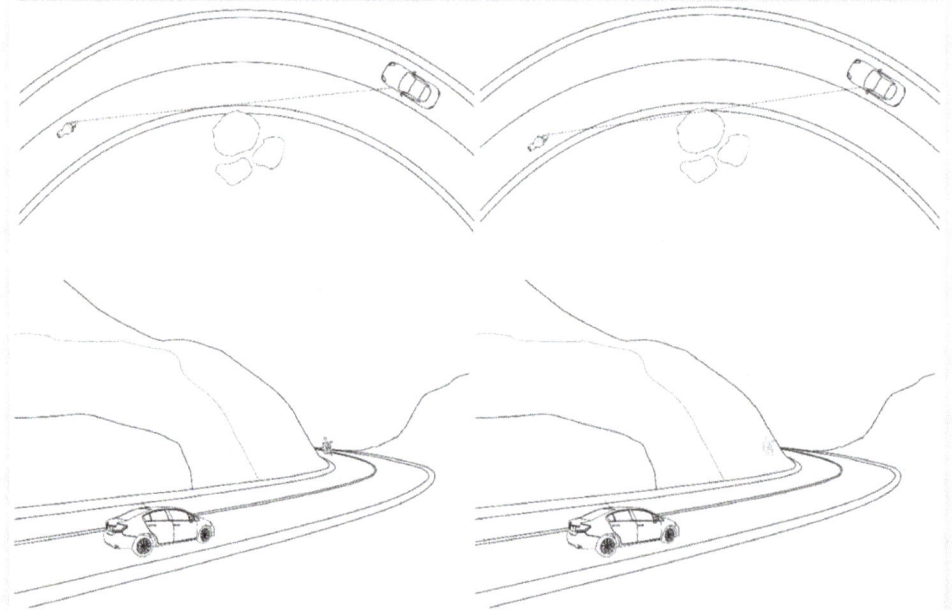

10.2 **Motorcycle Operation That Affects Visibility**

FIGURE 10.9 Lane positions available to motorcyclists.

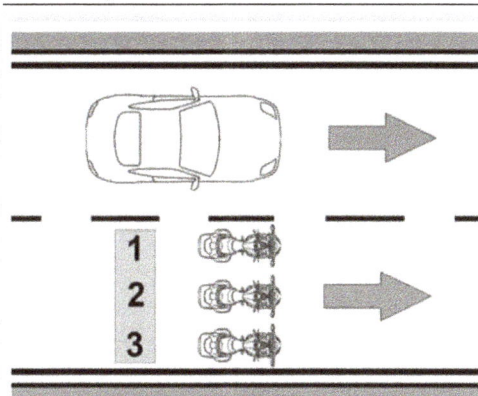

There are specific strategies that can be employed in the operation of a motorcycle to increase visibility. However, it is important to note that, in some circumstance, these strategies may compete with safe riding. For instance, one lane position may be more beneficial for the visibility of the motorcycle to other traffic, while a different lane position has better pavement conditions. Choosing a strategy to increase visibility also does not guarantee visibility, since the motorcyclist is dependent on other drivers to see them.

10.2.1 **Lane Position**

The ability of a motorcyclist to choose different positions within a single lane is unique to a motorcycle and stems from the narrow width of a motorcycle (Figure 10.9). A single lane of travel has three sections (left, middle, or right side) within which the motorcycle can travel. A motorcyclist's lane position can vary throughout their ride, depending on any number of factors, including roadway conditions, traffic conditions, rider skills and comfort level, presence of other riders, and the weather. Roadway conditions may include irregularities, cracks, potholes, and debris that make one lane position more advantageous than another. During inclement weather, certain parts of the lane may be more susceptible to oil and, therefore, have a slippery surface that should be avoided. Traffic patterns, too, can affect the lane position, as certain positions increase or decrease the visibility that a motorcyclist has of others and increase or decrease the ability of other motorists to see the motorcyclist.

Figure 10.10 illustrates the influence of lane position on the distance at which another motorist could see a motorcycle. In the image on the left, the motorcycle occupies the left side of the lane. In the image on the right, the motorcycle occupies the right side of the lane. These images illustrate that the motorcyclist becomes geometrically visible to the driver of the passenger car sooner when positioned to the left in the lane. The specific visibility distances could also be influenced by where the driver decides to stop.

FIGURE 10.10 Lane position and sight distance with a geometrical obstruction.

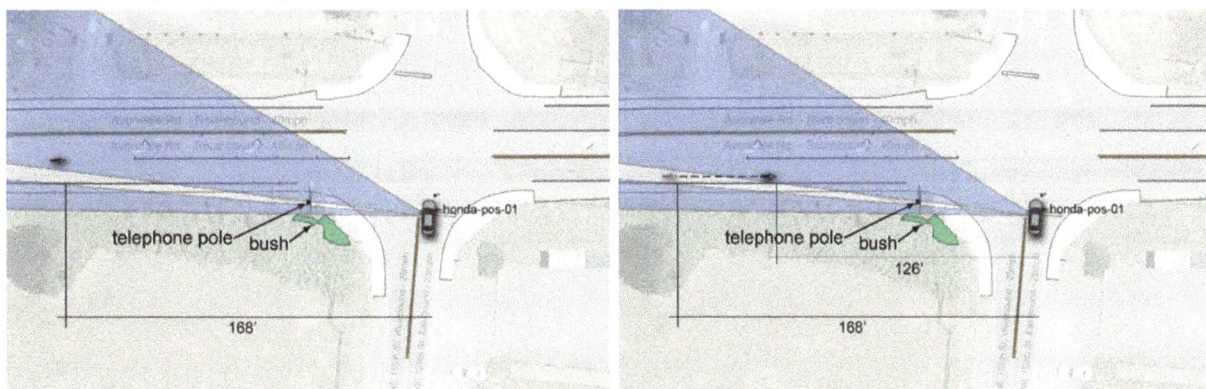

FIGURE 10.11 Motorcyclist moving side-to-side in the lane.

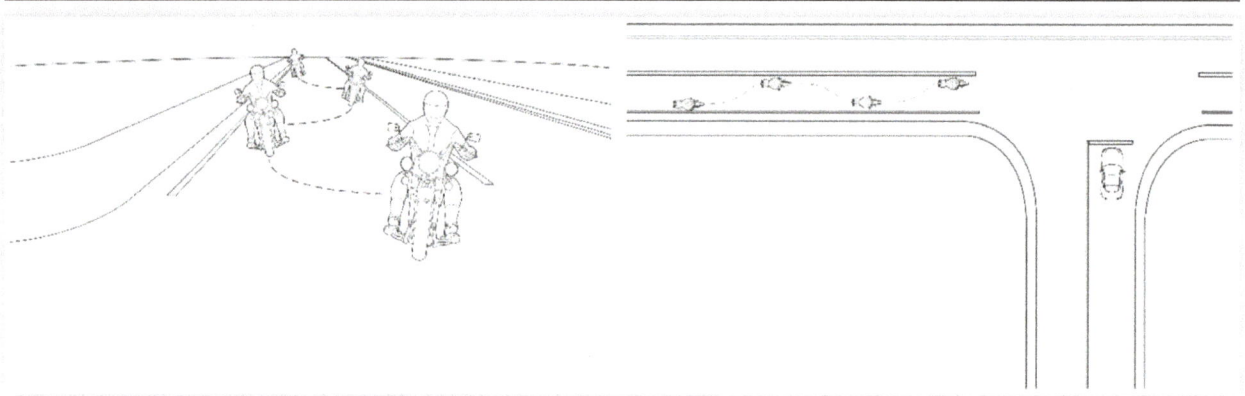

10.2.2 Maneuvering the Motorcycle within a Lane

A 2008 British miniseries called "Motorcycle Safety Videos" featured a pilot episode called "Crash Course – The SMIDSY." SMIDSY is an acronym for a common statement of drivers in a crash with a motorcyclist: "Sorry Mate, I Didn't See You." In this episode, a technique was described where a motorcyclist would move side-to-side in the lane as they approached an intersection to increase the likelihood of other drivers at the intersection seeing them (Figure 10.11). This motion is intended to make the motorcyclist more conspicuous to other drivers.

10.2.3 Headlamp and Brake Modulation

Modulation of the motorcycle headlamps between the high and low beams can also potentially attract the attention of other drivers. Brake lamps too can be modulated and flashed by mildly depressing the hand or foot brake repeatedly. This technique can be helpful when at a stop, or coming to a stop, and traffic is approaching from behind the rider. For some newer motorcycles, active and automatic design features have been added to modulate the lights. Some systems have pulsing rear brake lamps that automatically pulse when the brakes are applied. Some headlamps are modulated too, oscillating the intensity of the headlamp and changing its appearance for oncoming traffic.

10.3 Effectiveness of Daytime Running Lights on Motorcycles

A significant amount of research has been conducted related to the front lighting of motorcycles and its influence on the likelihood drivers will detect motorcycles during the day. In a 1985 study, for example, Zador examined the effectiveness—in terms of reducing fatal motorcycle accidents—of laws requiring the daytime and nighttime use of motorcycle headlights and taillights [1]. At the time of his study, 14 states in the United States had these laws. Zador used daytime motorcycle crash data from the Fatal Accident Reporting System (FARS) from 1975 to 1983. This study concluded that "the risk of daytime crashes was 13 percent lower in states with motorcycle daytime headlight laws than in states without such laws."

Hole and Tyrrell reported a study to examine if motorcyclists not utilizing a headlight in the day would be more at risk if most motorcyclists were utilizing a headlight [2]. They observed that "it has been suggested that drivers might scan for lights rather than for motorcyclists *per se.*" To explore this possibility, they conducted two experiments. In both experiments, test subjects viewed a series of slides depicting traffic, and they had to decide as quickly as possible if each image depicted a motorcyclist. In the first experiment, approximately half of the slides contained a motorcyclist. The final slide in the series shown to each subject always contained a motorcyclist, with the headlight either on or off. For the preceding slides that showed motorcyclists, the "headlight use was either consistent or inconsistent with that of the motorcyclist in the last slide." In the second experiment, Hole and Tyrrell "manipulated the probability with which motorcyclists with and without headlights were presented to the subjects." These researchers reported that the first experiment "showed that headlight-using motorcyclists were more quickly detected than unlit motorcyclists, especially when they were far away…[and] repeated exposure to headlight-using motorcyclists significantly delayed detection of an unlit motorcyclist." They further reported that the second experiment showed "that this delayed-detection effect occurred [even] when only 60% of the motorcyclists shown were using their headlight."

Yuan [3] reported a study of the effectiveness of the "ride-bright" legislation implemented in Singapore in November 1995. This legislation required motorcyclists to ride with their headlights on during the daytime. Yuan examined crash data for the years 1992 through 1996 and found that there was "a sharp decline in daytime fatalities compared with nighttime fatalities in 1996." Yuan observed that, "one possible reason why daytime headlights have successfully reduced fatal and serious injury accidents may be that the improved conspicuity gives time to the other motorists to react. It is reasonable to assume that if other motorists can be alerted earlier, they can stop their vehicles earlier and have a longer distance to travel before hitting the motorcycle or motorcyclist. The longer braking time available with daytime headlights may result in lower impact speeds, which in turn may lower the probability of fatal or serious injury accidents. If this is the case, then one way to make headlights more effective is to make them more conspicuous, say, by having 'multiple', 'more powerful' headlights to send even earlier warning signals."

Jenness et al. reported a daytime field experiment to determine if the gap acceptance behavior of drivers turning left in front of a motorcycle changed with forward lighting added to a motorcycle above and beyond the standard low beam headlamp that turns on automatically [4]. The intent of daytime running lights (DRL) on motorcycles is to increase conspicuity and thus, to overcome passenger car drivers' lack of expectancy and increase the likelihood passenger car drivers will recognize the presence of motorcycles. In his 1977 study, Hurt had noted that "one important countermeasure is the use of a lighted motorcycle headlamp during daylight…The data collected by the USC-DOT Motorcycle Accident Research Teams shows that the motorcycles NOT using the headlamp-on during daylight are overrepresented in the accident population. The bouncing, flickering headlamp of the moving motorcycle is a powerful attention-getting mechanism, which greatly improves motorcycle conspicuity in traffic" [5]. A study by Olson confirmed this finding, noting that "the most effective means of improving daytime conspicuity…is to require motorcyclists to drive during the day with their low-beam headlamp turned on" [6].

The study by Jenness et al. utilized 32 drivers (19 to 67 years old) and 5 experimental lighting systems with various configurations of auxiliary lighting. No experienced motorcycle riders or people with motorcycle riders in their immediate family were included as test subjects. Subjects viewed the approaching traffic on an active roadway (including a motorcycle) and indicated when it would and would not be safe to initiate their left turn across the approaching traffic. Jenness and his colleagues added a distracting element to the study by giving the subjects a secondary visual task that would, on occasion, occupy their attention. Jenness, et al. concluded that, *on average*, the safety margin that the test subjects gave the motorcycle did not differ significantly between any of the experimental lighting systems and the baseline lighting system. "However, having either low-mounted auxiliary lamps or modulated high beam lamps on the motorcycle significantly reduced the probability of obtaining a potentially unsafe short safety margin as compared to the baseline lighting treatment. Overall, the results suggest that enhancing the frontal conspicuity of motorcycles with lighting treatments beyond an illuminated low beam headlamp may be an effective countermeasure for daytime crashes involving right-of-way violations."

In another study, Jenness et al. examined the possibility that widespread use of DRL on passenger vehicles might make the use of DRL on motorcycles less effective at increasing the conspicuity of motorcycles [7]. They referred to this as the Fleet DRL Hypothesis. These authors examined crash data from Canada, where DRL use was mandatory for the entire vehicle population and compared it to crash data from 24 U.S. states where DRL use was not mandatory and "fleet penetration of DRL was modest." U.S. crash data was drawn from the Fatality Analysis Reporting System (FARS), and Canadian crash data was drawn from the Canadian National Collision Data Base (NCDB). Crashes in the years 2001 through 2007 were studied, and the authors stated that "crash scenarios that were plausibly relevant to frontal conspicuity of the involved vehicles were defined as DRL-relevant. The proportion of DRL-relevant crashes was modeled by country, year, and whether the crash involved a motorcycle." Jenness et al. concluded that "the Fleet DRL Hypothesis may be true for urban roadways (but may not true for rural roadways). These results suggest that there could be negative consequences for motorcycle riders of widespread DRL use in the vehicle fleet. For urban roadways especially, the proportion of two-vehicle fatal motorcycle crashes that are relevant to frontal conspicuity of the vehicles (DRL relevant) is higher in Canada than in the USA. This result and other related predictions verified by the modeling results support the Fleet DRL Hypothesis for urban roadways, that *widespread use of DRL in the vehicle fleet increases the relative risk for certain types of multi-vehicle motorcycle crashes*" (emphasis in original).

Cavallo and Pinto [8] also examined the influence of DRL on cars on the conspicuity of motorcycles. They showed 24 adult licensed drivers' color photographs representing complex urban traffic scenes with low-luminosity conditions (overcast skies). The photographs were displayed for 250 ms, and the subjects had to identify vulnerable road users (motorcyclists, cyclists, and pedestrians). The vulnerable road users were located at varying distances and eccentricities from the vantage point of the camera. The motorcycles in the scenes always had their front light on, whereas the researchers varied if the other vehicles in the scene had DRL on or not. Only half of the photographs contained a vulnerable road user. The limited viewing time given to the subjects was intended to resolve a methodological weakness Cavalla and Pinto point out in other studies. Namely, "we contend that the sensorial conspicuity of motorcycles should be assessed in complex environments, with a time-limited task where the observer has to 'notice' a motorcycle, not look for one. In short, the situation must call upon selective attention, in such a way that attentional conspicuity rather than search conspicuity is at stake." Cavallo and Pinto concluded that "the present study revealed a detrimental effect of car DRLs on the perception of vulnerable road users: motorcyclists, cyclists, and pedestrians were less well detected when the headlights of cars in their vicinity were on…The car-DRL effect tended to occur when the motorcycle was far away, and when it was located in the center of the visual scene. The negative effect of car DRLs at greater distances suggests that the

DRLs generated competing light patterns in conditions where the motorcycles were hard to see because of their small angular size. At shorter distances, where the angular size of the motorcycle and thus its inherent conspicuity were greater, car DRLs had little or no impact."

Rößger et al. reported a study in which they aimed "to identify a front signal pattern created by additional light sources that would make motorcycles clearly and quickly distinguishable from other vehicles…" [9]. They conducted two experiments. In the first, they presented a set of 40 photographs, one at a time, to the test subjects. Nine of these photographs contained a motorcycle and the other 31 did not. These other photographs showed other types of traffic or no traffic at all. The frontal appearance of the motorcycle was varied in the following configurations: (a) a single headlight on the front of the motorcycle, (b) a t-shaped pattern of lights on the front of the motorcycle, and (c) a t-shaped pattern of light on the motorcycle and additional lights on the operator's helmet. These researchers found that "motorcycles with a T-shaped light configuration are more quickly identified, particularly when the motorcycles are in visual competition with other motorized road users. Furthermore, analysis of gaze behavior showed that they were faster fixated by the subjects in the experiment, and the mean duration of fixations was shorter."

References

1. Zador, P.L., "Motorcycle Headlight-Use Laws and Fatal Motorcycle Crashes in the US, 1975-83," *Am J Pub Health* 75 (1985): 543-546.

2. Hole, G.J. and Tyrell, L., "The Influence of Perceptual 'Set' on the Detection of Motorcyclists Using Daytime Headlights," *Ergonomics* 38, no. 7 (1995): 1326-1341, doi:10.1080/00140139508925191.

3. Yuan, W., "The Effectiveness of Ride-Bright Legislation for Motorcycles in Singapore," *Accident Analysis and Prevention* 32 (2000): 559-563.

4. Jenness, J., Huey, R., McCloskey, S., Singer, J. et al., "Perception of Approaching Motorcycles by Distracted Drivers May Depend on Auxiliary Lighting Treatments: A Field Experiment," *Proceedings of the Sixth International Driving Symposium on Human Factors in Driver Assessment, Training and Vehicle Design*, Lake Tahoe, CA, 2011, 2–8.

5. Hurt, H.H. and DuPont, C.J., "Human Factors in Motorcycle Accidents," SAE Technical Paper 770103, 1977, doi:10.4271/770103.

6. Olson, P.L., Halstead-Nussloch, R., and Sivak, M., "The Effect of Improvements in Motorcycle/Motorcyclist Conspicuity on Driver Behavior," *Human Factors* 23, no. 2 (1981): 237–248.

7. Jenness, J., Jenkins, F., and Zador, P., "Motorcycle Conspicuity and the Effect of Fleet DRL: Analysis of Two-Vehicle Fatal Crashes in Canada and the United States 2001-2007," DOT HS 811 505, September 2011.

8. Cavallo, V. and Pinto, M., "Are Car Daytime Running Lights Detrimental to Motorcycle Conspicuity?," *Accident Analysis and Prevention* 49 (2012): 78-85, doi:10.1016/j.aap.2011.09.013.

9. Rößger, L., Hagen, K., Krzywinskib, J., and Schlag, B., "Recognisability of Different Configurations of Front Lights on Motorcycles," *Accident Analysis and Prevention* 44 (2012): 82-87.

Motorcycles at Night

Some of the variables that affect the visibility and conspicuity of motorcycles during the day also come into play at night. However, nighttime motorcycle crashes bring with them additional issues related to visibility and conspicuity that may need to be considered. For example, nighttime crashes often involve complex lighting conditions. The visibility of animals, pedestrians, cars, or other objects both on and off the road are affected by conditions such as the illumination provided by a vehicle's headlamps, by street lamps, by ambient lighting, by oncoming traffic, and by the characteristics of the weather. Also, the motorcycle operator's riding gear and the forward and signal lighting systems on the motorcycle can come into play. At night, riding gear can increase or decrease visibility, depending on the color and material properties of the gear, as well as its contrast to the environment. A rider's helmet and eye wear, which may be tinted, can reduce some transmission of light, diminishing the visibility of the roadway and objects in it to the motorcycle operator.

11.1 Clothing and Gear Worn by a Motorcyclist

The color and characteristics of a rider's clothing can add or detract from conspicuity, depending on the specific environmental characteristics. A motorcyclist will travel through a range of environments during any give ride and thus unlikely to select a single set of clothing that would optimize conspicuity for the full range of environments. Certain scenarios will create a situation where a highly reflective vest will be less conspicuous and visible than dark clothing. The images of Figure 11.1 illustrate this, showing that in some

FIGURE 11.1   Clothing and contrast with the background.

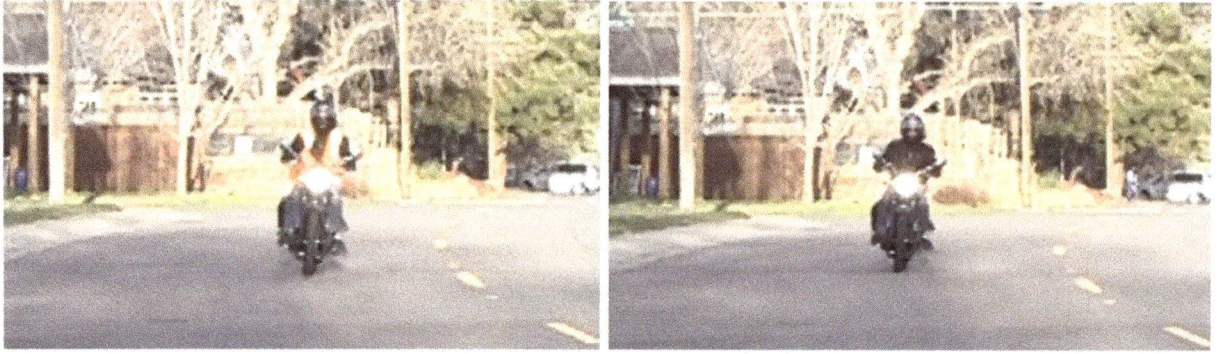

environments, black clothing can stand out better from the background than orange, reflective material. The image on the left shows the rider with a reflective orange vest. The image on the right shows the rider with a black jacket. The black clothing contrasts better with the background of this environment and is likely to make the motorcyclist more conspicuous and visible. The influence of a specific color, pattern, or material on visibility and conspicuity will depend on the time of day, the background, and the relative viewing position of the observer and position of the motorcycle.

Retroreflective vests are sometimes regarded as being more visible and conspicuous than black clothing in nighttime conditions. While this may be true in some nighttime circumstances, it is not necessarily true in all circumstances. As an example, consider the photographs in Figures 11.2 and 11.3. The first shows an approaching motorcycle and rider with a black leather jacket. The second shows a motorcycle and a rider with a reflective vest. Both photographs were taken from the perspective of a car driver approaching from the opposite direction with its headlamps on. In a situation where the motorcycle is approaching the driver from straight ahead, the rider is positioned behind the motorcycle's headlamp. As a result, much of the retroreflective benefit from the jacket tends to blend in with the headlamp. Retroreflective vests may be beneficial under other conditions where the motorcycle is approaching from the side or traveling away from the car. However, this issue would need to be considered on a case-by-case basis.

FIGURE 11.2   A rider approaching an oncoming car wearing a black leather jacket.

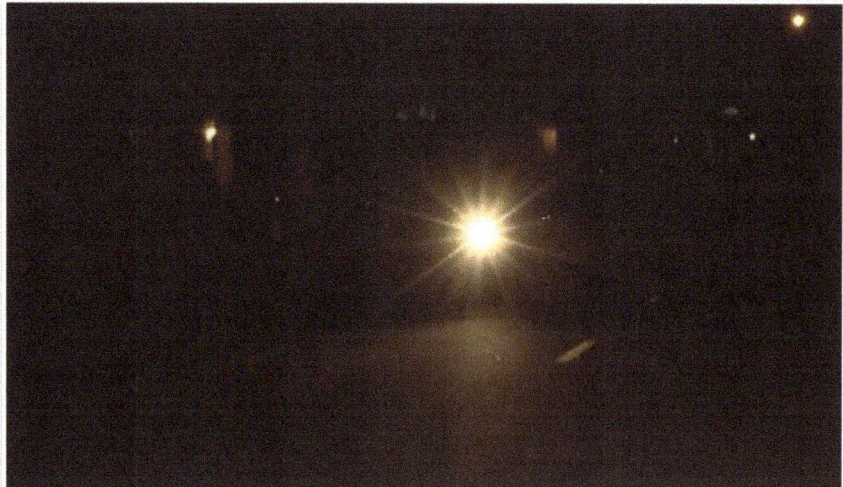

FIGURE 11.3 A rider approaching an oncoming car wearing a reflective vest.

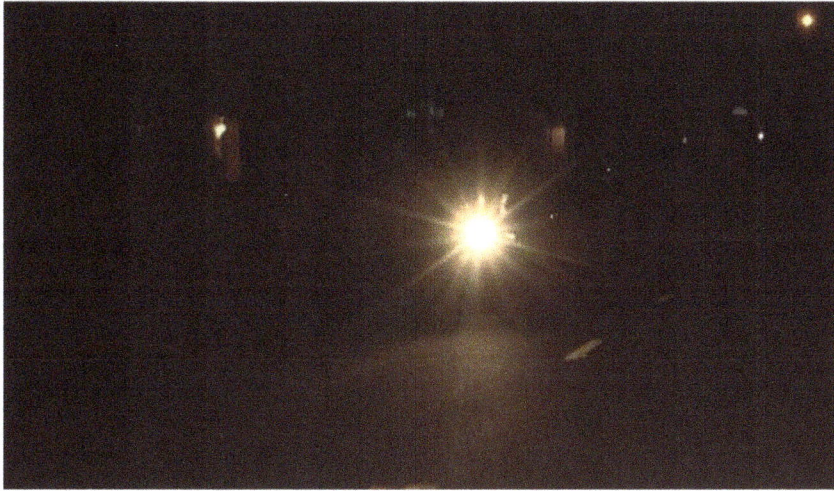

TABLE 11.1 Light transmission loss caused by different windshields, visors, and sunglasses

Filter	With (cd/m²)	Without (cd/m²)	Transmission loss (%)
Clear visor	1088	1143	5
Clear Oakley lens	1032	1094	6
SUV windshield (40°)	836	1090	23
Car windshield (35°)	761.4	1076	29
Truck windshield (40°)	692.7	1001	31
Gray Oakley lens	363.5	1097	67
Amber (VR28) Oakley lens	338.2	1104	69
Black iridium Oakley lens	269.5	1091	75
Tinted visor	286.2	1165	75
Blue piranha sunglasses	178.3	1086	84

Some state laws require that motorcyclists use eye protection while riding. This can be in the form of sunglasses, clear glasses, or helmet visors. Visors can be tinted like sunglasses, and if the rider has begun their trip during the day and continued riding into the night, the rider may end up in a situation where the eye wear is tinted under nighttime conditions. This additional tinting can have a dramatic effect on reducing the rider's ability to see other vehicles and objects at night. Table 11.1 shows test results of the reduction in light transmitted through windshield glass, tinted and clear helmet visors, and sunglasses.

In this testing, a gray scale chart of 40% reflectance was used as a standard object for measuring the reflectance. Luminance was measured in candela/meter² using a NIST certified Konica Minolta LS-110 luminance meter with an annual calibration. Measurements were taken during a 15-minute period during the day under cloudy conditions to make sure the lighting environment for all the different measurements remained constant. Measurements were taken of the 40% gray card for a baseline, and then from the same position, and measuring the same point on the gray scale card, different materials were placed in front of the luminance meter, and additional readings were taken. The photos in Figure 11.4 shows the general setup of the luminance meter, the vehicle representing a windshield, and the tripods that held the visors and sunglasses through which luminance measurements were taken. The percentages reported in this table do not directly correlate

FIGURE 11.4 Setup of testing for measuring light transmission loss from windshields, visors, and sunglasses.

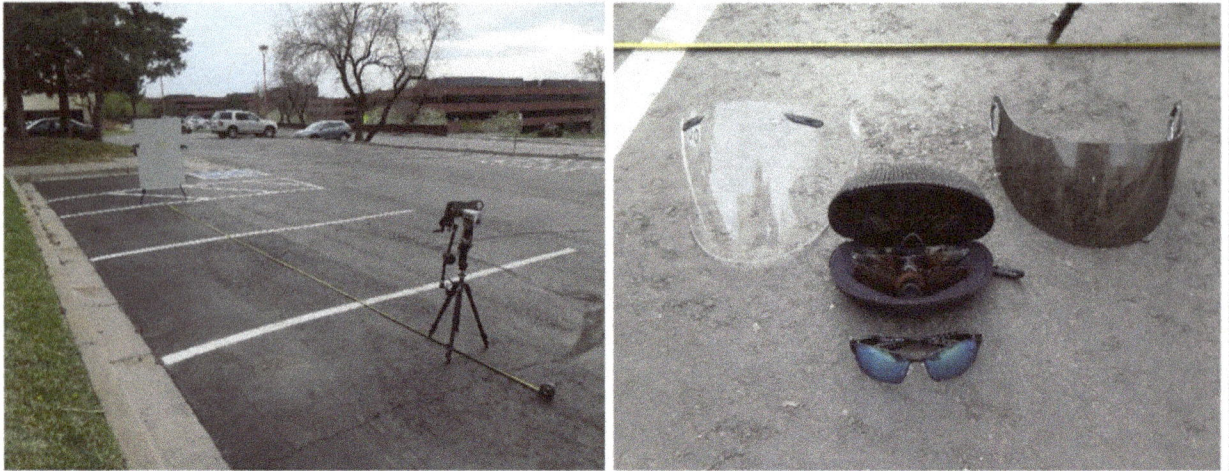

to a numerical loss of visibility. However, they do illustrate that operating a motorcycle at night with a tinted visor or with sunglasses could have a significant effect on visibility.

11.2 Motorcycle Headlamps and Signal Lighting

Motorcycles are typically equipped with forward lighting and signal lighting that differ from passenger cars and trucks. Turn signals, headlamps, and running lights are not spread as wide on the motorcycle as on a passenger car, since cars typically are much wider. The lamp housings are also limited in size on motorcycles and hence do not appear as large to other motorists. Headlamp designs vary between motorcycles, and some motorcycles have only a single headlamp, while others have three. The headlamps can be arranged in a row, like they are on a typical car, or in a triangle formation when there are three. Changes in the shape defined by the headlamps and placing the headlamps can increase the likelihood that a motorcycle will be detected.

Olson and Abrams [1] reported in 1982 that the Motorcycle Safety Foundation instructors that they surveyed "regarded motorcycle headlighting as inadequate." Specifically, those surveyed indicated "a need for more illumination in the foreground area and to the sides of the lane." Olson and Abrams also observed that "many motorcycle headlamps do not have the output of an automotive headlamp, and most motorcycles have but one headlamp." An earlier study by Sturgis found that improvements in the standardization of the aiming of headlamps were needed [2]. Because of the limited width of a motorcycle, generating a beam pattern on the roadway with two headlamps is not as effective as it would be on a car. The number of headlamp assemblies on a motorcycle may be limited to one and the lamp housing may be smaller in size, limiting some of the technology available.

Figure 11.5 shows various motorcycle headlamp design configurations ranging from one, two, or three headlamp designs. Gould studied the influence of different headlamp patterns and found that "the extent to which observers struggle to accurately judge motorcycle speed based on a solo headlight in nighttime conditions is rather alarming" [3]. Gould found that a triangle-shaped formation yielded better speed estimates by the

FIGURE 11.5 Different types of motorcycle headlamps.

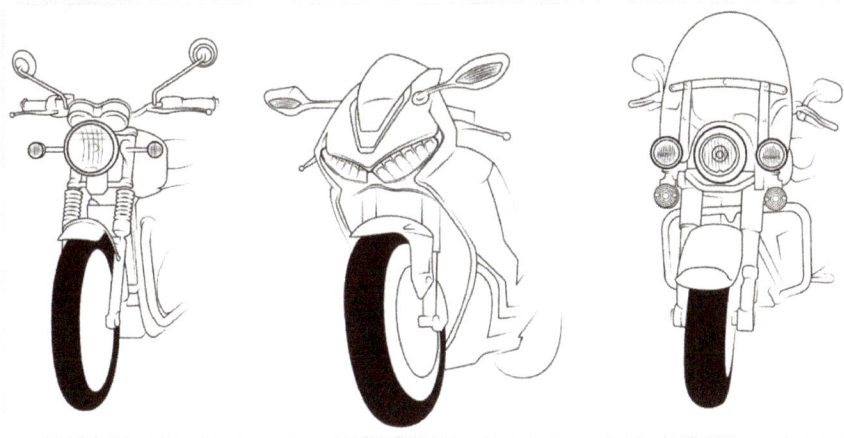

observers. In addition to these factors, the fact that motorcycles lean to traverse curves means that the distribution of light from their headlamps relative to the surrounding roadway will vary depending on the characteristics of the roadway and what maneuver the motorcycle is completing.

The visibility of an object at night is largely due to the luminance contrast between the object and its background. This contrast depends on many factors, one of which is the amount of illumination produced by the headlamps of the vehicle from which the object is being viewed [4]. Compared to typical passenger car headlamps, motorcycle headlamps typically provide less illumination. Thus, when evaluating a motorcyclist's ability to avoid an object, an animal crossing the road, for instance, the characteristics of the motorcycle headlamps come into play. When it comes to the ability of another driver to see a motorcycle at night, the headlamps also play a role, but this is not as dependent on the characteristics of the particular headlamp. The direction the motorcycle headlamps are facing also plays into whether other drivers see a motorcycle. Like daytime headlamps, modulation of the headlamp or brake lamp tends to increase the conspicuity of the motorcycle to other drivers.

11.3 Measuring Headlamp Performance

Neale presented testing of nine motorcycle headlamps that represented a wide variety of motorcycle styles and headlamp designs [5]. In addition, the performance of the headlamp in illuminating the roadway and illuminating the shoulder was evaluated. The motorcycles tested represented standard, sport, and cruiser models, and the headlamps tested include Fresnel-sealed beam, reflector optics, and projector optics. The testing was performed in an open area, where the only light source would be that of the tested headlamps. The roadway was flat and made of asphalt with a measured reflectivity of 8%. The setup included a grid consisting of 25 ft intervals extending out from the front of the motorcycle and 11 ft intervals to the right and left of center (Figure 11.6). At these locations, vertical lux measurements were taken at ground level and at 3 ft above the ground using a Konica Minolta T-10 illuminance meter. Measurements were taken left and right of center until the measurements reached approximately 1–3 lux, representing meaningful light level thresholds for detection of nonself-illuminated or retroreflective objects in the roadway [6].

FIGURE 11.6   Layout for headlamp testing.

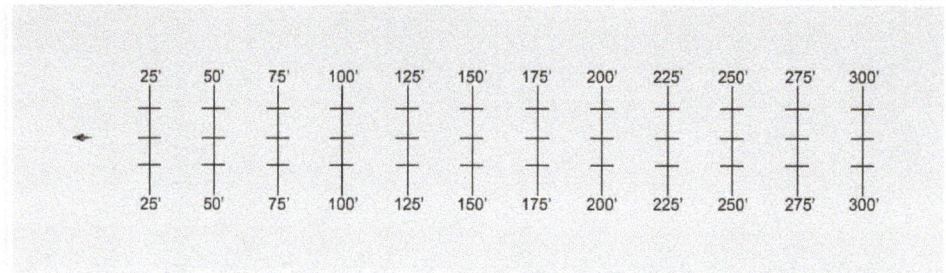

In testing the headlamps, two different setups were utilized-one with the headlamp in its normal mounting on the motorcycle and another with the headlamp mounted on a separate rig. On the rig, the headlamp was powered by two standard car batteries wired in parallel so that a steady and consistent power was supplied. These batteries were monitored by a battery charger to ensure that their charge did not get too low. This setup was tested with a multimeter at 13.8–14.2 V, which is a similar power supply to that of the motorcycles' systems. The service manual for each motorcycle specified the electrical system as a 12 V system and the charging voltages between 14 and 15.5 V. Each motorcycle that was tested was checked with a multimeter and showed voltages between 13.4 and 14.5 V during the tests. To determine the height of the headlamp on the rig and to adjust the aim, an exemplar motorcycle that used the headlamp as a specified part was examined. From this examination, the aiming and height were determined. The aiming was further confirmed at the site, visually, to make sure that the headlamp beam pattern was generally downward, and slightly to the right, with as much visibility of the road way as possible. For all the setups, the headlamp was warmed up for several minutes prior to taking measurements. Figure 11.7 shows the two setups used in this testing.

To validate the process of using a headlamp rig, a test was preformed where a headlamp was mapped both in the rig setup and on its motorcycle. The headlamp tested in these two configurations was from the 2010 Honda Fury (VT1300CXA). The average difference between lux measurements of the rig setup and the headlamp in the motorcycle

FIGURE 11.7   Two setups utilized in mapping motorcycle headlamps.

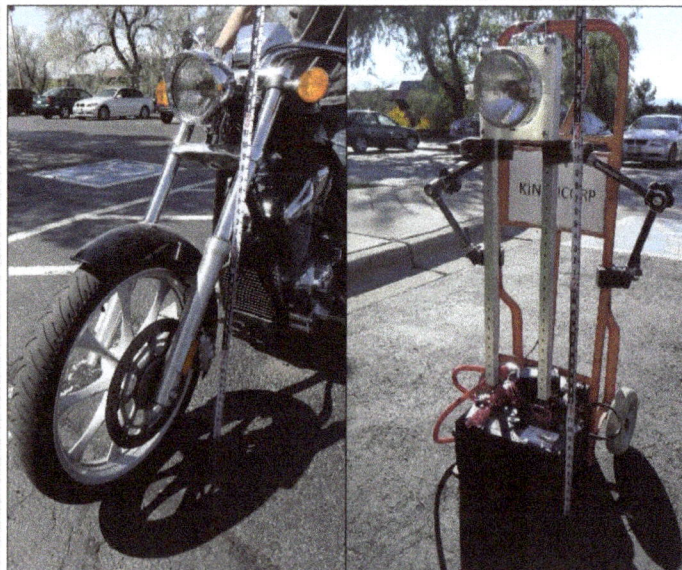

was about 3%, with the highest error being about 8% at one discrete position. This test showed that between the rig setup and motorcycle setup, the headlamp performance was reasonably close. Of the nine headlamps that were mapped, four were mounted on the motorcycles, and five were mounted on rigs. Figure 11.8 shows the motorcycles that were tested, and Figure 11.9 shows the headlamps that were tested on a rig. Further detail related to these headlamps is provided in Table 11.2.

FIGURE 11.8 Tested motorcycles.

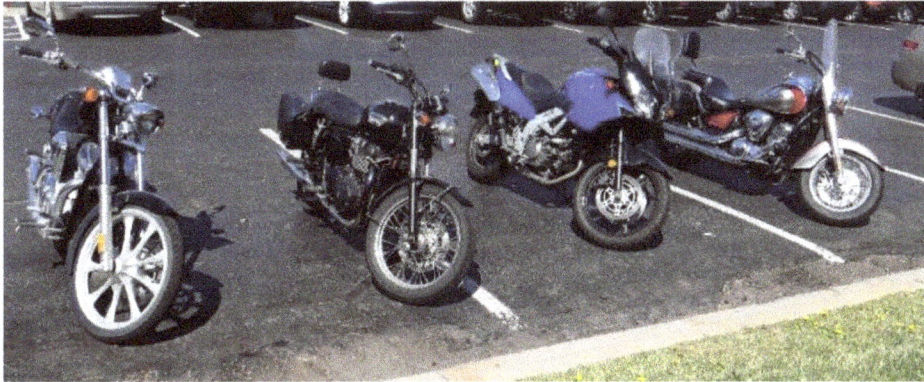

FIGURE 11.9 Headlamps tested on rigs.

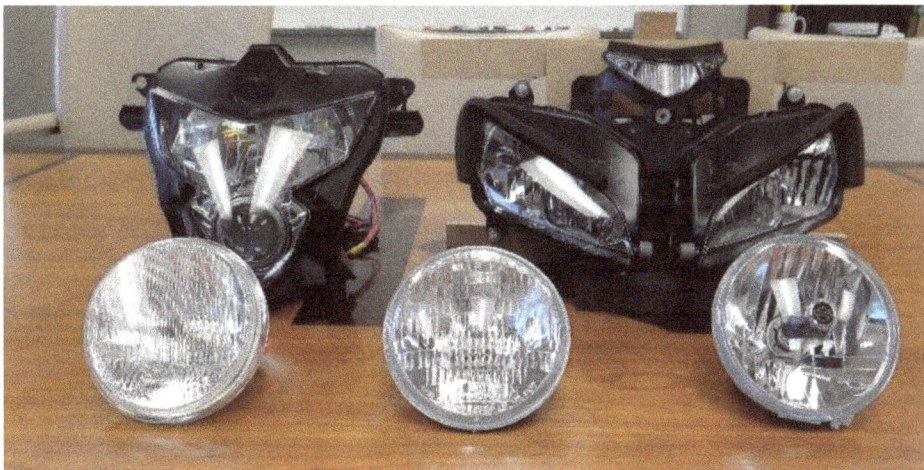

TABLE 11.2 Motorcycles and headlamps tested

Year	Make	Model	Category	Headlamp	Test setup
1993	Harley-Davidson	FXR	Cruiser	Fresnel	Rig
2004	Suzuki	DL650	Dual sport	Reflector	Motorcycle
2004	Harley-Davidson	FXSTDI	Cruiser	Fresnel	Rig
2004	Honda	CBR 1000RR	Sport	Reflector	Rig
2005	Harley-Davidson	FXSTSI	Cruiser	Reflector	Rig
2005	Suzuki	GSXR-600	Sport	Projector	Rig
2007	Kawasaki	VN900-D	Cruiser	Reflector	Motorcycle
2007	Triumph	Bonneville	Standard	Fresnel	Motorcycle
2010	Honda	Fury	Cruiser	Fresnel	Motorcycle

FIGURE 11.10 Iso-illuminance diagram of the 2004 Suzuki DL650.

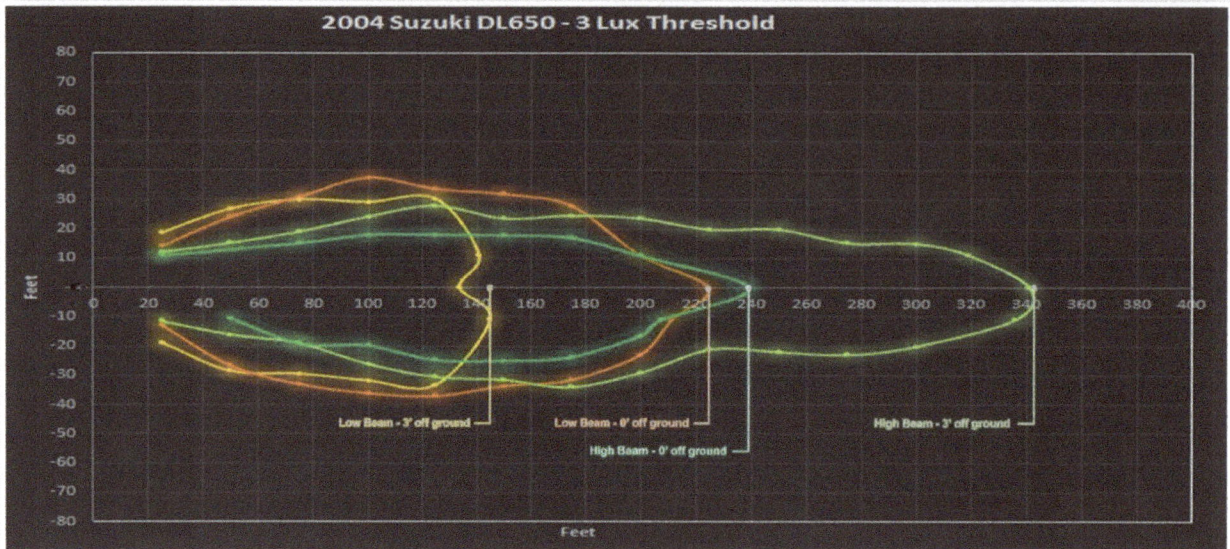

The illuminance measurements for these headlamps were plotted to a scaled iso-illuminance diagram. Figure 11.10 shows an example. This is the iso-illuminance diagram from the mapping of the 2004 Suzuki DL650 motorcycle headlamp. In this figure, low-beam and high-beam measurements are depicted.

For discussion purposes, the headlamp measurements were separated into two groups. One group contained those headlamps which had the shortest distance to a 3 lux level on the ground surface. The second group contained the half that had the farthest distance to a 3 lux level on the ground. Figure 11.11 shows the measurements for the farthest performing low-beam headlamps. Figure 11.12 shows the shortest performing low-beam headlamps, also measured at the 3 lux level at the road surface.

FIGURE 11.11 Beam patterns for the farthest performing headlamps, low beam, 3 lux at the road surface.

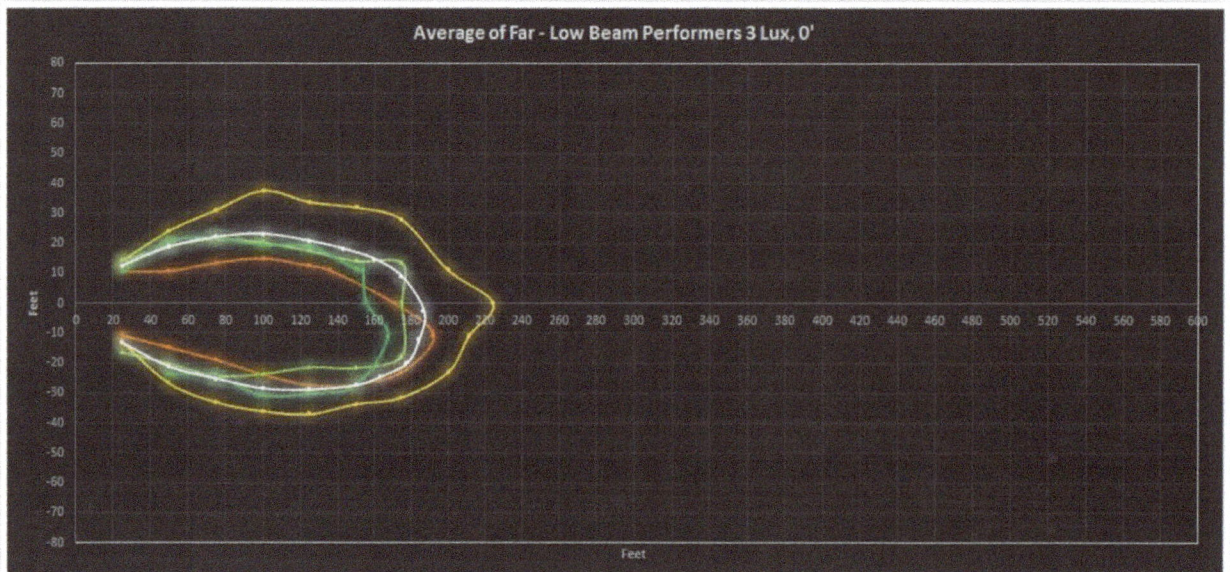

FIGURE 11.12 Beam patterns for the shortest performing headlamps, low beam, 3 lux at the road surface.

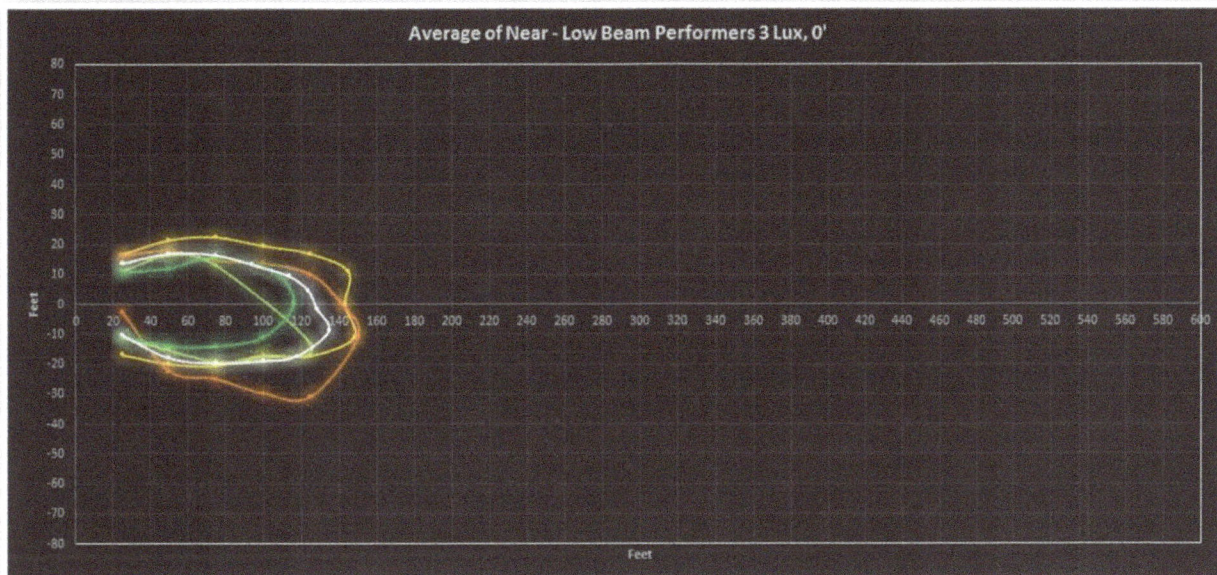

FIGURE 11.13 Low-beam comparison of farthest and shortest performing headlamps, 3 lux at the road surface.

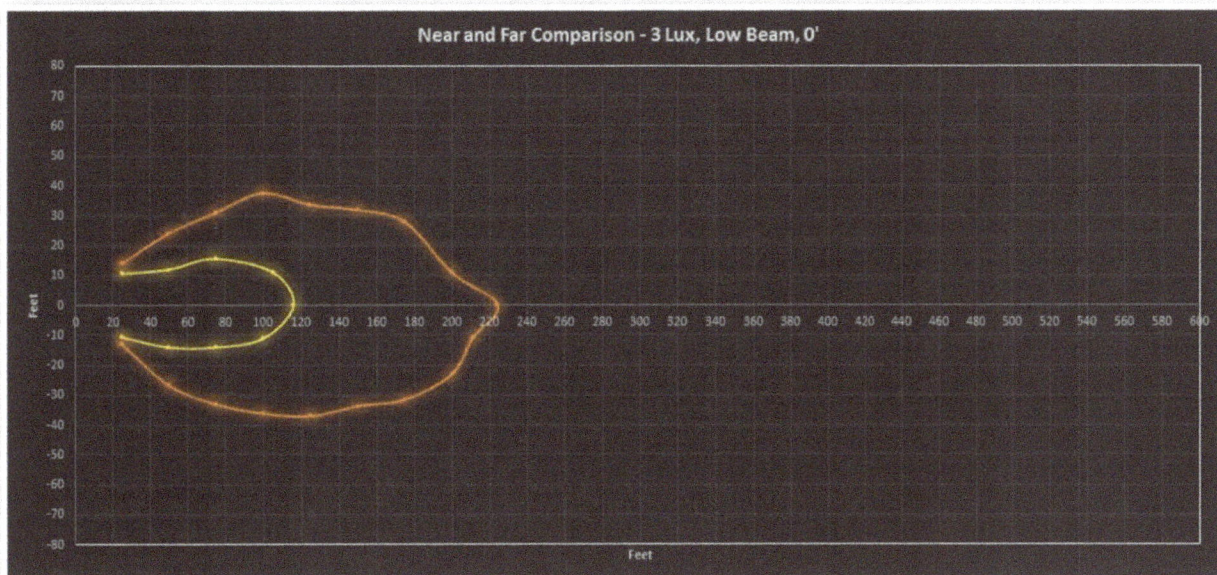

A profile was created that represents an average headlamp performance for the entire group. This average profile is shown in white.

There was a significant range in the performance of the various headlamps, for both the low-beam and high-beam samples. Figure 11.13 shows the shortest and farthest performing low-beam headlamps, and Figure 11.14 shows the shortest and farthest performing high-beam headlamps. Between the farthest and shortest low-beam performers, there was a difference of 109 ft. For high beams, the difference was around 228 ft. The low-beam headlamp patterns shown in Figure 11.13 are the 2004 Suzuki DL650 (farthest performer) and the 2004 H-D FXSTDI (shortest performer). For the high-beam comparison in Figure 11.14, the high-beam headlamp patterns shown are

FIGURE 11.14 High-beam comparison of farthest and shortest performing headlamps, 3 lux at the road surface.

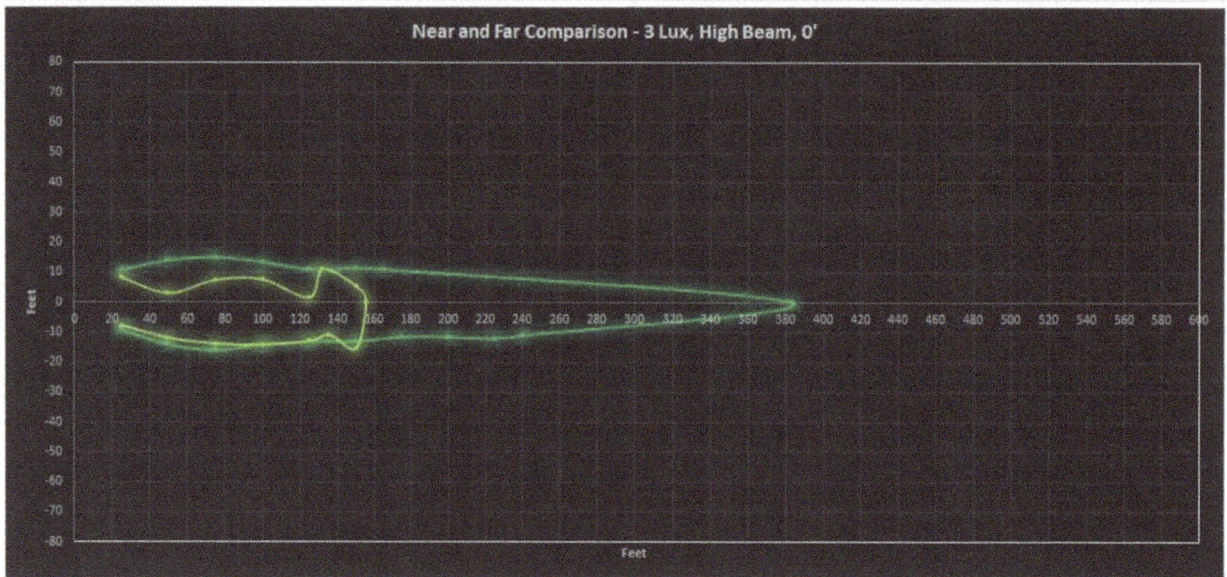

Near and Far Comparison - 3 Lux, High Beam, 0'

TABLE 11.3 Comparison of 3 lux maximum distance at road surface, low and high beams

Motorcycle	3 lux at ground level		
	Low beam (ft)	High beam (ft)	Difference (ft)
1993 Harley Davidson FXR	116	340	224
2004 Harley-Davidson FXSTDI	116	292	176
2004 Honda CBR1000RR	146	156	10
2004 Suzuki DL650	225	239	14
2005 Harley-Davidson FXSTSI	90	304	214
2005 Suzuki GSXR600	190	216	26
2006 Triumph Bonneville	192	148	−44
2007 Kawasaki VN900D	160	225	65
2010 Honda Fury	148	384	236

the 2010 Honda Fury (farthest performer) and the 2004 Honda CBR1000RR (shortest performer). Table 11.3 shows the maximum illumination distance for the low and high beams of each motorcycle (3 lux at the road surface).

For many of the headlamps, the high beam increased the level of light a significant distance beyond the low beam. However, for other headlamps, the high beam did not provide a significant increase in the illumination, and, for one of the headlamps tested, the light level on the ground on high beam was less than the low beam. It was determined that the angle of the high-beam pattern was oriented such that the light was projected forward rather than down toward the roadway. Table 11.4 lists the low-beam headlamps that were tested, ordered according to their performance (farthest to shortest). Table 11.5 lists the high-beam headlamps that were tested, ordered according to their performance (again, farthest to shortest).

Roadways may contain shoulders that are made of a different material than the roadway itself, including gravel, dirt, or grass. Since the reflectivity of the material on the shoulder can be different than the paved asphalt of the roadway, a comparison was conducted to examine how the headlamp performance might change due to the difference in surface

TABLE 11.4 Tested headlamps listed in order of performance—low beam

Year make model	Headlamp type	Bulb type	Low beam 3 lux at 0' (ft)
2004 Suzuki DL650	Reflector	Left, H4 12V 60/55W E13, right, H4 12V 60/55W E13	225
2006 Triumph Bonneville	Fresnel	H4 12V 60/55W E13	192
2005 Suzuki GSXR600	Projector	Upper—H4 12V 60/55W Lower—E520 H7 12V 55W DOT 12972LL E1	190
2007 Kawasaki VN900D	Reflector	H4 12342 LL 12V 60/55W E1 2C3 U	160
2010 Honda Fury	Fresnel	H4 ED 12V 50/55W U E1 2C3	148
2004 Honda CBR1000RR	Reflector	Left—J903 H7 12V 55W DOT 12972LL E1	146
1993 Harley-Davidson FXR	Fresnel	H4 12V 60/55W E13 2B9	116
2004 Harley-Davidson FXSTDI	Fresnel	HB2 DOT 9035 BiLux 12V 60/55W H4 U 37R E1 0080	116
2005 Harley-Davidson FXSTSI	Reflector	HB2 DOT 9003 L BiLux 12V 60/55W H4 U 37R E1	90

TABLE 11.5 Tested headlamps listed in order of performance—high beam

Year make model	Headlamp type	Bulb type	High beam 3 lux at 0' (ft)
2010 Honda Fury	Fresnel	H4 ED 12V 50/55W U E1 2C3	384
1993 Harley-Davidson FXR	Fresnel	H4 12V 60/55W E13 2B9	340
2005 HD FXSTSI	Reflector	HB2 DOT 9003 L BiLux 12V 60/55W H4 U 37R E1	304
2004 Harley-Davidson FXSTDI	Fresnel	HB2 DOT 9035 BiLux 12V 60/55W H4 U 37R E1 0080	292
2004 Suzuki DL650	Reflector	Left, H4 12V 60/55W E13, right, H4 12V 60/55W E13	239
2009 Kawasaki VN900D	Reflector	H4 12342 LL 12V 60/55W E1 2C3 U	225
2005 Suzuki GSXR600	Projector	Upper—H4 12V 60/55W Lower—E520 H7 12V 55W DOT 12972LL E1	216
2004 Honda CBR1000RR	Reflector	Left—J903 H7 12V 55W DOT 12972LL E1 Right—J903 H7 12V 55W DOT 12972LL E1	156
2006 Triumph Bonneville	Fresnel	H4 12V 60/55W E13	148

material of the shoulder. The 2010 Honda Fury was used for this comparison, and measurements were taken for this motorcycle at two different locations. The first location was a roadway that was entirely paved with asphalt and had no shoulder within the testing area (Figure 11.15). The second location included a two-lane asphalt paved roadway with a dirt and grass shoulder (Figure 11.16). The first location was used to establish a baseline measurement with no contribution from a material change on the shoulder. The flat asphalt pavement had 8% reflectivity. A single yellow lane line with an average reflectivity of 50% served as a station line for points of measurement. Headlamp lux measurements were taken at 25 ft intervals away from the motorcycle and 5 ft lateral intervals away from the centerline of the motorcycle toward the right shoulder of the roadway (Figure 11.17).

The site containing a shoulder was also tested. This site also had a yellow lane line that served as a station line from which measurements were taken. In addition to asphalt and yellow lane lines, the roadway contained a shoulder with gravel, grass, and dirt. The reflectivity measurements of the asphalt roadway and yellow lane line were the same as the baseline testing site—8% and 50%. Additionally, the reflectivity of the white line measured 50%, the gravel 20%, and the grass/dirt mix was 15%.

Headlamp lux measurements were gathered on this second site in the same manner as at the first site. After gathering the measurements, the numbers were compared. In the area where the roadway surface was the same between tests, the measurements remained consistent. However, on the gravel, dirt, and grass shoulder, the measurements

FIGURE 11.15   First test site.

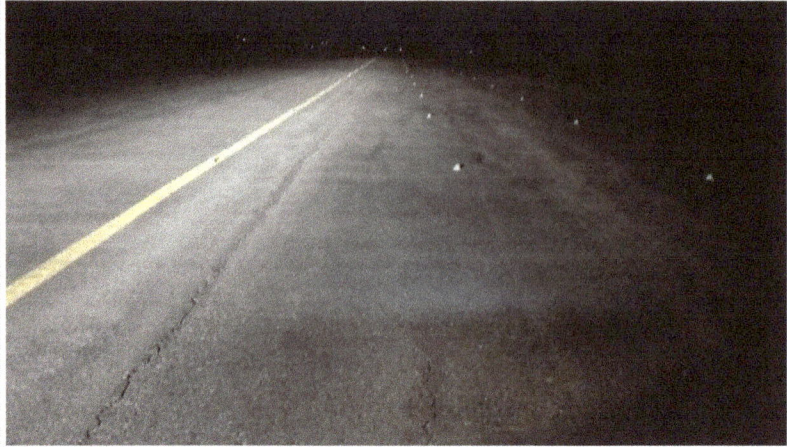

FIGURE 11.16   Second test site.

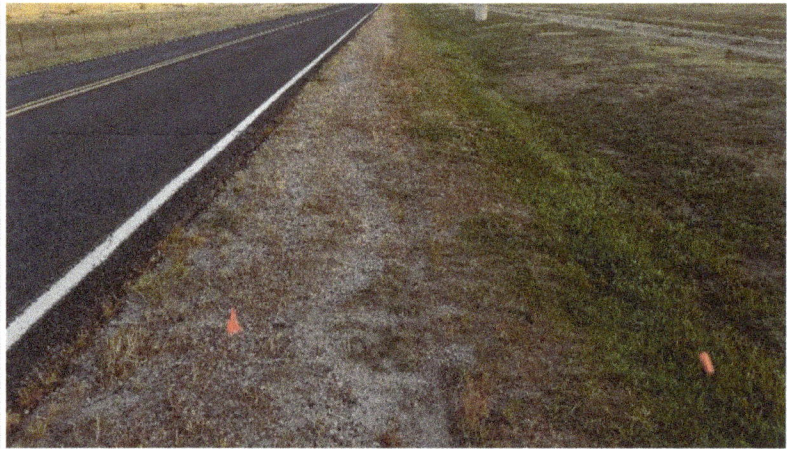

FIGURE 11.17   Iso-illuminance of testing at first site.

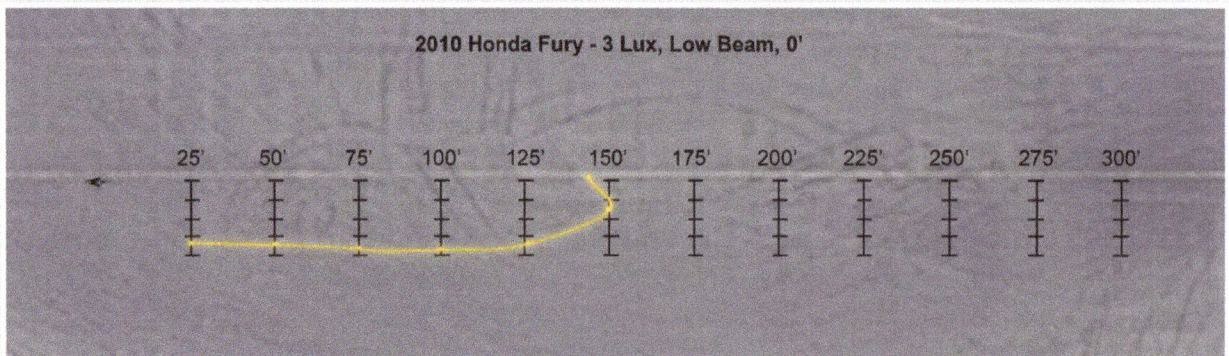

2010 Honda Fury - 3 Lux, Low Beam, 0'

differed. Not surprisingly, shoulder areas with higher reflective material than that of the asphalt produced higher illuminance values. Figure 11.18 shows the percentage increase in the measured lux value for each of the measured locations. The reflectance of the surface material is not the only factor influencing the measured lux values. The surface texture can also affect the overall light measurements.

FIGURE 11.18 Effects of shoulder on the measured illuminance.

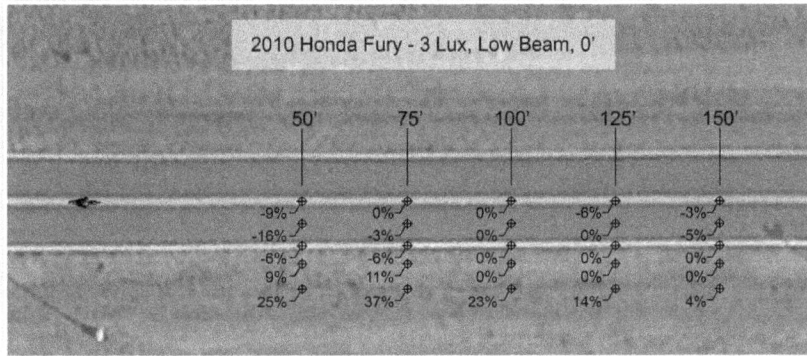

11.4 **Computer Modeling of Headlamps**

Neale also developed a methodology for simulating the illumination from a headlamp in a computer environment [4]. In developing this method, he noted that headlamp illumination depends on design factors such as the beam pattern of the projected lamp, its orientation relative to the object it is illuminating, and the intensity of the light. Environmental factors such as the atmosphere between the headlight and the object or dirt and debris on the headlamp lens can also affect the illumination. Neale simulated a new and clean, high-beam headlamp, measuring the accuracy of the computer model by calculating photometry values in the simulated lighting environment and comparing these to the actual photometric values measured in a real-world environment. The results demonstrated that despite the complexity of the light patterns and distributions of a headlamp, an accurate headlamp simulation could be produced.

Lighting simulation for nighttime environments has advanced along with advances in rendering technology and the widespread inclusion of rendering engines and light models in publicly available computer modeling and animation programs. Specifically, nighttime lighting simulation benefits from two main advancements: global illumination and photometric light files. Global illumination addresses the problem of how light behaves after it exits a light source and interacts with surfaces. By accounting for the effect of light interacting with surfaces that vary in texture, color, translucency, and reflectivity, the overall impact of light in an environment becomes much more realistic than previous lighting models that did not account for propagation and bouncing of light off surfaces. In addition to global illumination, the standardization of photometric light data also advanced light simulation since this step introduced digital data files that are specific to a light source, defining the lights intensity and distribution pattern.

When combined, global illumination and photometric light files enable light simulation and rendering programs to generate photorealistic images that visually represent the light conditions in an environment with physically accurate light values. Currently, light simulation programs utilize standardized photometric files for interior lighting and exterior lighting where street lights and area lights provide much of the lighting for parking lots, security lighting, roadways, highways, illuminated signs, and recreation areas.

The concept behind a simulated photometric light cluster is that the unique light distribution pattern can be created by shining light through a digital projection map, which properly displays the values from light to dark across the spectrum of the headlamp beam spread. A projection map is a digital image that acts much like a filter for a computer-generated light source, controlling the light rays that the computer light source emits. As a digital image, the projection map contains pixel values from light to dark, and as the

FIGURE 11.19 Photograph of projected headlamp of canvas.

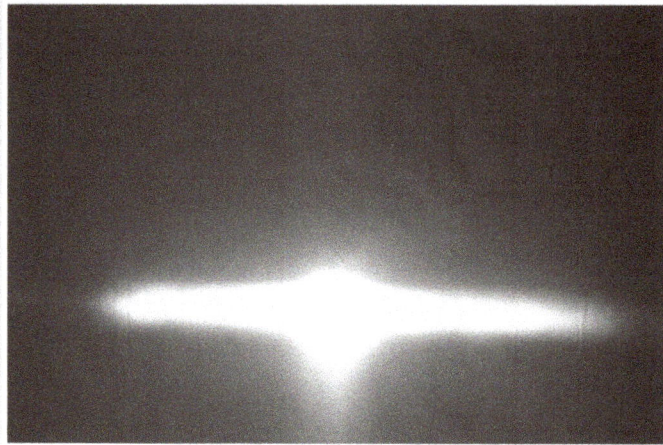

computer-generated light source passes through the map, the pixels of darker value allow less light than those pixels of lighter. It is in this general manner that the projection map combined with a computer-generated light source can approximate actual light source since the light from an actual lamp manifests its own filters as it projects onto a surface.

Figure 11.19 is a photograph of a typical light pattern produced by a headlamp projected onto a canvas mounted on the wall of a darkroom. This light pattern contains a hotspot, where the intensity of the light energy is most concentrated. The light spreads out from the hotspot in a horizontal and oblong pattern. The light intensity decreases toward the edges. As the headlamp moves forward or back from the surface on which it's projecting, the oblong shape changes, as does the location of the hotspot. In digitally modeling a headlamp, it is essential to capture this dynamic nature of the headlamp spread over distance.

If the photograph of Figure 11.19 were a projection map, the areas in dark would prevent light from shining through, while the areas in white would allow it. The values that fall between white or black would allow a percentage of light through, equal to the percent of whiteness or blackness of that area of the projection map. This concept is illustrated in Figure 11.20. In this illustration, a light source sits behind a projection map through which the light passes to project an image further away. The projection through this map results in the light being filtered to match the actual light spread and intensity of the photographed headlamp. In the actual computer environment, this map is not separate from a light source but rather an algorithm assigned to a light source, defining the distribution of light emitted from the light source according to the specific pattern of light and dark.

FIGURE 11.20 Illustration of using a projection map to match a headlamp beam pattern.

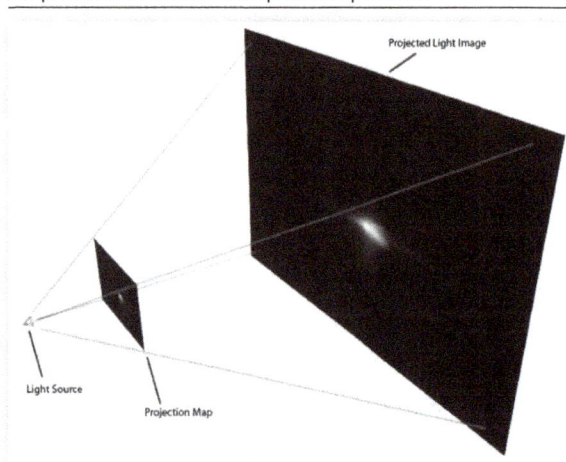

The illustration in Figure 11.20 shows a single light source and projection map. However, multiple light sources and projection maps are typically needed to accommodate a headlamp's parabolic shape and sophisticated lenses that direct and focus the light in complex ways. The hotspot, for instance, is created from a combination of light coming from both the left and right sides of the headlamp. For example, Figure 11.21 below shows the lens on a truck headlamp. There are several patterns that emerge on the surface of the headlamp that control the spread and distribution of the light.

FIGURE 11.21 Lens of a truck headlight.

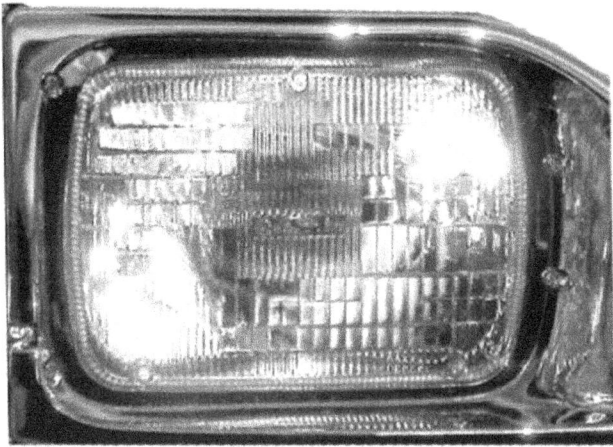

FIGURE 11.22 Illustration of using multiple light sources and projection maps to model a beam pattern.

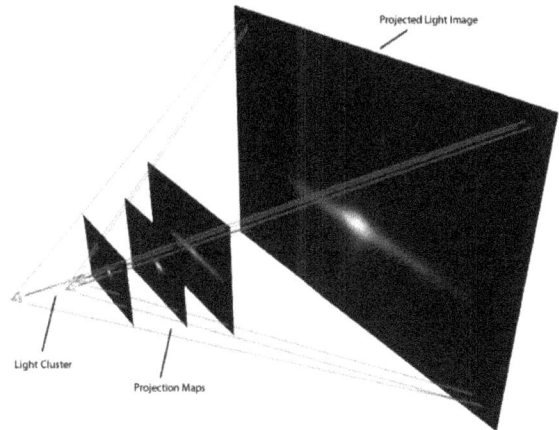

A series of rectangles of varying sizes can be seen on the surface of this headlamp. The size and location of these rectangles direct light in different ways to achieve a final light distribution. For the rectangle areas that control the hotspot, a pattern can be seen that is similar on both the right and left sides of the headlamp, represented in rectangles larger than the surrounding areas. These similar lens configurations on both sides of the lamp contribute to creating a focused hotspot in the center of the photograph in Figure 11.19. To simulate an effect such as this, it would then require two light sources, projecting through two maps to create an accurate hotspot.

This may seem counterintuitive since there is only one light source inside the headlamp assembly (the halogen bulb in this case). However, the parabolic reflectors and lens on the surface of the headlamp focus, redirect, and reflect the single light in ways that make it exit the headlamp assembly from different locations, giving the impression of more than one light source. Neale found that a total of three light sources and three maps were required to properly generate an accurate simulation of this headlamp. The conceptual illustration in Figure 11.22 demonstrates how the three light sources project through image maps to create a single headlamp simulation.

Neale also evaluated the validity of using photometric files for simulating headlamp light distributions of several different headlamp types [7]. Headlamps were sent to a light laboratory to have photometric files created. Photometric light files represent the light intensity value for measured light sources and use real-world units and values to enable their application in light simulation software. Photometric data files contain information in candela values that describe how light from a light source or light assembly is distributed, and, because photometric data are recorded in real world units, they can be used to predict light values in a computer-generated environment. Photometric data is used in light simulation programs to provide physically accurate representation of the propagation of light energy in an environment from lamps, luminaries, and other light assemblies or light sources. The light intensity distribution (or LID) of a light source or lamp assembly is measured using photometry equipment such as spectrometers or goniometers that are designed to measure light intensity at specific angles on photocells. The data collected on the cells represents the light intensity at a given angle and is presented in a digital format of values in standardized ASCII format defined by standards created by IESNA.

A test was setup by Neale to compare the real-world luminance values from the headlamps to the light values obtained in the simulation program with the photometric files. To test the headlamps in a real-world environment, a site with a typical paved

TABLE 11.6 Vehicles and headlamp types evaluated by Neale [7]

Vehicle make	Model	Year	Class	Lamp type
Toyota	Land Cruiser	1994	SUV	Lens optics
Cooper	Mini	2005	Passenger	Projector optics
Nissan	Pickup Truck	2006	Pickup	Reflector optics

FIGURE 11.23 Photographs of the vehicles and headlamps evaluated by Neale [7].

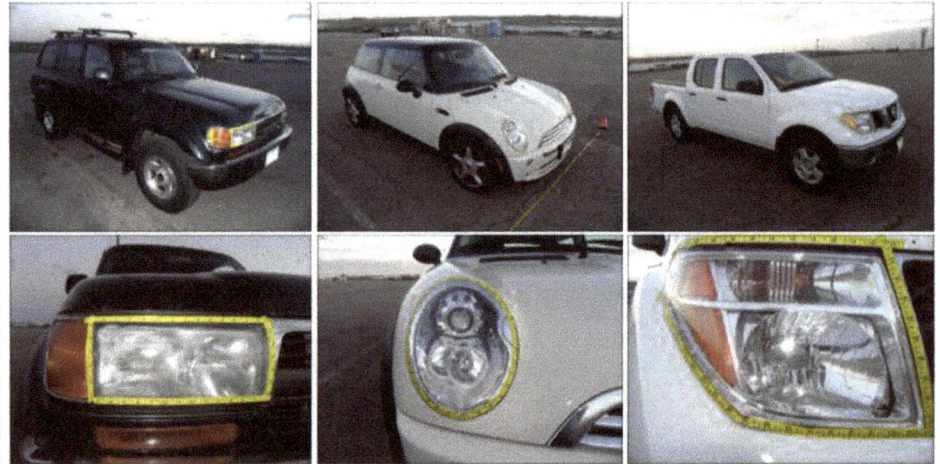

roadway surface was chosen that contained no ambient lighting. To include several basic headlamp design types, three different vehicles were used, each representing a different class of vehicle. Table 11.6 and Figure 11.23 list and show the make and model of the vehicles used in this study and the headlamp designs for each vehicle.

In addition to representing three different classes of vehicles, each vehicle in this study had a different optic system. The lens optics, projector, and reflector optics headlamp designs (shown from left to right in Figure 11.23) account for most of the vehicle headlamp types used on passenger vehicles. After mapping these headlamp systems, Neale then simulated their light distributions using photometric files in Autodesk's 3DS Max Design 2009 Exposure Technology light simulation tool. This light simulation package is widely used in light simulation environments, and the accuracy of the light simulation model has been widely published and validated.

Neale found that the behavior and pattern of light distribution from an actual headlamp were different than the behavior of light emitted by a photometric file of a headlamp in a simulation program. This is because headlamps contain sophisticated optics that result in a headlamp assembly projecting light more like several light sources than one. The design of this optics system in headlamps renders a photometric data file of the headlamp inadequate in representing light intensity and distribution in a simulation environment. While photometric light files are accurate for some types of light sources and luminaries, the photometric file does not represent the complex reflector and lens assemblies of the headlamp that collect and distribute headlamp light such that the projection of the light changes over distance.

Headlamps are not static lights like a street lamps or building, since the vehicles move within the environment. Also, the stringent design requirements for headlamps to both illuminate objects ahead for better visibility while reducing glare for oncoming traffic result in complex optics. The beam formation of a headlamp may not occur until 30 to 50 ft from the headlamp itself, and this beam pattern is a central light contributing component of the headlamp for far field distances. The reflectors and lenses of headlamps direct the light from the light source to achieve a hotspot in the distance by focusing light from both horizontal sides of the headlamp. Because these two beams are crossing in the distance, it is not possible for a photometric file to record the direction the light is crossing and how this crossing affects the hotspot close or farther away from the headlamp.

11.5 Terminology for Nighttime Visibility Analysis

Adapting Luminance Level: Phillips et al. [8] note that "the luminance level to which the observer adapts just prior to and during viewing the object of interest is a very important factor in determining the visibility of the object. The contrast sensitivity of the human visual system changes with adaptation level, becoming less sensitive to contrast at lower light levels. This is why a book that is quite easy to read under a bright lamp can become nearly impossible to read under dim illumination. The contrast of the letters and the page may be exactly the same, but our eyes are much less sensitive to this contrast at lower light levels."

Illuminance: The amount of light reaching a surface [8, 9]. This is dependent on the distance from the source, and this dependence is governed by the following equation:

$$I = \frac{c}{d^2} \qquad (12.1)$$

In this equation,

I is the illuminance in foot-candles or lux
c is the source output in lumens or candelas
d is the distance from the source to the surface in feet or meters

Luminance: Light reflected from a surface that yields the sensation of brightness [9]. Objects with a higher luminance will appear brighter than objects with a lower luminance [8]. Luminance is measured in units of candelas per meter squared (cd/m²).

Luminance Contrast: A difference between the luminance of an object and the luminance of its background. Krauss and Olson [9] note that "seeing requires that contrast be created by means of differential reflectivity within the object and between the object and its background. The contrast may come from such things a color, brightness, pattern and shading, or any combination of these." The following formula is used to calculate the luminance contrast [8]:

$$C = \frac{L_o - L_b}{L_b} \qquad (12.2)$$

In this equation,

C is the contrast
L_o is the luminance of the object
L_b is the luminance of the background

If the luminance of the object is greater than the background, the result is positive contrast. If the luminance of the object is less than the background, the result is negative contrast (silhouette). The greater the contrast, the greater the visibility of the object.

Luminance Contrast Sensitivity: The difference in luminance between an object and its background that is necessary for the object to be detected.

Luminous Intensity: The output of a light source, measured in candelas (cd) or lumens (lm) [9]. A lumen is the total light output from a source per unit time. Krauss and Olson note that "lumen is the term generally used to describe the output of area sources of illumination such as streetlamps. When dealing with directional sources such as automotive headlamps the preferred term is candela."

Lux: The illuminance 1 meter from a light source with a luminous intensity of 1 cd.

Photometry: The measurement of light [9].

Psychophysical Validation of a Photographic Representation: A process for validating the accuracy of the visibility conditions depicted in a photographic image. According to Ayres [10], "the key is to base evaluation of the print on observations made the scene. Baker & Fricke (1986) briefly describe a procedure in which a test target or pattern, such as grey numbers on a black background, are slowly moved from a dark area to a lighted area to find the point at which the numbers are just barely readable at the observer's position; then the viewing conditions for the picture are to be adjusted so that the numbers are barely readable. This is the essence of a psychophysical or subjective validation procedure...An important feature of this approach is its conceptual simplicity. Given the complexity of photography – characteristics of cameras and lenses and films, the chemistry of the developing process, the nonlinearities of printing – it is very difficult to place confidence in the visibility represented by a photographic print based solely on good photographic technique. Instead, if the visibility of some aspect of a print reproduces the visibility recorded at the scene, then the details of the photographic process do not need to be considered."

Threshold Contrast: The contrast at which an object will be detected 50% of the time [8].

Veiling Luminance: Contrast-reducing glare [8].

Visual Acuity: Sharpness of vision.

References

1. Olson, P. and Abrams, R., "Improved Motorcycle and Moped Headlamps," UM-HSRI-82-18, May 1982.

2. Sturgis, S.P., "Motorcycle Headlighting Research," UM-HSRI-HF-75-3, August 1975.

3. Gould, M. et al., "Judgments of Approach Speed for Motorcycles across Different Lighting Levels and the Effect of an Improved Tri-Headlight Configuration," *Accident Analysis and Prevention* (2012), doi:10.1016/j.aap.2012.02.002.

4. Neale, W.T.C. and Hessel, D., "Simulating Headlamp Illumination Using Photometric Light Clusters," SAE Technical Paper 2009-01-0110, 2009, doi:10.4271/2009-01-0110.

5. Neale, W.T.C., McKelvey, N., Pentecost, D., and Koch, D., "Motorcycle Headlamp Distribution Comparison," SAE Technical Paper 2018-01-0112, 2018, doi:10.4271/2018-01-0112.

6. Muttart, J. et al., "Determining when an Object Enters the Headlight Beam Pattern of a Vehicle," SAE Technical Paper 2013-01-0787, 2013, doi:10.4271/2013-01-0787.

7. Neale, W.T.C., Hessel, D., and Marr, J., "Evaluation of Photometric Data Files for Use in Headlamp Light Distribution," SAE Technical Paper 2010-01-0292, 2010, doi:10.4271/2010-01-0292.

8. Phillips, E.S., Khatua, T., Kost, G., and Piziali, R., "Vision and Visibility in Vehicular Accident Reconstruction," SAE Technical Paper 900369, 1990, doi:10.4271/900369.

9. Krauss, D. and Olson, P., *Forensic Aspects of Driver Perception and Response*, 4th ed., (Tucson, AZ: Lawyers and Judges Publishing Company, 2015), ISBN:978-1-936360-333-8.

10. Ayres, T.J., "Psychophysical Validation of Photographic Representations, *Safety Engineering and Risk Analysis* (SERA-Vol. 6), *1996 American Society of Mechanical Engineers (ASME) International Mechanical Engineering Congress and Exposition*, Atlanta, GA, November 17-22, 1996.

12

Human Factors in Motorcycle Crashes

This chapter addresses human factors issues relevant to motorcycle crashes, including perception-response times for motorcyclists and drivers and the physical and willingness limits on accident avoidance maneuvers by motorcyclists and drivers. Earlier chapters began to address some human limits relevant to motorcycle crash analysis. For instance, Chapter 3 summarized studies related to the braking capabilities of motorcyclists and concluded that, by utilizing their front brakes, motorcyclists should reasonably be able to achieve a deceleration of 0.5 g. Many motorcyclists will be able to achieve more than this. Chapter 4 summarized studies related to the turn-away and swerving capabilities of motorcyclists. All the motorcyclists involved in these studies executed swerves that exceeded a lateral acceleration of 0.3 g (when analyzed within the framework of Equation (3.31)). Chapter 4 also cited data showing that many riders reach a limit on their willingness to continue to lean their motorcycle before reaching the motorcycle's maximum lean angle. Watanabe and Yoshida found that the maximum lean angles utilized by novice riders were typically in the range of 15° to 25°, and those used by experienced riders were in the range of 34° to 40°. These results imply that the experienced riders in the study by Watanabe and Yoshida used maximum lean angles that would approach the lean angle limits of many motorcycles, whereas novice riders stopped well short of the motorcycle limits.

Beyond this basic information, a reconstructionist may need to calculate or estimate the time required for a motorcyclist or a driver to perceive and respond to a hazard. Also, since there is often a need to evaluate how the driver of a passenger vehicle could have avoided a motorcyclist, there is a need to define some of the performance limits of passenger vehicle drivers, as well. Finally, the reconstructionist will benefit from understanding factors that may come into play in specific situations, such as motorcycle conspicuity, rider skill level and the influence of training, protective equipment for motorcyclists, and group riding. This chapter develops each of these topics.

In discussing the human factors issues that arise when reconstructing motorcycle crashes, several epidemiological studies are cited. In the context of crash reconstruction, epidemiological studies are useful in illuminating factors that may have contributed to a crash, but they cannot reveal which of these factors *actually* contributed to any particular crash. Determining which factors contributed to a particular crash must come out of an evaluation of the evidence and facts specific to that particular crash. For example, epidemiological studies related to motorcycle crashes have demonstrated that, after being involved in a crash with a motorcycle, passenger car drivers often report not having seen the motorcycle. Researchers have identified many factors that could contribute to the motorcycle not being seen-the small and narrow profile of motorcycles, the passenger car driver not expecting to see a motorcyclist, the motorcycle being occluded by other traffic or some geometric feature of the site, a lack of lighting to make the motorcycle detectable, or a lack of contrast between the rider and surrounding environment. For any particular crash, though, each of these factors should be evaluated in relationship to the evidence rather than simply assuming that any of these factors contributed to the crash. It is possible that none of them contributed to a particular crash and that the physical evidence will show that the driver actually did see the motorcyclist. For example, there may be pre-impact skid marks from the car, even though the driver reported not having seen the motorcyclist.

General categories of factors that can lead to a crash emerge from epidemiological studies. Treat, et al., for instance, found that human factors contributed to the occurrence of the crash in 92.6% of their crash investigations [1]. Environmental factors contributed in 33.8% of the crashes and vehicular factors contributed in 12.6% of the crashes. Treat noted that "the major human direct causes were improper lookout, excessive speed, inattention, improper evasive action, and internal distraction. Leading environmental causes were view obstructions and slick roads. The major vehicular causes were brake failure, inadequate tread depth, side-to-side brake imbalance, under-inflation, and vehicle-related vision obstructions. Vision (especially poor dynamic visual acuity) and personality (especially poor personal and social adjustment) were found related to accident-involvement." The principle, though, is that an accident reconstructionist's conclusions should be driven by the evidence and facts related to the particular crash being analyzed.

Hurt and Dupont [2] reported research they conducted as a part of the Traffic Safety Center at the University of Southern California, under the sponsorship of the National Highway Traffic Safety Administration of the U.S. Department of Transportation. They reported that this research was to involve "on-scene, in-depth multidisciplinary investigation of at least 900 motorcycle accidents, and the acquisition of at least 3600 police traffic accident reports for comparison." At the time of their 1977 report, 300 of the on-scene investigations had been completed, and 900 traffic crash reports had been gathered. Based on this data, Hurt and Dupont offered a number of observations, including that "the motorcycle is particularly sensitive to environmental problems such as animals in the roadway, oil, water, and gravel contamination of the roadway, grooved freeways, railroad tracks, etc. Also, it is clear from the accident investigations that vehicle mechanical problems have far more serious consequences for the motorcycle than for the contemporary passenger automobile. A puncture flat on the freeway essentially guarantees a disaster for the motorcycle rider while the same occurrence in a passenger car would only cause anxious moments...Of course, in the study of any system of motor vehicle accidents, the problems of inattention, alcohol, risk-taking behavior, etc., will appear and contribute to accident causation. However, the purpose of this paper is to describe those human factors problems that are peculiar to the motorcycle accident. These special motorcycle problems are those of motorcycle conspicuity, rider skill, training and licensing, and protective equipment." While any of these factors might contribute to the occurrence of motorcycle crashes in a general sense, determining which factors actually contributed to a motorcycle crash requires analysis of the evidence.

A more recent study-referred to as the Motorcycle Accidents In Depth Study (MAIDS)-examined the causes of motorcycle accidents in five European countries (France, Germany, the Netherlands, Spain, and Italy) [3]. This study was conducted by the Association of European Motorcycle Manufacturers (ACEM), and, as the final report (Version 2.0) for this study indicates, 921 accidents were investigated and reconstructed. The study concluded that the cause of most motorcycle accidents "was found to be human error. The most frequent human error was a failure to see the [motorcycle] within the traffic environment, due to lack of driver attention, temporary view obstructions or the low conspicuity of the [motorcycle]…When the accident riders were compared to the exposure population, the data demonstrated that the use of alcohol increased the risk of being in an accident, although the percentage was lower than in other studies. Unlicensed [motorcycle] operators who were illegally riding…were also found to be at greater risk of being involved in an accident when compared to licensed [motorcycle] riders."

12.1 Why Do Drivers Pull Out in Front of Motorcyclists?

Hurt and Dupont [2] noted that "the most likely comment of an automobile driver involved in a traffic collision with a motorcycle is that he, or she, did not SEE the motorcycle…" (emphasis in original). Hurt continued: "The origin of this problem seems to be related to the element of conspicuity (or conspicuousness) of the motorcycle; in other words, how easy it is to see the motorcycle. When the motorcycle and the automobile are on collision paths, or when the vehicles are in opposing traffic, the conspicuity due to motion is very low, if it exists at all. Consequently, recognition of the motorcycle by the automobile driver will depend entirely upon the conspicuity due to contrast. If the approaching motorcycle and rider blend well with the background scene, and if the automobile driver has not developed improved visual search habits which include low-threat targets…the motorcycle will not be recognized as a vehicle and a traffic hazard exists."* Without discounting the factors listed by Hurt, it should be recognized that his statements go too far, discount too much, and are not fully supported by later research. Though he acknowledges it elsewhere, physical obstructions from other traffic, inattention and distraction on the part of a passenger car driver, a driver conducting a visual search of inadequate duration, a lack of expectation to encounter a motorcycle, and excessive speed on the part of a motorcyclist are other factors that may account for (or at least play into) a driver not seeing a motorcyclist.

* Helman [4] cited a number of sources and noted that conspicuity can be defined as "the extent to which an object stands out from its surroundings. Conspicuity is different than visibility (although in practice the same factors affect both) which is usually defined as the ease with which an object can be detected when an observer is aware of its location. It is generally acknowledged that the most important determinant of an object's conspicuity/visibility is its contrast with its surroundings, although other features such as an object's movement relative to its background also play a role."

In 1989, Olson examined the literature related to why passenger car drivers sometimes fail to detect motorcyclists [5]. Although he noted that "considered logically, it seems reasonable that motorcycles should be less conspicuous than cars because they are smaller," Olson questions motorcycle conspicuity as the likely explanation for car drivers missing motorcycles. He observed that "the strongest support for the conspicuity hypothesis may be that the offending operator often reports a failure to detect the other vehicle." However, Olson noted that "the conspicuity hypothesis has not been seriously challenged. Almost all investigators have accepted it as fact, concentrating their efforts on means to improve conspicuity rather than on asking whether the hypothesis is correct. This is unfortunate because alternative hypotheses can be advanced. Some have research data to support them; some are speculative. All are consistent with the known facts..." Olson noted that drivers claiming to have <u>not</u> seen another vehicle is <u>not</u> unique to motorcycle-car intersection collisions.* He stated: "Violations of right of way are a common cause of collisions between automobiles, and afterward the errant driver often claims not to have seen the other vehicle. This should not be surprising. Of all the reasons that someone would deliberately move into the path of an oncoming vehicle, failure to detect it must be high on the list. But if the claimed failure to detect is not unique to motorcycle collisions, then it is not evidence for a special conspicuity problem with motorcycles." Olson discussed other explanations for why passenger car drivers sometimes miss motorcyclists, including visual obstructions and errors in the drivers' estimates of how far away a motorcycle is and how fast it is traveling.

Olson's observations are consistent with other studies. Pai, for example, published a literature review related to motorcycle right-of-way accidents in 2011 [7]. He reported that "two major causes of such a crash scenario are the lack of motorcycle conspicuity and motorist's speed/distance judgment error, respectively." This appears to be imprecise language that means that some motorists <u>did not</u> see the motorcycles prior to the accident and other motorists <u>did</u> but misjudged the timing of its approach. Pai continued: "A substantial number of studies have manipulated physical characteristics of motorcycles and motorcyclists to enhance conspicuity... Although various conspicuity aids have proven effective, some researchers reported that motorcyclist's/motorcycle's brightness per se may be less important as a determinant of conspicuity than brightness contrast between the motorcyclists and the surroundings...Research examining the effects of conspicuity measures on motorists' speed/distance judgments when confronting motorcycles has been rather inconclusive." In relationship to motorists' judgments of approaching vehicles, Pai noted that "larger vehicles tended to be judged to arrive sooner than motorcycles. Such a speed/distance judgment error is likely attributable to some psychological effects such that larger automobiles appear more threatening than motorcycles. Older motorists particularly have difficulties in accurately estimating the distance and the speed of an approaching motorcycle."

Along these same lines, Sager [8] and his colleagues noted in 2014 that "much previous research has focused on motorcycle properties, such as size, shape, and color to explain its inconspicuousness...Much of the motorcycle safety research conducted since has focused on making motorcycles more conspicuous, generally through various lighting treatments such as headlight modulators, additional lights, and bright reflective garments...There is some debate, however, regarding the effectiveness of these measures... it has been suggested that the problem may not be one of conspicuity at all...collision statistics remain largely unchanged, suggesting that the issue may <u>not</u> be related solely

* Herslund and Jørgensen [6], for instance, reported a study of crashes in which drivers reported that they failed to see approaching bicyclists. They reported that experienced drivers may be more likely to make these errors than inexperienced drivers, and they suggested that this may relate to the expectations and search patterns drivers develop over time.

to the motorcycle's static properties." Sager's research suggests that the motorcycle and rider's dynamic properties, such as lane position, also make a difference to the likelihood a motorcyclist will be detected.

Sager and his colleagues demonstrated this using a driving simulator to examine the motorcyclist's lane position as a factor in crashes where a passenger car driver turns left and violates the right-of-way of the motorcycle. They used a North American driving configuration with cars driving on the right (rather than left) side of the road. He described their experiment as follows: "Seventeen participants faced oncoming traffic in a high-fidelity driving simulator and indicated when gaps were safe enough for them to turn left at an intersection. We manipulated the size of the gaps and the type of oncoming vehicle over 135 trials, with gap sizes varying from 3 to 5 s, and vehicles consisting of either a car, a motorcycle in the left-of-lane position, or a motorcycle in the right-of-lane position. Our results show that drivers are more likely to turn in front of an oncoming motorcycle when it travels in the left-of-lane position than when it travels in the right-of-lane position." Sager and his colleagues had determined, based on the intersection geometry and the acceleration capabilities of the vehicle, that "a three-second gap in a stream of oncoming traffic would not allow for the safe execution of a left turn, that a four-second gap would allow for the safe execution of a left turn, but leave very little safety margin, and that a five-second or more gap in the stream of traffic would allow for the execution of a left turn and leave a reasonable safety margin."

For each of the three gap sizes—3, 4, and 5 s—participants chose to turn more frequently when the motorcyclist was in the left-of-lane position than when the motorcycle was approaching in the right-of-lane position. Sager concludes that, "these results are consistent with our hypothesis that the right-of-lane position offers more motion cues to an oncoming driver and is therefore more likely to deter oncoming drivers from crossing in front of a motorcyclist's path as they approach an intersection. However, our findings are inconsistent with some motorcycle rider training which motorcyclists generally leave with the belief that they should always ride in the left portion of the lane. Our results suggest that the right-of-lane position may be a safer riding position when entering an intersection."

Unfortunately, however, the crash scenario studied by Sager is not the only one likely to be encountered by motorcyclists. Drawing general conclusions about the optimum lane position for a motorcyclist, who may encounter multiple hazards simultaneously, seems unwarranted based on Sager's research alone. There are scenarios a motorcyclist could encounter where their choice of lane position, and how it might or might not affect visibility and conspicuity, may compete with other crash avoidance factors. Ouellet [9], for example, examined the optimal lane positioning for motorcyclists in terms of the time they had available for collision avoidance, noting that "lane positioning as the rider approaches a potentially threatening situation is a simpler, more reliable and more effective means of reducing collision risk than reliance on emergency braking." His study revealed that "the motorcycle rider can do more to avoid a collision by moving laterally away from a threatening vehicle, putting at least one lane-width between them, before a vehicle begins to violate his right-of-way, than he can be effective braking after the other vehicle has begun to violate his right-of-way" (emphasis in original). Depending on the intersection geometry and what other vehicles are present, these statements could dictate a left-of-lane, right-of-lane, or center-of-lane positioning.

In 1996, Hole, Tyrrell, and Langham reported three experiments related to motorcycle conspicuity [10]. These experiments involved showing the test subjects a series of images containing traffic. Less than half of the images contained motorcyclists, so that the test subjects could not assume there would be a motorcyclist in each image. Hole and his colleagues recorded the time it took the subjects to determine if a motorcyclist was present in each image. They varied if the motorcycle headlight was on or not, the type of clothing worn by the motorcyclists (plain dark, plain bright, patterned dark, and patterned bright), the distance of the motorcycles from the viewer, and the driving situation (urban or semirural). They also examined the influence of background clutter on the conspicuity of the motorcyclists. These researchers reported that "the effectiveness of the conspicuity aids used, especially clothing, may depend on the situation in which the motorcyclist was located: bright clothing and headlight use may not be infallible aids to conspicuity. Brightness contrast between the motorcyclist and the surroundings may be more important as a determinant of conspicuity than the motorcyclist's brightness *per se*. Motorcyclists' conspicuity is a more complex issue than has hitherto been acknowledged."

Specific findings by these researchers included the fact that "motorcyclists were detected more quickly the nearer they were to the viewer, and in both locations the biggest difference between the headlight-off and headlight-on conditions was at the furthest viewing distance"; "the effectiveness of the headlight as a conspicuity aid was much less clear-cut in the urban setting than in the semi-rural environment...headlight use in the urban location enhanced conspicuity only when the motorcyclist was wearing plain bright or patterned dark clothing: when patterned-bright or plain dark clothing were worn, subjects responded faster when the headlight was off than when it was on. In the urban setting, a consistent advantage for headlight use was demonstrated only when the motorcyclist was wearing patterned-dark clothing"; "in both locations, many more motorcyclists were undetected at the furthest distance from the viewer than when the motorcyclist was nearby...for the semi-rural location, at all three distances, there error-rate for the slides in which the motorcyclist's headlight was lit was half that for the slides in which the headlight was unlit...For the urban location, at all three distances, the error-rate for the slides in which the motorcyclist's headlight was lit was lower than that for the slides in which the headlight was unlit, but not markedly so"; "in both locations, there was little effect of clothing type except possibly at the furthest distance."

Reconstructionists should be careful about an overly literal application of these findings, but they do demonstrate the interplay between several factors in the visual environment a driver can encounter. Hole, Tyrrell, and Langham noted several limitations of their study. Among these was their observation that "problems are also caused by the fact that instructing subjects to look for motorcyclists may cause them to process a traffic scene in ways that are different to those used in normal driving...Cole and Hughes distinguish between two types of conspicuity. 'Attention conspicuity' refers to the capacity of a stimulus to be noticed when the observer is not actively looking for it. 'Search conspicuity' refers to the capacity of a stimulus to be noticed when the observer is specifically looking for it. The experiments reported here have examined factors affecting motorcyclists' search conspicuity, but in real life, attention conspicuity may also be important." Helman [4] further clarified the relationship between visibility, search conspicuity, and attention conspicuity with the following three statements:

- If the observers are directed to look *at* the location of the motorcycle to see if they can detect it, we are measuring visibility.

- If the observers are directed to look *for* the motorcycle in the scene but are not told where it is, we are measuring search conspicuity.

- If the observers are simply asked to report the things in the road scene that grab their attention, we are measuring attention conspicuity.

Finally, Hole, Tyrrell, and Langham observed that "the fact that there were few differences between conditions when the motorcyclist was nearby implies that motorcyclists' conspicuity *at the close range within which accidents often occur* might be relatively unaffected by such factors: within this range, it is possible that the psychological state of the driver may play a more important role than the physical characteristics of the motorcyclist...inappropriate expectancies may be more important in accident causation than the motorcyclist's physical properties."

Horswill, Helman, Ardiles, and Wann [11] noted that "drivers adopt smaller safety margins when pulling out in front of motorcycles compared with cars. This could partly account for why the most common motorcycle/car accident involves a car violating a motorcyclist's right of way. One possible explanation is the size-arrival effect in which smaller objects are perceived to arrive later than larger objects. That is, drivers may estimate the time to arrival of motorcycles to be later than cars because motorcycles are smaller." These authors conducted two experiments to test this hypothesis. In the first experiment, test subjects (28 drivers who had never ridden a motorcycle) were shown video footage of traffic approaching the viewing position of the camera. Four vehicles were used to create the video footage—a small motorcycle, a large motorcycle, a car, and a van—and these vehicles were driven toward the scene at speeds of ether 30 or 40 mph. The scene blacked out 4 s before the vehicle reached the camera's position. Subjects were asked to press a response button when they estimated the vehicle would have reached the viewing position of the camera. This experiment resulted in the conclusion, consistent with the authors' hypothesis, that "time-to-arrival estimations were significantly longer for motorcycles than for the larger vehicles...."

In the second experiment, Horswill et al. varied the time at which the video was blacked out (1, 2, 4, and 7 s prior to arrival). For these scenarios, each subject viewed the approaching vehicle for 4 s prior to the screen going black, but the starting position of the vehicle varied. From this experiment, the authors concluded that the "motorcycles were estimated to arrive significantly later than cars, and this was significant when vehicles disappeared 1 s before they arrived (both at 30 and 40 mph). This indicated that vehicle differences were unlikely to be a result of threshold differences in detecting object expansion as all vehicles in the 1-s condition would be well above threshold before occlusion." From both experiments, these authors concluded that "one reason that motorcyclists could be at greater risk of being hit at road junctions is because of an unfortunate optical illusion. People estimated that motorcycles reached them later than cars when time-to-arrival was actually the same...This effect is consistent with the size-arrival effect...in which participants judge, incorrectly, that approaching smaller objects will arrive later than larger objects." In 2003, Horswill and Helman had examined motorcyclists' behavior in comparison to that of car drivers and reported that "motorcyclists chose faster speeds than the car drivers, overtook more, and pulled into smaller gaps in traffic, though they did not travel any closer to the vehicle in front" [12]. If a motorcyclist does choose to approach an intersection at a high speed, this will exacerbate the size-arrival effect and make it harder for a left-turning driver to judge the gap available for to complete their turn.

Brenac, Clabaux, Perrin, and Van Elslande [13] observe that "the hypothesis of a link between motorcycle speed and low conspicuity may indeed be advanced: for a given time to potential collision, the higher the motorcyclist's speed, the greater is the distance from the other vehicle. And therefore, for a given time to potential collision, the higher the motorcyclist's speed, the smaller is the motorcyclist's apparent size in the field of vision of the other driver." The other implication, of course, is that the slower the motorcyclist is traveling, the greater the time available for the intruding driver to clear the intersection before the motorcyclist arrives. Brenac and his colleagues conducted in-depth investigations of 22 collisions occurring in urban areas between motorcycles and other vehicles, many of which were situations where drivers pulled out into the path of an approaching motorcycle. Based on these reconstructions, Branac and his colleagues concluded that there was "a significant relation between problems of conspicuity and the motorcyclist's high level of speed in accident cases occurring in urban areas."

A 2006 study by Labbett and Langham examined the visual search patterns of drivers at two intersections using a hidden video camera [14]. One of the intersections had a visibility obstruction on the corner, and the other did not and allowed for an unobstructed view of several hundred meters. The intersections were on the campus of the University of Sussex, and the video footage enabled these researchers to determine which vehicles had a university parking pass and which did not. This was used to determine which drivers were likely familiar with the intersections and which were not. Labbett and Langham concluded that, on average, "the drivers observed spent less than 0.5 seconds searching for hazards." They also found that the drivers tended to only search in one direction. Labbett and Langham also did an experiment in which participants were shown video clips of approaching traffic. They found different search patterns between novice and experienced drivers. "The experienced drivers tended to fixate on only small areas of the screen whilst novice drivers tended to search many parts of the scene."

In 2010, Gershon reported two experiments related to motorcycle conspicuity [15]. The first experiment "evaluated the influence of [the motorcycle and rider's] attention conspicuity on the ability of un-alerted viewers to detect it." The second experiment "evaluated the [motorcycle and rider's] search conspicuity to alerted viewers." Gershon and his colleagues varied the driving scenario (urban and interurban), the motorcycle rider's outfit (black, white, and reflective), and the distance of the motorcycle from the viewer. In the first experiment, 66 students were individually presented with a series of pictures. They viewed each picture for 0.6 s and then were asked to report all the vehicle types they observed in each picture. In the second experiment, 64 participants viewed the same pictures utilized in the previous experiment. In the second experiment, though, the participants were instructed to look for motorcycles and to report if each photograph showed a motorcycle.

For the first experiment, Gershon reported that the detection of the motorcycles "depended on the interaction between its distance from the viewer, the driving scenario and [the] rider's outfit...when the [motorcycle] was distant the different outfit conditions affected its' attention conspicuity. In urban roads, where the background surrounding the [motorcycle and rider] was more complex and multi-colored, the reflective and white outfits increased its attention conspicuity compared to the black outfit condition. In contrast, in inter-urban roads, where the background was solely a bright sky, the black outfit provided an advantage for the [motorcycle's] detectability."

For the second experiment, Gershon reported that the "detection rate of the alerted viewers was very high and the average reaction time to identify the presence of a [motorcycle] was the shortest in the inter-urban environment. Like the results of experiment 1, in urban environments the reflective and white clothing provided an advantage to the detection of the [motorcycle and rider], while in the inter-urban environment the black outfit presented an advantage. Comparing the results of the two experiments revealed that at the farthest distance, the increased awareness in the search conspicuity detection rates were three times higher than in the attention conspicuity." In other words, the rider's clothing made a difference, but the driver's awareness or expectation that there would be motorcyclists in some of the pictures made a bigger difference. As Gershon noted, "unfortunately, detectability - especially attention conspicuity - is compromised by the perceptual characteristics of the environment that change continuously along a route. Thus, to increase detectability, [motorcycle] riders need to be aware of the perceptual aspects of their riding environment. In parallel, the results of the second experiment with alerted viewers demonstrate that other road users (e.g., car drivers) can improve their detection performance when they increase their level of expectancy and awareness concerning a possible existence of a [motorcycle] on the road (as drivers with high expectation obtained nearly 100% detection rates)."

Helman [4] and Rogé [16] both referred to a driver's expectation to see motorcyclists as cognitive conspicuity. That a lack of expectancy (a lack of cognitive conspicuity) may play a significant role in car drivers failing to recognize the presence of a motorcycle is consistent with the fact that motorcycles make up a relatively small percentage of the vehicle population and therefore, may not be encountered that frequently by passenger car drivers. For example, in 2015, motorcycles made up only 3% of all registered vehicles in the United States [17]. Layer on top of that the weather conditions that can limit the riding season in many states and motorcycles end up accounting for only 0.6% of all vehicle miles traveled in the United States. Thus, the typical passenger car driver will encounter motorcycles less frequently than they encounter other passenger cars. The lack of expectancy that this low frequency may cause is targeted by advertising campaigns in some states with slogans such as "Share the Road: Look Twice for Motorcyclists."

Lenné and Mitsopoulos-Rubens [18] reported a study in which they subjected 43 experienced drivers to a series of trials in a driving simulator. The task given to these subjects was to "turn ahead of an oncoming vehicle if they felt that they had sufficient room to do so safely." In some trials, subjects had to turn in front of a motorcycle with its headlight on, and, in other trials, the headlight was off. The gap available for the turn was also varied (short, medium, long). Lenné and Mitsopoulos-Rubens reported that "at short time gaps low-beam headlights may confer some benefit in gap acceptance by encouraging drivers to accept fewer gaps ahead of a motorcycle with headlights on than ahead of a motorcycle with headlights off. No statistically significant differences in gap acceptance between the headlight conditions were found at either the medium or long time gaps."

Crundall et al. [19] noted that the most common cause of motorcycle collisions in the United Kingdom "was that of another vehicle pulling into the path of a motorcycle when exiting from a side road onto the main carriageway." These authors observed that the statistics related to the number of look-but-fail-to-see collisions with motorcyclists may be inflated "by self-report biases. One could imagine alternative causes: a failure to look in the appropriate direction; or having looked and perceived the approaching motorcycle, the car driver might fail to judge the level of risk that the conflicting motorcycle presents." To further examine these issues, they developed a test in which subjects viewed video of an intersection on multiple screens simultaneously. The video was from the vantage point of a driver wanting to pull out at a T-junction, and the screens were set up such that the subjects could turn their heads to the left and right to look for conflicting traffic. Crundall noted that "Mirror information was edited into the forward-facing video footage, providing a left-side mirror in the bottom-right of the left screen, a right-side mirror in the bottom-left of the right screen, and a rear-view mirror at the top of the central screen. The three televisions were angled from each other at 120 degrees providing an immersive video, wherein participants could look to the left and right, as if looking through the side windows of their car, to check for conflicting vehicles on the main carriageway." Both novice and experienced drivers were tested, as was a group of drivers with considerable experience driving both cars and motorcycles. "Specifically, we were interested in when drivers first fixate the conflicting vehicles approaching the T-junction (when they look), how long they looked for (a measure of whether they perceive) and when they press a button to pull out from the junction (which, given that the necessary - but not sufficient - preconditions of looking and perceiving are met, can be considered a measure of appraisal)."

Crundall's study included 74 test subjects-25 novice car drivers with a mean age of 20.6 years and a mean experience level of 1.6 years, 25 experienced car drivers with a mean age of 33.4 years and a mean experience level of 14.8 years, and 24 drivers with significant experience with both cars and motorcycles (dual drivers) with a mean age of 44.9 years and a mean experience level of 25.7 years with cars and 20.0 years with a motorcycle. The videos used in the study include 10 scenarios with conflicting motorcycles, 10 with conflicting cars, and 10 with no conflicting vehicles. Conflicting vehicles could appear from either the right or the left. The clips included the approach phase to the T-junction, the stop, and then the time for the participants to make a decision about when they would pull out. Crundall also noted that "a further 42 clips (not analysed in the current paper) were randomly interspersed which required a different response; either a lane-change decision...or a hazard perception response. Participants could not predict when a hazard might appear, and thus had to remain vigilant to hazards even during the T-junction scenarios. Response times reflecting when the participants thought it was safe to pull out were recorded, along with the participants' eye movements."

Crundall reported that "the most immediate finding from the analyses was the greater caution given to conflicting motorcycles than to conflicting cars. Both the percentage of safe responses and the [reaction times] reflect a greater safety margin in responding to motorcycles... In regard to group differences, dual drivers were more cautious than the novice drivers, with the experienced group falling in between. This pattern held regardless of whether or not there was conflicting traffic. While the overall means improved with experience, the differentiation between motorcycle clips and car clips seemed greatest for the dual drivers followed by the novice drivers...dual drivers were the most sensitive to the presence of a conflicting motorcycle, while experienced drivers appeared the least sensitive."

Crundall's research suggests that car drivers who also ride motorcycles are more aware of approaching motorcycles and less likely to violate their right-of-way. This is consistent with the findings of other researchers. Magazzù et al., for instance, found that "having gained experience in riding any motorcycle...results in drivers being less prone to cause crashes with motorcycles with respect to drivers with no motorcycle license. It is reasonable to assume that car drivers who hold a motorcycle license have acquired more ability in riding and controlling two wheeled vehicles than drivers without a license. Therefore, it is possible to infer that some riding ability and knowledge of the risk annexed to riding, could protect drivers, maybe by helping them in the detection of oncoming motorcycles and the prediction of their manoeuvres" [20].

Rogé et al. [16] reported a study aimed at determining "whether the low visibility of motorcycles is the result of their low cognitive conspicuity and/or their low sensory conspicuity for car drivers." These authors defined sensory conspicuity as "the extent to which an object can be distinguished from its environment because of its physical characteristics: angular size, eccentricity in relation to the point of gaze, brightness against the background, color, and so on...in other words, sensory conspicuity reflects an object's ability to attract visual attention and to be precisely located as a result of its physical properties." Rogé relates cognitive conspicuity to driver expectations, noting that "an observer's focus of attention is strongly influenced by his or her expectations, objectives, and knowledge...in many cases, inappropriate expectations may be more important in accident causation than the motorcyclist's physical properties." These authors tested a sample of 42 car drivers in a simulator. Half of the drivers were motorcyclists, and the other half were not. These subjects were subjected to three test sessions lasting 12 min each, with a break in between sessions. During each session, the subjects drove on roads with a speed limit of 90 kph and on a highway with a speed limit of 130 kph. They also passed through junctions and roundabouts where the speed limit was 50 and 30 kph. The traffic encountered by the test subjects in the simulator included 49 vehicles-small cars, vans, buses, tractor-trailers, and motorcycles. The authors noted that "the participants could not anticipate when and from where a motorcycle might appear because they never came back to the same section of the circuit and had to detect a motorcycle in several different situations." The authors of this study concluded that both sensory and cognitive conspicuity had an influence on drivers' detection of motorcyclists. Specifically, "a high level of color contrast between the motorcycles and the road surface enhanced the visibility of motorcycles," and car drivers who were also motorcyclists detected the motorcyclists sooner than car drivers who were not motorcyclists.

Helman et al. [4] identified and reviewed 27 studies (including some of those reviewed above) that sought to improve motorcyclists' visibility or conspicuity or to improve the accuracy of judgments of motorcyclists' speed or time to contact by other road users. These authors reported that "both [bright clothing and daytime running lights] seem to be capable of improving conspicuity, when this is measured in terms of detection (under search and attention conspicuity conditions), and when measured in terms of a behavioural response (such as size of gap accepted in front of a given motorcycle). The majority of studies covered in this review support this conclusion, although there are limitations… due to the number of different visual contexts in which motorcyclists find themselves when riding. For example, coloured clothing is more effective when viewed against a contrasting background. In terms of lighting, although it appears that dedicated daytime lighting on motorcycles is effective in increasing conspicuity, this effect may be smaller when other vehicles have their lights on…When lighting is arranged in such a way as to accentuate the form of the motorcycle (and to provide greater information for judging approach speed), this aids the observer in determining the time to arrival of the approaching bike (especially at night)…Across all treatments there is evidence that colour can play a role in effectiveness; this may be especially true in settings where coloured motorcycle lights aid in the motorcycle standing out from surrounding vehicles which have white lights. Although most studies reviewed show benefits of bright clothing, dark clothing may be better if the background is also brightly coloured. In line with the underlying mechanisms proposed, higher contrast with background surroundings to enable better visibility, search conspicuity, and attention conspicuity would be beneficial. Given that environments may differ over even fairly small changes in time or location, there is not likely to be a one-size-fits-all solution, meaning that motorcyclists need to be aware of the limitations of whichever interventions they use."

Review of these studies leads to the following observations related to collisions where a passenger car driver violates a motorcyclist's right-of-way and then states that they did not see the motorcyclists. First, for a driver to avoid making an unsafe turn in front of a motorcyclist, they need to <u>detect</u> the motorcyclists. If they do detect the motorcyclist, they will then need to make a reasonable judgment about the time available to complete their turn before the motorcyclist arrives at the intersection. The following factors may contribute to drivers failing to detect approaching motorcyclists: (a) inattention and distraction on the part of the driver; (b) occlusion of the motorcycle caused by the geometry of the intersection, by other traffic, by the geometry of the driver's vehicle, or by the small size of the motorcycle relative to a passenger car; (c) drivers not expecting to see motorcyclists on the road; and (d) a lack of conspicuity of the motorcycle and rider. The influence of the motorcycle headlight and the color and characteristics of the rider's clothing on the likelihood the motorcycle will be detected depends on the specific environment in which the accident unfolds and on how far away the motorcycle is when it needed to be detected. The following factors may contribute to drivers misjudging the time it will take for a motorcyclist to arrive at the intersection after they have detected them: (a) excessive speed on the part of the motorcyclist [12] and (b) the small size and narrowness of the motorcycle and rider relative to other vehicles on the roadway.

12.2 The Perception-Response Process

To determine how a crash could have been avoided, it may be necessary to analyze a range of reasonable perception-response times for a motorcyclist or driver. Olson [21] divided the perception-response process into four steps: detection, identification, decision, and response. According to Olson, "perception-response time begins when some object or condition of concern enters the driver's field of vision…[detection] concludes when the driver develops a conscious awareness that 'something' is present. The something may be within the field of view of the driver for some time before it is detected. Hence, there is the potential for a significant delay between the presentation of the stimulus and its being detected." During the identification step, "sufficient information is acquired about the object or condition to be able to reach a decision as to what action, if any, is required." During the decision step, the driver decides whether to change their speed or direction in response to the hazard, and during the response step, they enact that decision by moving their hands or feet to operate the controls of the vehicle. Consistent with Olson's definition, Ayres and Kubose [22] state that the perception-response time is the time that elapses from "perceptual availability" of a hazard until the "onset of a visible useful response" (such as braking or steering). Muttart [23], on the other hand, asserts that the perception-response time should not begin at the point of first perceptual availability or at the first point of detection but rather at the first point a detectable object or situation becomes an immediate hazard. He states, "perception-response should be from perception as an immediate hazard up until first *vehicle* response."

Research by Muttart over the last two decades has done much to advance the way that accident reconstructionists evaluate perception-response times [23, 24, 25, 26]. In the past, it was common for reconstructionists to cite rules of thumb-for instance, to assume that a reasonable perception-response time for a driver was always 1½ s, regardless of the situation. Muttart's work has demonstrated that perception-response times are situation dependent and that there is variability in the response times within a population of drivers. These facts were perhaps obvious but not often used by reconstructionists in practice. Muttart's work has given reconstructionists the ability to apply these ideas to their practice by developing mathematical equations for predicting driver perception-response times for various situations and implementing these equations in his software, I.DRR (Interactive Driver Response Research).

These equations are based on data from more than 200 driver response studies. The following scenarios are addressed within I.DRR: (1) drivers responding to lead vehicles that were either stopped or moving slowly, (2) drivers responding to being cut off, (3) drivers responding to vehicles intruding into their path, and (4) drivers responding to traffic signals. Within each of these categories, Muttart has demonstrated that apparent discrepancies between the results of various studies can be explained in terms of differences in methodology. He noted that, "in general, as the methodology of the experiment became closer to that of real life, the response times increased." Also, "response times increased from laboratory to simulator to closed course and then to road studies."

As an example, Figure 12.1 depicts some sample data obtained from I.DRR for a path intrusion scenario. The orange bars are average perception-response times for car drivers responding to a path intrusion in the daytime. The blue bars are average perception-response times for motorcyclists responding to a path intrusion in the daytime. These values are approximately 0.1 s longer than those for the car drivers. In his 4-h webinar related to the path intrusion scenario, Muttart indicates that motorcyclists' perception-response times are generally about 0.1 s longer than passenger car drivers'

FIGURE 12.1 Path intrusion perception-response times from I.DRR.

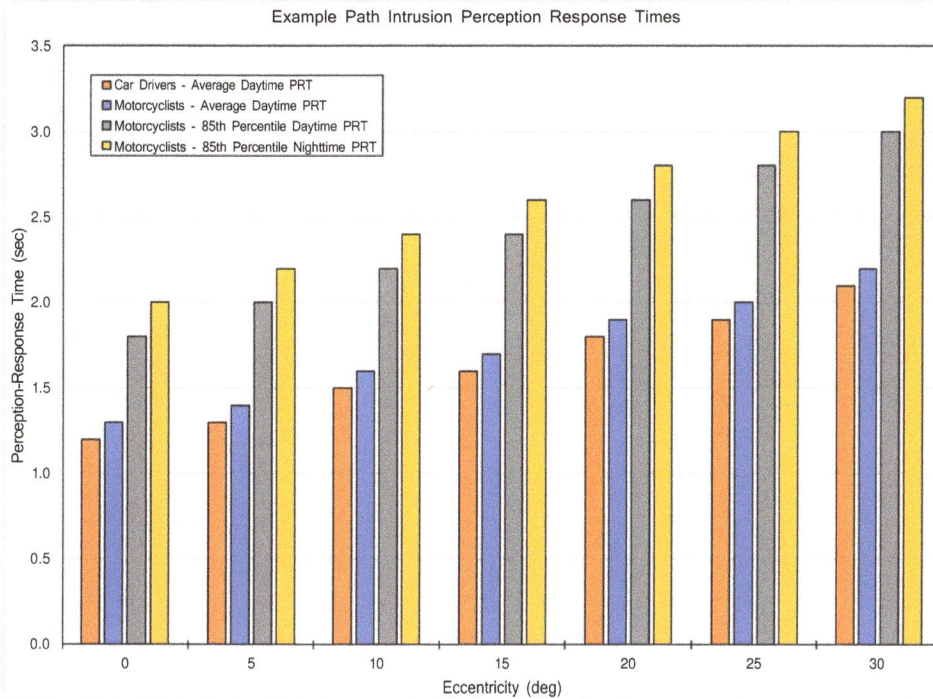

perception-response times. These slightly longer perception-response times for motor-cyclists occur even though some studies have shown motorcyclists to be more skilled at hazard perception than car drivers [27]. Muttart appears to attribute this to the number and complexity of the avoidance responses that motorcyclists can have.

The gray bars in Figure 12.1 are 85th percentile perception-response times for motorcyclists responding to a path intrusion in the daytime. These values vary from 0.5 to 0.8 s longer than the average values. The yellow bars are 85th percentile perception-response times for motorcyclists responding to a path intrusion at night. These values are 0.2 s longer than the daytime values. This graph also shows that the perception-response times depend on the eccentricity, which is the angle between the heading of the through vehicle and the area from which the intruding vehicle is coming (the stop bar of an intersection roadway, for instance). As this angle increases, the perception-response times increase. In practice, this angle depends on the geometry of the roadway and on the relative positions of the vehicles when the intruding vehicle begins pulling out. This is only a single example, and the reconstructionist can conduct their own analysis with I.DRR for specific situations.

Another important point is made by Ayres and Kubose [22], who noted that "it has long been understood that faster responses tend to be less accurate…Clearly there is no single value that can be said to represent the reaction time of even one person for one task, without considering the accuracy of task performance." This is relevant to crash avoidance because "a driver would tend to respond quickly although perhaps not very accurately when a collision is imminent, but would take a more careful approach (accurate, appropriate) with more time available. There is some evidence that drivers are sensitive to the immediacy of a hazard and can adjust accordingly." Thus, "one should not expect…that drivers will efficiently use all time available to make an optimum avoidance maneuver…it is unreasonable to expect optimal response timing and maneuver performance by drivers faced with emergencies."

12.3 Motorcyclists' Responses to a Laterally Incurring Vehicle

Hurt's 1977 report noted that, when a passenger car driver fails to see the motorcyclist, this will not likely be apparent to the motorcyclist, "because of the rider's apparent eye contact with the automobile driver. The motorcyclist believes, until the collision, that the automobile driver sees him and knows the motorcycle is there. A likely comment by the motorcycle rider involved in a collision in such a situation is that the automobile driver LOOKED directly at the motorcycle and then promptly turned in front of the motorcycle…" (emphasis in original).

In evaluating the responses of drivers to laterally incurring vehicles, Ising et al. observed that, in accident reconstruction, "there has traditionally been an assumption that full braking is occurring upon completion of the mechanical brake lag. This assumption is challenged by a growing body of research indicating a concurrent driver-related delay between brake application and full braking. Such a delay would have upstream consequences on the calculated relative positions and speeds of the vehicles at the moment of hazard onset" [28]. Other authors make similar observations. Prynne and Martin noted that "accident studies have shown that the full braking capability of vehicles is not often used in emergencies…Emergency braking, therefore, is often a two-stage process with drivers rapidly depressing the brake pedal to the normal limit of depression (about a third of the full range available) and then depressing the pedal further to some lower position after they have thought about the situation." [29]. Prynne and Martin also note that "as a general rule drivers brake if the obstacle is some distance away and swerve if the obstacle is very close…these are automatic reactions."

Ising examined this issue through analysis of data from Mazzae et al. [30]. The Mazzae study included both dry and wet road testing. The dry road testing utilized 104 male and 88 female drivers between the ages of 25 and 55 years old. The wet road testing utilized 26 males and 27 females. Test subjects were told that the study was to assess steering and speed maintenance in typical driving conditions. They drove several laps on a track, passing through a simulated intersection several times. Initially, real vehicles were situated at this intersection as if waiting to travel across the road on which the subjects were driving. Between the third and fourth laps, the real vehicles were replaced with foam replicas, and as the subjects approached the intersection on their fourth lap, the foam vehicle to the right was towed rapidly into their path, blocking half of their lane. This study is discussed in greater detail in the next section.

Ising analyzed Mazzae's data and observed that "there is a driver-related braking delay occurring after initial brake application and prior to full emergency braking. In the first phase of brake application, lasting approximately 0.3 seconds, the vehicle reaches a moderate deceleration (about 0.4g). Thereafter, the vehicle deceleration profile is dependent on [time-to-intersection (TTI)] with those drivers that did ultimately apply full braking taking approximately 0.4 to 0.8 seconds longer to do so…this interpretation of our TTI data is consistent with the suggestion of Prynne and Martin who hypothesized a two-phase braking process in which drivers monitored their approach and adjusted their braking accordingly. However, if drivers were capable of rapidly incorporating visual feedback of hazard distance into their braking behavior, it is not clear why there was no difference found between drivers whose braking attempts resulted in a crash and those who avoided impact. Relative vehicle position perceived after braking is initiated may play only a modest role in braking behavior." Ising concludes his article with this important statement related to crash avoidance analysis: "Finally, while the calculated braking profile can be applied when full braking is known to have been applied, this study showed that many drivers never achieved full, or even moderate, braking in this lateral incursion scenario."

12.4 **Motorcyclists' Braking Responses**

Hurt and Thom [31] examined the influence of hand position on motorcyclist's brake response times. This study utilized a Kawasaki KH100 that was equipped with "an electromechanical timer to record response times in brake actuation. A red light of approximately 25 in.² surface was mounted on the front of the test motorcycle in the central visual space of normal motorcycle operation. The timer was coupled with controls so that the timing would start simultaneously with the illumination of the red signal light, and the timer would stop as the participant applied the front brake by lever actuation." The motorcycle was stationary during the tests, and the participants knew that they were to apply the brake lever when the light became illuminated. Each of the 100 subjects was tested in two initial hand positions—full grip on the throttle and with fingers pre-positioned on the brake lever. The mean response time for all subjects with a full grip on the throttle was 0.433 s, and with fingers pre-positioned on the brake lever, it was 0.219 s. There was also less variability in the response times with the fingers pre-positioned on the brake lever ($\sigma = 0.053$ s versus $\sigma = 0.086$ s). This study demonstrates that a motorcyclist's hand position can make a difference to their perception-response time. However, the specific numbers reported by this study would not be applicable within accident reconstruction since the riders were pre-alerted to the scenario and the correct response.

Prem [32] conducted emergency, straight-line braking tests with 59 volunteer riders. He used the Motorcycle Operator Skill Test (MOST) to provide a quantitative assessment of the riders' skill level. The MOST takes the riders through a series of tasks designed to test their steering and braking performance. The braking maneuver analyzed by Prem was a part of the MOST, and it was a task that required the riders to brake aggressively to a stop from a speed of 32 kph. A red signal light was activated to indicate to the riders when they should begin braking. The motorcycles used by the volunteers were instrumented to record the rider's front and rear brake-lever force inputs and motorcycle speed. Prem was interested in assessing the differences in braking technique between skilled and less-skilled riders. Prem found that skilled riders applied higher levels of front brake force than the less-skilled riders. Less-skilled riders preferred the use of the rear brake. The skilled riders also modulated the level of front and rear-wheel braking to maintain optimum braking as weight shifted toward the front of the motorcycle during heavy braking. The less-skilled riders maintained a generally constant level of pressure independent of the weight shift. More skilled riders also exhibited shorter braking reaction times.

Ecker [33] examined the brake reaction times of Austrian motorcyclists by testing more than 300 individuals. He noted that most of the volunteer riders were participants in the motorcycle safety courses offered by the Austrian Automobile Association. A Honda CB500 motorcycle was utilized, which was equipped with two digital timers to measure brake reaction times on both the front and rear brakes. Ecker reported that "A red signal light was mounted on the instrument panel of the motorcycle, being positioned on the peripheral of the visual field for motorcycle operation…The light could be activated at any time by the test coordinator via remote control. Thereby the trigger signal for starting the braking maneuver was rather unexpected for the riders. At the same moment the signal light was triggered, the digital timers also were started." The test subjects were instructed to drive at a speed of approximately 60 kph (37 mph) and to make a "full stop emergency braking maneuver when the bright red flare of the signal light went on." Thus, while the riders may not have been able to predict when the light would turn on, they knew it would turn on and what the appropriate response was. The "brake reaction time" was defined as "the period of time that starts with the trigger signal and ends when the brake light switch registered a brake application...It was neither feasible nor advisable to detect the first contact with the brake lever because some riders already had minimal contact prior to the trigger signal. However, the electrical switches at the front-wheel brake and the rear-wheel brake were adjusted for minimal travel of the respective lever...."

Ecker found that "hand- and foot-position during riding can have a significant effect on the brake reaction time." He also found that riding experience, measured by "total driven distance" and "number of years of motorcycle use" influenced the average BRT. "Both parameters show a negative correlation coefficient with BRT on the front wheel brake (and on the rear wheel) ranging from −8% to −16%...it can be concluded that riding experience improves the brake reaction time and (at least) compensates adverse effects of age. Since the latency period can hardly be shortened by experience (i.e. training) it can be supposed that the movement period is shorter for experienced riders. A possible explanation could be that experienced riders are more frequently in a 'ready-to-brake' position, it might also be that these riders have better trained muscular actions and therefore a faster response."

Davoodi reported two road experiments in Malaysia in which motorcyclists responded by braking to expected and unexpected objects [34, 35]. In the expected condition, motorcyclists applied their brakes as quickly as possible after a light was activated on the roadside. There were 89 motorcyclists that were subjected to this condition. In the unexpected condition, motorcyclists applied their brakes in response to a 1 m by 3 m obstacle (constructed of yellow fabric and imprinted with the word "STOP" in two places) that "suddenly" appeared in their lane. There were 16 riders that were subjected to this condition. The mean perception-response time in the expected condition was 0.71 s. The mean perception-response time in to the unexpected object was 1.29 s and the 85th percentile perception-response time was 2.12 s. Davoodi concluded that "the results of this study showed that motorcyclist PRTs on the road in expected and unexpected scenarios were approximately the same as that for driver PRT in the same situation."

Lenkeit, Hagoski, and Bakker [36] utilized a motorcycle riding simulator with conventional brakes to study the braking responses of non-expert riders in emergency braking situations. This testing utilized sport-touring and cruiser motorcycle configurations. The 68 subjects were tested on the type of motorcycle they would typically ride. The subjects were exposed to situations requiring a range of deceleration, from normal slowing to emergency braking. The emergency braking behavior of the subjects was tested with two scenarios involving an opposing vehicle "moving rapidly into the rider-subject's lane" from the right, requiring a braking response to avoid a collision. The authors noted that "a previous 1981 NHTSA motorcycle study indicated that as many as 83% of US motorcycle riders involved in crashes did not use their front brakes prior to the crash." However, Lenkeit et al. reported that "over the range of scenarios there were some cases of a rider-subject using just the rear brake, though many more where just the front brake was used. There were a few riders who, essentially, never used the rear brake. When the focus was narrowed to the two emergency situations, there were no cases where the rider-subject used just the rear brake, though again, some riders used only the front brake."

12.5 **Are Training and Licensing Effective?**

In relationship to rider skill, licensing, and training, Hurt noted that "riding a motorcycle demands the development of a particular set of skills...If the new motorcycle rider begins the learning process in traffic, there is a real threat to survival. The attention required to the details of coordinating clutch, throttle, shifter, steering, front brake, rear brake, etc., quickly saturates the inexperienced rider and leaves little attention to the surrounding traffic...Lack of experience is a difficult thing for the new motorcycle rider to overcome, or survive. The motorcycle rider with low experience is clearly overrepresented in the accident population...The accident-involved motorcycle rider generally demonstrates a high level of primary control failure in the pre-crash circumstances. Usually the hazard is detected, but the rider is not capable of making the vehicle respond as wanted." Sometimes, a question arises about the degree to which training and licensing improve this situation.

Jonah, Dawson, and Bragg [37] reported a study that sought to determine whether graduates of the 20-h Motorcycle Training Program (MTP) in Ontario, Canada, were less likely to have had an accident or committed a traffic violation on their motorcycles when compared to informally trained (IT) riders. The MTP included training in the following: brake applications, cold starting, moving off and stopping, gear shifting, hand signals, slow speed control, traffic behavior on a riding range, emergency braking, collision avoidance, emergency decision-making, advanced skills, obstacles, rules of the road, mechanical and electrical knowledge, and defensive riding. A sample of MTP graduates and IT riders were interviewed about their riding experiences in the previous 4 years. The interviews were carried out in 1978 and related to the motorcyclists' experiences between the beginning of 1974 and the end of 1977. These authors found that the MTP graduates were less likely than IT riders to have had accidents and violations during this 4-year period. However, they noted that "the graduates and IT riders differed in sex, age, time licensed, distance travelled, education and riding after drinking, all characteristics significantly related to accident and violation likelihood. Multivariate analyses, *controlling for the differences in these characteristics*, revealed that the MTP graduates and IT riders did not differ in accident likelihood but the MTP graduates were significantly less likely to have committed a traffic violation than the IT riders. Although the lower incidence of traffic violations among graduates could be attributed to the training program, it is possible that the graduates sought formal training because they were safety conscious and this attitude also influenced their riding behavior" (emphasis added). They further noted that "MTP riders were more likely to be female, older, better educated, have higher family incomes and be married that IT riders. Although the MTP graduates were more likely to own their own motorcycle, they were licensed for a shorter period and had travelled less distance on a motorcycle in the last 4 yr...Finally, IT motorcyclists were more likely to have ridden a motorcycle after drinking alcohol than MTP graduates which is, perhaps, indicative of greater risk-taking among the IT motorcyclists. Riding after drinking was therefore used as a proxy variable for safety consciousness such that riders reporting that they rode a motorcycle after drinking were assumed to have a poorer attitude toward safety than those reporting never having ridden after drinking."

Mortimer reported similar findings in 1984 [38]. He examined samples of riders who had and had not taken the 20-h Motorcycle Safety Foundation's motorcycle rider course within the prior 3 years. Mortimer reported that "when controlling for age and years licensed, those who took the course did not have a lower accident rate than the control group." There were also no differences in the violation rate between the two populations.

Mortimer did report that "those who had taken the motorcycle rider course made significantly more use of boots, gloves and shirts or jackets with long sleeves when riding." Satten [39] had also reported that motorcyclists who had taken a motorcycle rider course made more use of protective clothing but did not have lower accident rates. Osga [40] similarly did not find that motorcyclists that took a motorcycle rider course had lower accident rates. Mortimer concluded that "there is apparently no evidence that the motorcycle rider course is effective in reducing accidents, but [some studies showed] graduates of the course had fewer traffic violations and made more use of safety clothing, which could be important in reducing the severity of injuries in the event of a crash." Mortimer also observed that "there may also be another, intangible benefit of the course...44% of those who had passed the course did not ride a motorcycle. Perhaps, having learned to ride they decided against the use of this mode of transportation. If they had learned to ride on streets and highways, some of them would have become involved in accidents."

McDavid et al. [41] reported a study of the effectiveness of the British Columbia Safety Council's 37-h motorcycle safety training program. This study compared the driving records of two groups of riders from 1979 to 1984—one group that obtained their motorcycle license by taking the training course and the other that obtained their license without taking the Safety Council's training course or any other formal training. McDavid observed that "a common methodological problem in previous studies is the lack of similarity between persons who seek motorcycle training and those who do not. Age and sex differences, as well as other uncontrolled differences between trained and untrained groups, could account for differences in key dependent variables (principally accident rates) ...multivariate analysis does not necessarily compensate for selection biases and should not be used as a substitute for more rigorous research designs...In looking for the effects of training on motorcycle accidents, matching on age and sex is clearly desirable. In addition, matching on other variables that predict accident behavior after training, such as accident behavior before training, is important." McDavid's point can perhaps be summarized by noting that an important question not addressed by some of the other studies is whether the likelihood a young, male motorcyclist (or any other category one might choose to look at) being involved in an accident is reduced by *that* young, male motorcyclist receiving formal training.

McDavid addressed these issues by pairing each formally trained rider with an untrained or IT rider of similar age, sex, and driving record. He noted that "by controlling for differences in pretraining driving records, it is more likely that the two groups of riders are matched in driving attitudes, permitting a fairer comparison of trained and untrained riders after they are licensed." With this shift in methodology, McDavid reported that there were "observable differences in the frequency and severity of accidents between the two groups. Trained riders tend to have fewer accidents of all kinds (all motor vehicle accidents combined), fewer motorcycle accidents, and less severe motorcycle accidents. Although these differences are not large in a statistical sense, they suggest that when care is taken to carefully match trained and untrained riders, training is associated with a reduction in accidents. Given that motorcycle accidents tend to be much more severe than automobile accidents, the evidence from the study supports the use of training as a means of reducing the human and material costs of motorcycle accidents."

Billheimer [42] examined the effectiveness of the California Motorcyclist Safety Program (CMSP). At the time he published his study, this program had been in use for more than 10 years and had trained more than 100,000 motorcyclists. Billheimer found that "fatal motorcycle accidents have dropped 69 percent since the introduction of the CMSP, falling from 840 fatal accidents per year in 1986 to 263 in 1995. If accident trends in California had paralleled those in the rest of the United States over this period, the state would have experienced an additional 124 fatalities per year." Billheimer noted that another factor that influenced this statistic was the introduction of a mandatory helmet law in 1992. He did not quantify the relative influence of training versus helmet use. For novice riders with less than 500 miles of experience prior to their training, Billheimer found that "trained riders experience fewer than half the accident rates of their untrained counterparts for at least 6 months after training. Beyond 6 months, riding experience begins to have a leveling effect on the differences between the two groups." For more experienced riders with more than 500 miles of experience prior to their training, "no significant differences in accident rates were detected between the two groups, either before or after riders took the basic training course. There was no evidence that riders electing to enter a safety course voluntarily rode any more safely than their untrained counterparts before taking training."

Daniello, Gabler, and Mehta published a literature review of studies that examined the effectiveness of motorcycle training programs and the influence of licensing [43]. In commenting on these studies, these authors make several observations relevant to interpreting the reviewed studies. For example, they observed that "accident rates are a common, but not necessarily ideal, measure of training effectiveness. Accidents are infrequent and may have many causes besides training or rider skill." They also noted that several studies have shown that "riders who choose training tend to be more conscious of safety than those who do not seek formal training." However, they also observe that "it is also possible that those who seek training are inherently not as good at motorcycling as those who do not seek training. Seeking training may then be a result of a lesser skill level, favoring the notion that those who are trained are more likely to be involved in an accident."

Daniello, Gabler, and Mehta also reported that "accident rates and the licensing system in place in a locality are correlated…states requiring a training course for licensing tended to have lower fatality rates based on the estimated vehicle miles traveled…the number of fatal accidents per mile traveled was significantly lower in states where a system with a restricted permit was implemented as opposed to states with an unrestricted permit. Also, states that (a) require a skills test to attain a permit, (b) mandate a longer duration of time between receiving a permit and obtaining a license, or (c) place three or more restrictions on permit holders have a lower motorcycle fatality rate than other states when the number of accidents per mile traveled is compared…"

12.6 **Crash Injury Protection**

In relationship to crash injury protection, Hurt and DuPont stated that "even the most advanced modern motorcycle contributes little, if anything, to the crash injury protection of the rider…for example, in the typical motorcycle accident with front impact, the rider slides forward. His body hits the motorcycle fuel tank, steering head and handlebars, and then impacts the adjacent area of the automobile involved in the collision…While the front suspension has suffered great deformation, this energy absorption has served to decelerate only the motorcycle and has contributed little to any safe arrestment of the rider. Arrestment of the rider is accomplished only by direct contact and injuries are so associated. If the body parts impact relatively soft automobile surfaces of low curvature, injuries are correspondingly reduced; if body parts contact relatively hard or sharp surfaces, the motorcycle rider's injuries are correspondingly increased…At this point it is obvious that crash injury protection and crashworthiness are things that the motorcycle rider must provide for himself. The vehicle configuration does not conveniently incorporate features which provide crash protection. The combined environment of abrasive pavement and hard metal automobiles is hostile to the motorcyclist and capable of causing him severe injury. Of course, the most severe injury associated with motorcycle accident is due to impact of the unprotected head…" In a 1989 study, Wilson reported that "motorcycle helmets are estimated to be 29% effective in preventing fatalities" [44]. Wilson utilized data from the Fatal Accident Reporting System (FARS) for the years 1982 through 1987. The effectiveness of a helmet for a specific crash will, of course, depend on the specifics of the crash. In some crashes, a helmet will help, and in others it will not. As with any other factor related to crash or injury causation, a reconstructionist will need to account for features of the specific crash.

12.7 Group Riding

Some motorcycle crashes occur while motorcyclists are riding in a group. In evaluating the cause of such a crash, it may be relevant to consider the group riding dynamics and the ways in which the group may have interacted. Variables worth considering include the group size, the riding formation of the group, the experience level of those in the group, the hierarchical structure of the group, and the means through which the group was communicating. When riding in a group, lane position and formation can be important issues, since two motorcycles riding in the same lane may create a constraint on the ability of the riders to maneuver and avoid obstacles or respond to hazards. When riding in a group, communication is required since the group will be entering and exiting various roadways and traveling the designated route as a unit. Communication may also be important if a rider has an issue with their bike or needs to attend to a condition that would remove their bike from the formation and route taken by the other riders.

In some way, riding in groups can be safer. For example, a group of riders may be more conspicuous and visible than a single rider. However, there are also safety risks associated with riding in groups. For example, an inexperienced rider traveling with a group of more experienced riders may push themselves beyond their skill level to keep up with the group. Groups can safely range in size from 2 to 8 riders, but if the group becomes larger than that, the total distance of roadway the group consumes can become quite long making a safe maneuver as a unit challenging and potentially, making the group too large for the front and back of the group to stay together and to communicate.

Figure 12.2 depicts the riding formations that groups of motorcyclists should use for straight roadways (left image) and for curves (right image). As these images show, groups should utilize a single-file formation for curves or when the full width of the lane cannot be used for staggering riders, such as roads with street car tracks, roads with construction or deteriorated sections, and narrow bridges. The single-file formation is also helpful

FIGURE 12.2 Proper riding formations for groups.

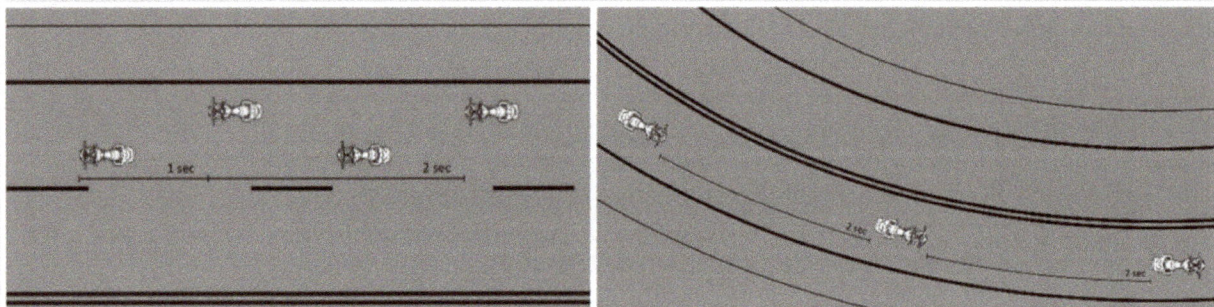

FIGURE 12.3 Hand signals used in group riding.

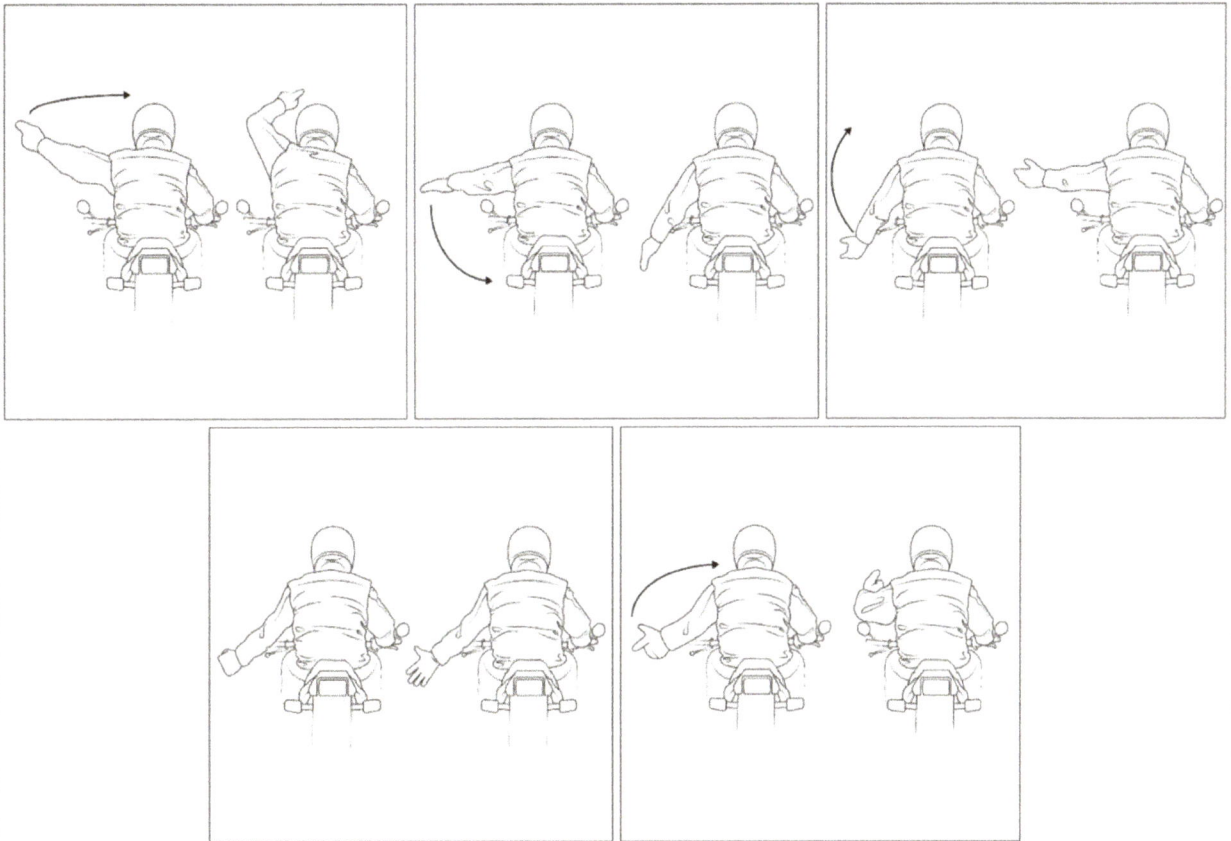

when passing slower vehicles or exiting and entering the highway. Riding single file allows the full width of the lane to be used by a rider but also increases the length of the group, since subsequent riders must maintain a safety cushion from the rider in front. The staggered formation shown in the left image below results in a more compact group than the single-file formation. Single-file riding of groups of even four riders on roadways with higher speed limits can create a long line of riders. Thus, staggered riding should be used on relatively straight roadways and most highways with gentle curves. The staggered riding formation allows riders to be closer together, thus riding as a unit, but still maintain a safety cushion between vehicle behind and in front, and without reducing the lateral space needed to maneuver the motorcycle left and right during the ride.

The experience and training in the group may vary. For this reason, riders may occupy different positions in the group. The lead rider sets the pace, determines when the group enters and exits and passes vehicles. The last rider is referred to as the chase rider and has a duty to keep an eye on riders in front. If a rider in the group departs, encounters a mechanical problem, or is in a crash or emergency, the chase rider is there to assist. Because of the responsibility of the lead rider and the chase rider, both positions require skill, awareness, communication, and experience.

Riding groups can communicate with hand signals or with connected headsets. Both options can allow riders to inform each other of potential hazards, emergency, and disabled vehicles along the roadside, and to take breaks and get gas or any number of other needs that an individual might have. Some of the basic hand signals that a group might use are shown in Figure 12.3. The signals have the following meaning: (1) pull over; (2) slow down; (3) speed up; (4) blinker is on; (5) you lead.

12.8 **Passenger Vehicle Driver Capabilities**

Often, reconstruction of a motorcycle crash will include evaluating the ability of a passenger vehicle driver to avoid the crash. For such analysis, the reconstructionist may need to consider reasonable physical and psychological limits for the passenger vehicle driver—limits on longitudinal and lateral acceleration, on steering rate, and on steering magnitude. Depending on the circumstances, these limits may be a characteristic of the vehicle or a characteristic of the driver. Regardless of the source of these characteristics, limits on these variables (along with the driver's perception-response time) define the driver's ability to avoid a crash.

In a 1976 study, Rice conducted testing with 90 nonprofessional drivers [45]. These drivers were instructed to drive as aggressively as they could through a driving course while successfully traversing the course. The driving course, which included elements such as an off-road recovery, large radius arcs, an avoidance maneuver, and a surprise intrusion, was setup to require steering inputs greater than what would be required for typical driving. Rice reported steering rates for drivers traversing the avoidance maneuver portion of the course. He indicated that, for successful runs through this section, the average maximum steering rate was 520 degrees per second. For unsuccessful runs through this section, the average maximum steering rate was 850 degrees per second. Rice also studied 11 runs involving loss of control in other parts of the course and reported that these runs exhibited steering rates in excess of 1000 degrees per second.

Mazzae [46, 47] examined driver crash avoidance behavior in an intersection incursion scenario using field testing at a test track with actual vehicles and using the Iowa driving simulator. The field testing was conducted in the vehicle dynamics area (VDA) at the Transportation Research Center (TRC) in East Liberty, Ohio. The study included 245 test subjects between the ages of 25 and 55 years, with 192 participating in dry pavement testing and 53 participating in wet pavement testing. Participants drove either a 1995 Chevrolet Lumina or a 1996 Ford Taurus. Unexpectedly, during each participant's drive, an artificial full-scale vehicle was pushed 6 ft into the path of their vehicle from the right. In the dry pavement study, 94% of the subjects attempted both steering and braking inputs, and in the wet pavement study, 98% of the subject attempted both steering and braking inputs. In both the dry and wet pavement studies, roughly half steered first and half braked first. The average maximum steering rate observed during the avoidance maneuvers was 262 degrees per second for the dry pavement and 294 degrees per second for the wet pavement. The highest observed steering rates were 1159 degrees per second for the dry pavement and 1335 degrees per second for the wet pavement study. Mazzae noted that "ninety-five percent of the steering rates observed were less than 600 degrees per second in the dry pavement study and less than 643 degrees per second in the wet pavement study."

The simulator study utilized 60 males and 60 females between the ages of 25 and 55 years. All 120 subjects steered and braked to avoid a collision with a vehicle coming into their lane. Seventy-nine percent of the subjects applied the brakes first, prior to steering. Seventeen percent steered first. The remaining 4% steered and braked simultaneously. The average magnitude of the avoidance steering input was around 148 degrees, and the average maximum steering rate was 514 degrees per second. Ninety-five percent of the steering rates were less than 981 degrees per second. Around 35% of the subjects crashed in their attempt to avoid. Mazzae noted that, "steering inputs exhibited by subjects in this IDS study were larger and quicker than those observed in the related test track studies…This difference is believed to be attributable to the lack of 'road feel' present on the IDA as well as the limited range of travel of the simulator motion base." Nonetheless, Mazzae's results further establish the speed with which normal human drivers can turn a steering wheel.

Carr [48] conducted additional analysis of the data sets produced by Mazzae. For the dry pavement data, with ABS-equipped vehicles, Carr reported a 95th percentile peak steering input of 136° and a 95th percentile peak steering rate of 661 degrees per second. Carr observed that the "driver choice of steering appears to be influenced by the amount of lateral acceleration experienced…The drivers seem to limit the amount of steering demand when the vehicle responds with moderate lateral acceleration or movement. When the vehicle does not have significant response, as in the situation of locked wheel braking [without ABS], the drivers seem to continue to apply more steering to try to achieve a desired lateral response." Carr observed that "all of the yaw rates created as a result of the drivers' demands are well below the capacity of modern vehicles which generally exceed 35 to 45 degrees per second with no challenges to lateral stability on dry pavement surfaces." Carr stated that the "subject drivers chose to utilize a very high percentage of the vehicle's braking capacity as a part of their crash avoidance behavior." He reported a median peak longitudinal deceleration rate of 0.71 g and a 95th percentile of 1.05 g. The willingness limits of the drivers in relationship to lateral acceleration were not as great. Carr reported a median peak lateral acceleration of 0.23 g and a 95th percentile of 0.59 g.

Bartlett [49] reported a study of driver capabilities documented in a dry asphalt, closed, cone-marked course. This study used 467 drivers (418 males and 49 females) who drove one of two police vehicles—a front-wheel drive 1996 Chevrolet Lumina and a rear-wheel drive 1992 Chevrolet Caprice. The drivers were instructed to drive "as if they were responding to assist another officer in trouble, with approval from their supervisors to drive as quickly as they could to facilitate his rescue." The participants drove through a series of maneuvers including a 100 ft radius circle, a decreasing radius turn, and a slalom course. Bartlett reported an average maximum steering rate of 828 degrees per second (calculated over 100 ms). The maximum steering rate observed over 100 ms was 1199 degrees per second for the male drivers and 919 for the female drivers.

In 2005, Forkenbrock presented data related to the steering rates of drivers during double-lane-change tests conducted as a part of the National Highway Traffic Safety Administration's (NHTSA) Light Vehicle Handling and ESC Effectiveness Research Program [50]. These tests utilized five vehicles, all of which were equipped with electronic stability control (ESC). Testing was conducted with and without the ESC enabled. In examining this data, Forkenbrock documented instantaneous steering rates as high as 1819 degrees per second. Even when averaged over a 1-s interval, Forkenbrock found that one driver sustained a steering wheel rate of 963 degrees per second.

Forkenbrock noted that when NHTSA conducted the double-lane-change tests, it had not been anticipated that the data would be used to examine the steering capabilities of human drivers. He stated that the "emphasis was on path following…For this reason, the results…should not be taken to represent the absolute limit of a human performance." The magnitude of the steering inputs and rates observed by Forkenbrock could also have been affected by the physical characteristics and experience level of the drivers. Forkenbrock reported that the double-lane-change maneuvers were performed by four experienced drivers, all four of which were male and of average build. Two of the drivers were in their 20s, one was in his 30s, and the fourth was in his 60s. Each driver had experience as a test driver.

References

1. Treat, J.R., Tumbas, N.S., McDonald, S.T. et al., "Tri-Level Study of the Causes of Traffic Accidents," DOT HS-034-3-535, May 1979.

2. Hurt, H.H. and DuPont, C.J., "Human Factors in Motorcycle Accidents," SAE Technical Paper 770103, 1977, doi:10.4271/770103.

3. Association of European Motorcycle Manufacturers (ACEM), "MAIDS: Motorcycle Accidents in Depth Study," Final Report 2.0, April 2009, http://www.maids-study.eu/pdf/MAIDS2.pdf.

4. Helman, S., Weare, A., Palmer, M., and Fernandez-Medina, K., "Literature Review of Interventions to Improve the Conspicuity of Motorcyclists and Help Avoid 'Looked But Failed to See' Accidents," Published Project Report PPR638, Transportation Research Laboratory, 2012, http://smarter-usa.org/wp-content/uploads/2017/05/12.-literature-review-of-interventions-to-improve-conspicuity-of-motorcyclists-new-zealand.pdf.

5. Olson, P.L., "Motorcycle Conspicuity Revisited," *Hum. Factors* 31, no. 2 (1989): 141–146.

6. Herslund, M.-B. and Jørgensen, N.O., "Looked-but-Failed-to-See Errors in Traffic," *Accident Analysis and Prevention* 35 (2003): 885-891, https://doi.org/10.1016/S0001-4575(02)00095-7.

7. Pai, C.W., Motorcycle Right-of-Way Accidents – A Literature Review. *Accid. Anal. Prev.* 43, no. 3 (2011): 971–982.

8. Sager, B., Yanko, M.R., Spalek, T.M., Froc, D.J. et al., "Motorcyclist's Lane Position as a Factor in Right-of-Way Violation Collisions: A Driving Simulator Study," *Accident Analysis and Prevention* 72 (2014): 325-329.

9. Ouellet, J.V., "Lane Positioning for Collision Avoidance: An Hypothesis," *Proceedings: The Human Element: 1990 International Motorcycle Safety Conference*, Orlando, FL, 1990, vol. 2, 9.58–9.80.

10. Hole, G.J., Tyrrell, L., and Langham, M., "Some Factors Affecting Motorcyclists' Conspicuity," *Ergonomics* 39, no. 7, (1996): 946–965, http://smarter-usa.org/wp-content/uploads/2017/05/2.-some-factors-affecting-motorcyclists-conspicuity-1996.pdf.

11. Horswill, M.S., Helman, S., Ardiles, P., Ardiles, W. et al., "Motorcycle Accident Risk Could Be Inflated by a Time to Arrive Illusion," *Optometry and Vision Science* 82, no. 8 (2005): 740-746.

12. Horswill, M.S. and Helman, S., "A Behavioral Comparison between Motorcyclists and a Matched Group of Non-Motorcycling Car Drivers: Factors Influencing Accident Risk," *Accident Analysis and Prevention* 35 (2003): 589–597, https://doi.org/10.1016/S0001-4575(02)00039-8.

13. Brenac, T., Clabaux, N., Perrin, C., and Van Elslande, P., "Motorcyclist Conspicuity Related Accidents in Urban Areas: A Speed Problem?," *Advances in Transportation Studies* 8 (2006): 23–29, http://worldcat.org/issn/18245463.

14. Labbett, S. and Langham, M., "What Do Drivers Do at Junctions?," *Road Safety Congress*, 2006.

15. Gershon, P., Ben-Asher, N., and Shinar, D., "Attention and Search Conspicuity of Motorcycles as a Function of Their Visual Context," *Accid. Anal. Prev.* 44, no. 1 (2012): 97–103, http://dx.doi.org/10.1016/j.aap.2010.12.015.

16. Rogé, J., Douissembekov, E., and Vienne, F., "Low Conspicuity of Motorcycles for Car Drivers: Dominant Role of Bottom-Up Control of Visual Attention or Deficit of Tow-Down Control?," *Human Factors* 54, no. 1 (February 2012): 14-25, doi:10.1177/0018720811427033.

17. National Highway Traffic Safety Administration, "Traffic Safety Facts – 2015 Data – Motorcycles," DOT HS 812 353, March 2017, https://crashstats.nhtsa.dot.gov/Api/Public/ViewPublication/812353.

18. Lenné, M.G., and Mitsopoulos-Rubens, E., "Drivers' Decisions to Turn across the Path of a Motorcycle with Low Beam Headlights," *Proc. Hum. Factors Ergon. Soc. Annu. Meet.* 55, no. 1 (2011): 1850–1854, http://dx.doi.org/10.1177/1071181311551385.

19. Crundall, D., Crundall, E., Clarke, D., and Shahar, A., "Why Do Car Drivers Fail to Give Way to Motorcycles at T-Junctions?" *Accid. Anal. Prev.* 44, no. 1 (2012): 88–96, doi:10.1016/j.aap.2010.10.017.

20. Magazzù, D., Comelli, M., and Marinoni, A., "Are Car Drivers Holding a Motorcycle License Less Responsible for Motorcycle – Car Crash Occurrence? A Non-Parametric Approach," *Accid. Anal. Prev.* 38, no. 2 (2006): 365–370, http://dx.doi.org/10.1016/j.aap.2005.10.007.

21. Olson, P.L., "Driver Perception Response Time," SAE Technical Paper 890731, 1989, doi:10.4271/890731.

22. Ayres, T. and Kubose, T., "Speed and Accuracy in Driver Emergency Avoidance," *56th Annual Meeting of the Human Factors and Ergonomics Society*, Boston, 2012, ISBN:978-0-945289-41-8.

23. Muttart, J.W., "Chapter 14: Estimating Driver Response Times," *Handbook of Human Factors in Litigation*, (CRC Press, 2005).

24. Muttart, J.W., "Evaluation of the Influence of Several Variables upon Driver Perception Response Times," *Proceedings of the 5th International Conference of the Institute of Traffic Accident Investigators*, York, England, 2001.

25. Muttart, J., "Development and Evaluation of Driver Response Time Predictors Based upon Meta-Analysis," SAE Technical Paper 2003-01-0885, 2003, doi:10.4271/2003-01-0885.

26. Muttart, J.W., "Quantifying Driver Response Times Based upon Research and Real Life Data," *Proceedings of the Third International Driving Symposium on Human Factors in Driver Assessment, Training and Vehicle Design*, June 2005.

27. Rosenbloom, T., Perlman, A., and Pereg, A., "Hazard Perception of Motorcyclists and Car Drivers," *Accident Analysis and Prevention* 43 (2011): 601-604.

28. Ising, K.W., Droll, J.A., Kroeker, S.G., D'Addario, P.M. et al., "Driver-Related Delay in Emergency Responses to a Laterally Incurring Hazard," *Proceedings of the Human Factors and Ergonomics Society 56th Annual Meeting*, 2012.

29. Prynne, K. and Martin, P., "Braking Behaviour in Emergencies," SAE Technical Paper 950969, 1995, doi:10.4271/950969.

30. Mazzae, E.N., Barickman, F.S., Forkenbrock, G., and Baldwin, G.H.S., "NHTSA Light Vehicle Antilock Brake System Research Program Task 5.2/5.3: Test Track Examination of Drivers' Collision Avoidance Behavior Using Conventional and Antilock Brakes," DOT HS 809 561, National Highway Traffic Safety Administration, 2003.

31. Hurt, H., Thom, D., and Hancock, P., "The Effect of Hand Position on Motorcycle Brake Response Time," *28th Proceedings of the Human Factors Society*, 1984.

32. Prem, H., "The Emergency Straight-Path Braking Behaviour of Skilled versus Less-skilled Motorcycle Riders," SAE Technical Paper 871228, 1987, doi:10.4271/871228.

33. Ecker, H., Wasserman, J., Ruspekhofer, R., Hauer, G. et al., "Brake Reaction Times of Motorcycle Riders," *International Motorcycle Safety Conference*, Orlando, FL, 2001.

34. Davoodi, S.R., Hamid, H., Pazhouhanfar, M., and Jeffrey, W., "Motorcyclist Perception Response Time in Stopping Site Distance Situations," *Safety Science* 50, no. 3 (2012): 371-377, https://doi.org/10.1016/j.ssci.2011.09.004.

35. Davoodi, S.R. and Hamid, H., "Motorcyclist Braking Performance in Stopping Distance Situations," *Journal of Transportation Engineering* 139, no. 7, no. 7, (July 1, 2013): 660-666, https://doi.org/10.1061/(ASCE)TE.1943-5436.0000552.

36. Lenkeit, J.F., Hagoski, B.K., and Bakker, A.I., "A Study of Motorcycle Rider Braking Control Behavior," DOT HS 811 448, U.S. Department of Transportation, National Highway Traffic Safety Administration, March 2011.

37. Jonah, B., Dawson, N., and Bragg, B., "Are Formally Trained Motorcyclists Safer?," *Accident Analysis and Prevention* 14, no. 4 (1982): 247-255.

38. Mortimer, R., "Evaluation of the Motorcycle Rider Course," *Accident Analysis and Prevention* 16, no. 1 (1984): 63-71.

39. Satten, R.S., "Analysis and Evaluation of the Motorcycle Rider Courses in 13 Northern Illinois Counties," *Proceedings of the International Motorcycle Safety Conference*, Washington, DC, 1980.

40. Osga, G.A., "An Investigation of the Riding Experiences of MSF Rider Course Participants in South Dakota," Report HFL-80-2, University of South Dakota, August 1980.

41. McDavid, J.C., Lohrmann, B.A., and Lohrmann, G., "Does Motorcycle Training Reduce Accidents? Evidence from a Longitudinal Quasi-Experimental Study," *Journal of Safety Research* 20 (1989): 61-72.

42. Billheimer, J.W., "Evaluation of California Motorcyclist Safety Program," Transportation Research Record 1640, Paper No. 98-0652, 1998, doi:10.3141/1640-13.

43. Daniello, A., Gabler, H.C., and Mehta, Y.A., "Effectiveness of Motorcycle Training and Licensing," *Transportation Research Record: Journal of the Transportation Research Board*, no. 2140 (2009): 206-213, http://dx.doi.org/10.3141/2140-23.

44. Wilson, D.C., "The Effectiveness of Motorcycle Helmets in Preventing Fatalities," DOT HS 807 416, March 1989.

45. Rice, R.S., Dell'Amico, F., and Rasmussen, R.E., "Automobile Driver Characteristics and Capabilities – The Man-Off-The-Street," SAE Technical Paper 760777, 1976, doi:10.4271/760777.

46. Mazzae, E.N., Barickman, F., Baldwin, G.H.S., and Forkenbrock, G., "Driver Crash Avoidance Behavior with ABS in an Intersection Incursion Scenario on Dry versus Wet Pavement," SAE Technical Paper 1999-01-1288, 1999, doi:10.4271/1999-01-1288.

47. Mazzae, E.N., Baldwin, G.H.S., and McGehee, D.V., "Driver Crash Avoidance Behavior with ABS in an Intersection Incursion Scenario on the Iowa Driving Simulator," SAE Technical Paper 1999-01-1290, 1999, doi:10.4271/1999-01-1290.

48. Carr, L., Liebbe, R., Crimeni, J., and Johnston, M., "Motor Vehicle Driver Characteristics - Crash Avoidance Behavior," SAE Technical Paper 2007-01-0449, 2007, doi:10.4271/2007-01-0449.

49. Bartlett, W., Masory, O., and Wright, B., "Driver Abilities in Closed Course Testing," SAE Technical Paper 2000-01-0179, 2000, doi:10.4271/2000-01-0179.

50. Forkenbrock, G., "An Assessment of Human Driver Steering Capability," DOT HS 809 875, National Highway Traffic Safety Administration, June 2005.

13

Visualization of Motorcycle Crashes

13.1 View from the Motorcyclist's Perspective

Some reconstructions will require a visibility study, a video reenactment, or a visualization from the perspective of a motorcyclist, a driver, or witness. Documenting the view from a motorcyclist's perspective can have challenges that require a specific setup or procedure. For instance, a motorcycle in motion can experience significant vibration, especially at high speeds. In addition to that, equipment attached to a motorcycle can be exposed to ambient temperatures, winds, and adverse weather conditions. Also, the motorcyclist will typically use both hands to maneuver and control the motorcycle, and so, their hands will not be available for holding or monitoring equipment. Also, it may be difficult to find a flat surface on the motorcycle to securely mount equipment. There are essentially three mounting options for cameras and other equipment that will record the view from a motorcycle or its motion: (1) mounting equipment to the motorcycle, (2) mounting equipment to the operator, (3) or mounting equipment to another vehicle.

13.1.1 Mounting Equipment on the Motorcycle

Mounting cameras and other equipment on the motorcycle alleviates the need for the operator to handle or manage the equipment while riding. Camera equipment mounted on the motorcycle can have a fixed viewpoint, and with multiple cameras, a view ahead can be synchronized with a view of the speedometer. Figure 13.1 is a photograph showing

FIGURE 13.1 Sample mounting equipment for a motorcycle.

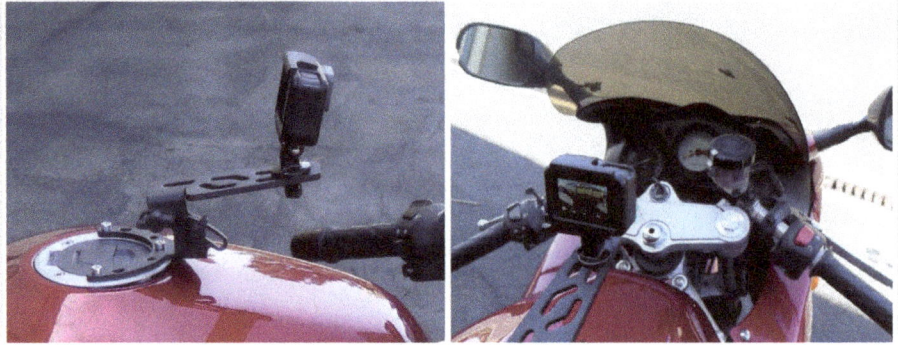

one option, which is to mount a camera on the fuel tank. This rigid mount is designed to fit onto sport-type motorcycles, including Suzuki, Yamaha, Ducati, and Triumph, that have similar gas tank metal flanges with mounting fixtures around the gas cap. There is a rigid metal mount designed to screw into the gas tank screw holes for secure tank-mounted connection.

Mounting equipment on a motorcycle can pose problems, though. There are many different types and styles of motorcycles, and the camera mounting hardware may need to be uniquely fitted to the specific make and model being tested. Generic mounts that are suctioned to the gas tank can be flexible enough to accommodate many motorcycles, but they may vibrate more, blurring the image, or even come detached. Suctioned mounts need to be further attached with adhesive or tape to make sure they are secure. Air, wind, moisture, and debris may further affect the performance of a suction mount. The achievable height with some mounts may also be limited, since the weight of a camera may put too much force on the mounting screws if the mount is too high. Typically, tank mounts are not suitable for larger cameras. They are better suited for lightweight, compact cameras, such as a GoPro. However, these compact action cameras may have limitations in focus, focal length, and field of view that higher-end cameras do not have. Controls on higher-end cameras allow the user to maximize the quality of the footage, specifying the settings that are most suitable for each specific photograph or video run. Compact action cameras can be especially limiting at night, when their limited control settings may be inadequate for calibrating the footage for the nighttime lighting.

13.1.2 Mounting Equipment on the Operator

Cameras can also be mounted to the motorcyclist via chest plates or helmet camera mounts. Examples are shown in Figure 13.2. One of the benefits of the chest plate is that it is more stationery than a helmet-mounted camera. The camera mounted on the helmet will turn and pivot as the operator turns his head, while the chest plate camera will continue facing generally forward. If a view straight ahead for the entire length of a motorcycle run is needed, then the chest plate camera can take care of this without interfering with the operation of the motorcycle. Since the video footage is on the body, there is a good opportunity to record smooth clear footage even on rougher roadways. The body acts like a shock absorber for the rough road, preventing vibrations from continuing into the mounting gear. As a result, footage from operator mounts is generally smooth. Like tank-mounted equipment, the operator-mounted equipment is easy to setup, lightweight, and simple to use.

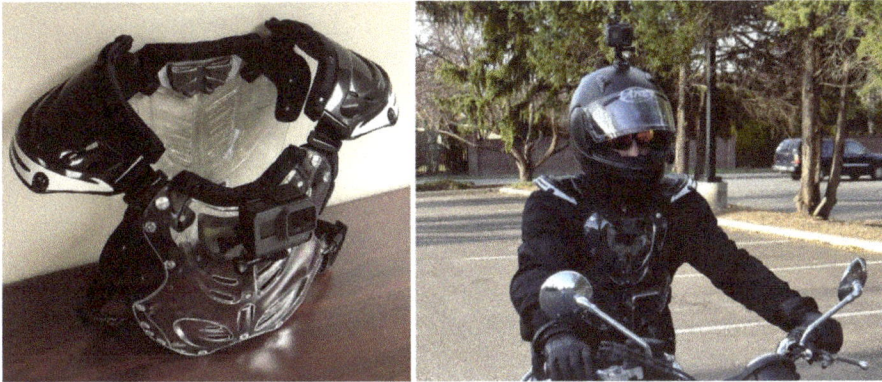

Mounting equipment on the operator poses some similar issues to mounting equipment on the motorcycle. Since the mounting gear is lightweight, the use of high-end cameras is typically not feasible. The mounts will typically be too small to accommodate the weight and size of high-end cameras. Also, heavier equipment can cause weight balance issues while riding. In addition, mounting a camera on the operator's chest or helmet puts the camera at a different height off the ground than their eyes. Depending on the issue being evaluated, this may or may not matter. In general, matching the exact eye height in a particular crash is irrelevant since the object or scene being viewed is far enough ahead that a change in eye height several inches up or down would not have any noticeable effect on the view. Nonetheless, there may be instances where this discrepancy between eye height and camera height matters.

13.1.3 Mounting Equipment on Another Vehicle

Often, high-quality footage can be obtained from the perspective of a motorcyclist without even utilizing a motorcycle. Typical issues with motorcycle or operated-mounted equipment can be remedied with a rig that is secured to a passenger vehicle. The photographs of Figure 13.3 show a sample set of equipment and subsequent mounting on a vehicle. The setup shown is for a nighttime visualization, and so, a special rig for the motorcycle headlamp is depicted. When using a setup like this, it will likely be important

FIGURE 13.3 Rig for a passenger vehicle for replicating a motorcyclist's view.

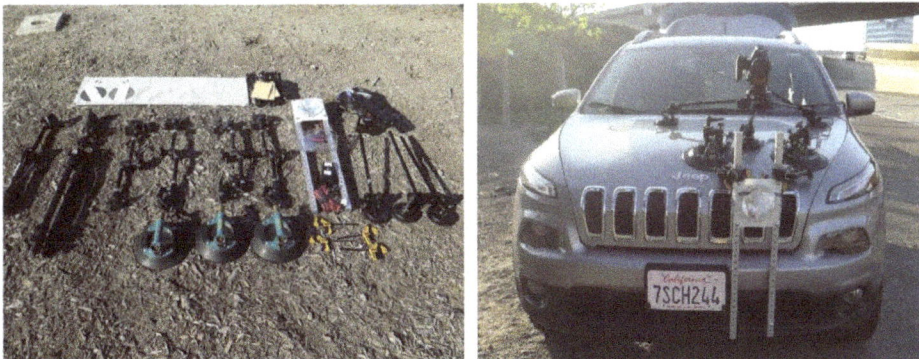

to use a vehicle that where the vehicle's headlamps can be turned off, so the only light source being recorded by the camera is from the headlamp rig.

The camera mounting rig depicted in Figure 13.3 includes three suction grips that are placed on the hood of the car to form a tripod for the camera. These suction grips have arm extensions that connect in the center of the tripod where a camera plate connects them together. This rig can be adjusted to various heights and distances behind the headlamp rig. When setting up a rig like this, be aware that many motorcycles position a rider with an eye height that is higher off the ground than that of a driver in a standard passenger car (Figure 13.4).

Another example of a camera mounting rig is shown in Figure 13.5. In this setup, an additional suction handle and extension arm were used to rigidly hold the back of the camera plate, as the plate sometimes tends to vibrate without the additional stiffening arm. If the view to be obtained is from a particular lane position, the camera mount could be set up on either side of the hood to accommodate this.

With the camera in place and adjusted, a headlamp rig can also be added to the vehicle. For nighttime motorcycle cases, it may be necessary to determine visibility using a substantially similar headlamp as the headlamp on the motorcycle in the accident. To accommodate this, a headlamp specific to the accident motorcycle can be obtained and

FIGURE 13.4 A motorcyclist will often have a higher eye height than a passenger car driver.

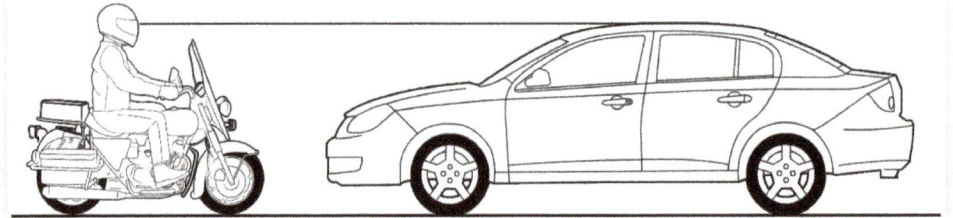

FIGURE 13.5 Camera mounting equipment.

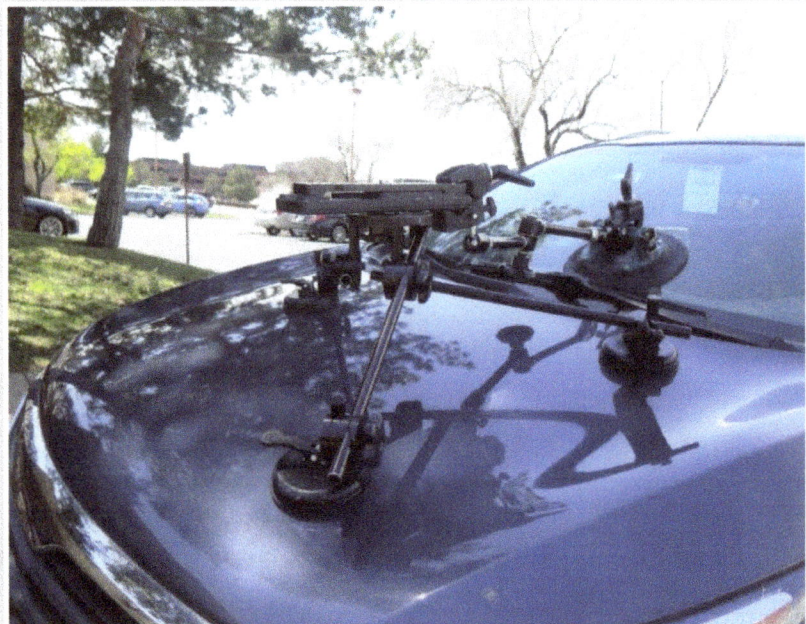

CHAPTER 13

FIGURE 13.6 Headlamp mounting equipment and comparison to exemplar motorcycle.

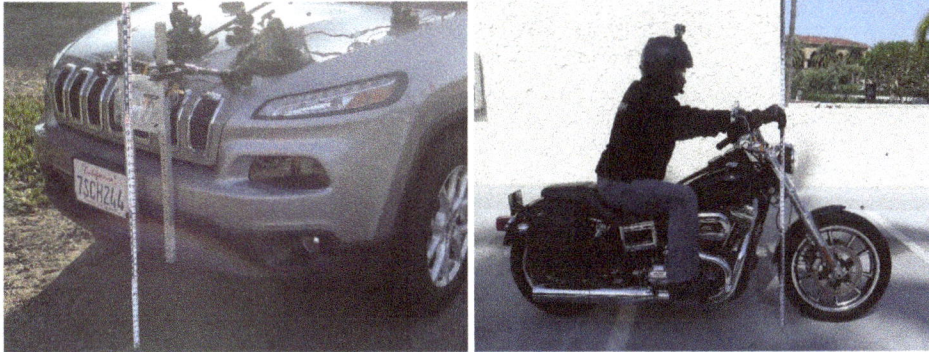

FIGURE 13.7 Motorcycle camera mount and frame from resulting footage.

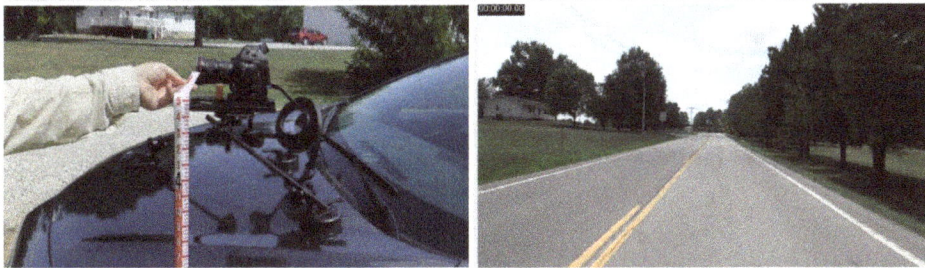

used in the rig. To determine the correct mounting height and aiming, a comparison can be made to an inspection of an exemplar motorcycle with the same stock headlamp. Figure 13.6 illustrates this type of comparison.

In this setup, the electrical power to the headlamp is supplied by the battery of the passenger vehicle. In the case of a motorcycle, a voltage level between 13.8 and 14.2 V would be typical. The actual voltage that is available from the car's battery can be verified using a voltage meter. The controls to turn the headlamp on and off and to start and stop the video recording are inside the vehicle and attached with extension controls and cables connecting the unit to the controls. This setup can also include a video monitor in the vehicle showing the image being recorded. This enables checking that good quality video was captured. Figure 13.7 shows another sample camera mount for a daytime situation, along with a frame of the resulting footage.

13.2 View of the Motorcycle from Other Vehicles

The views other drivers have of a motorcycle may also be relevant to a reconstruction. This may include a vehicle traveling behind or approaching from the opposite direction of the motorcycle, though the most common two-vehicle collision with a motorcycle involves a vehicle turning left across the motorcyclist's path. Documenting the perspectives of other drivers often requires different techniques and equipment than what is required for collecting the motorcyclist's perspective. Two basic setups are common for capturing footage of a forward-looking scenario. The first is a rigid mount inside the

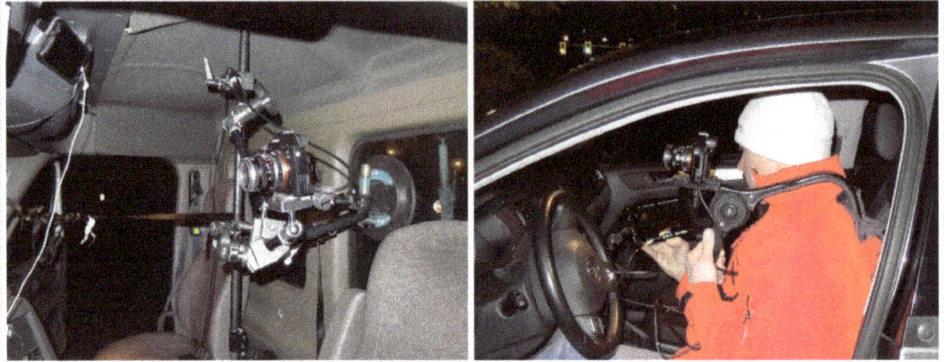

vehicle. The second is a shoulder-mounted camera harness that is lightweight and easy to setup and occupies a minimal amount of space. Photographs showing both types of setups are included in Figure 13.8.

Sometimes, a driver who pulls out in front of a motorcyclist later says that they looked left, then right, then back left again before pulling out. It can be difficult to represent this scanning pattern with standard camera mounting. Swivel heads can be added to camera mounts, but this can increase the height of the camera, and maneuvering the swivel head from inside the vehicle can be difficult. Rotating the camera head by hand in a smooth, natural way can also be difficult. These issues can be addressed using a handheld camera grip with a motorized swivel. This equipment can be used with a range of camera sizes. Motorized control of the swivel results in motion that is smooth and consistent. If the video footage is good quality and smooth, the timing of the swivel motion can be adjusted in post-processing video editing software. Figure 13.9 is an example of a handheld, motorized camera mount that can be positioned at the driver's height and used to mimic left and right glances.

A second technique is to use a 360° camera. These cameras are easy to setup and operate, but they require special processing software. The technique of capturing a 360° image sequence has been around for decades, starting in the 1990s with virtual reality software such as Apple's QuickTime VR. This 360° virtual reality imagery effectively stitches together overlapping photographs. A tripod is used that has a camera head that allows a consistent interval rotation of the head to obtain overlapping images around all 360°. The software is then used to stitch these images together into one seamless file that the user can open and virtually navigate around. Since the photographs were captured from a single position, though, the user can only stand in one spot and look around. Adding motion to the usability of this technology, the 360° video camera uses the same concept but stitches multiple frames from multiple positions. To do this, each frame of video must already contain imagery for 360° of information, so that every frame of video is a 360° field of view. Several systems exist that use multiple cameras mounted together, each camera pointing in a different direction with some overlap between each of the cameras to have full coverage of the 360° field of view. The video from

FIGURE 13.9   Motorized handheld camera mount.

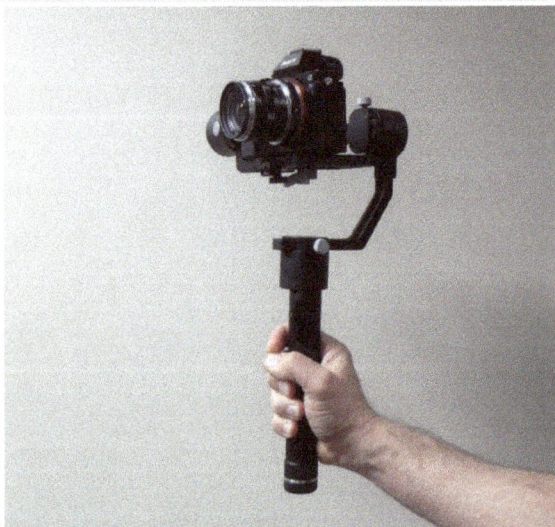

279

FIGURE 13.10 | 360° camera and setup within a vehicle.

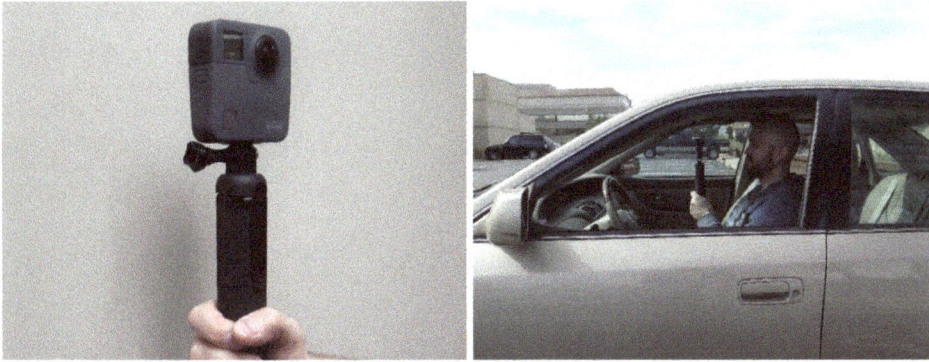

these mounted cameras could be stitched together using post-processing software to end up with a video file that has a 360° field of view. Figure 13.10 shows an example of a 360° camera—the GoPro Fusion. This camera incorporates two cameras, each taking half of the 360° image with a very wide-angle lens. The software stitches the images together to form a 360° field of view movie. The cameras are attached to a simple holding rod and because of the way it captures the image, there is no need to move or rotate the camera during filming. Rather, the appearance of a glance to the left and then to the right are processed from this 360° video later.

After the camera has recorded a drive-through or turn maneuver, the video can be post-processed and stitched together. In this case, the GoPro Fusion Studio 1.1 software that came with the camera was utilized. When the video file is processed, the movie is a single image containing all the imagery from 360° as shown in Figure 13.11. To simulate a glance to the left, right, and back, the video can be processed to only show portions of 360° image in the final video file. Figure 13.12 shows a concept drawing of how the 360° recorded video can be used to simulate a head glance back and forth. Figure 13.13 shows three images from the post-processed 360° video file, demonstrating the ability to represent head movement where there is first a glance left, then to the middle, then to the right.

FIGURE 13.11 | Unmodified image from a 360° camera.

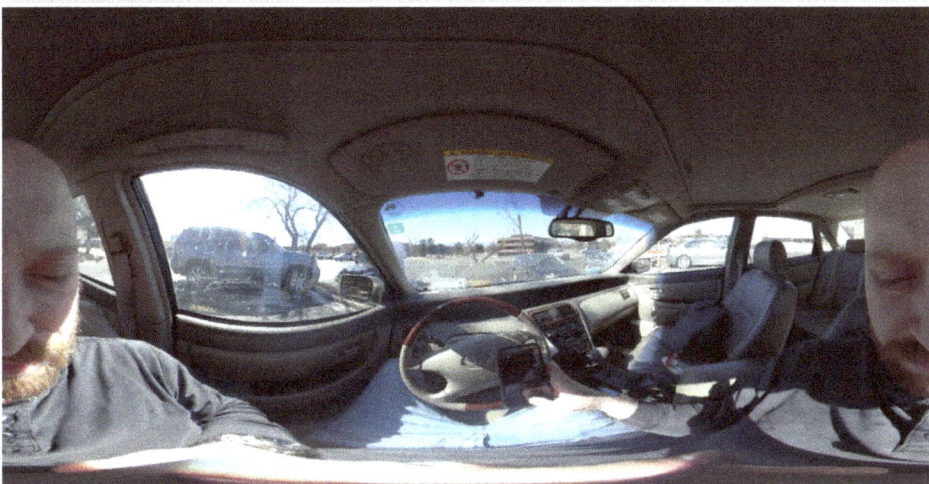

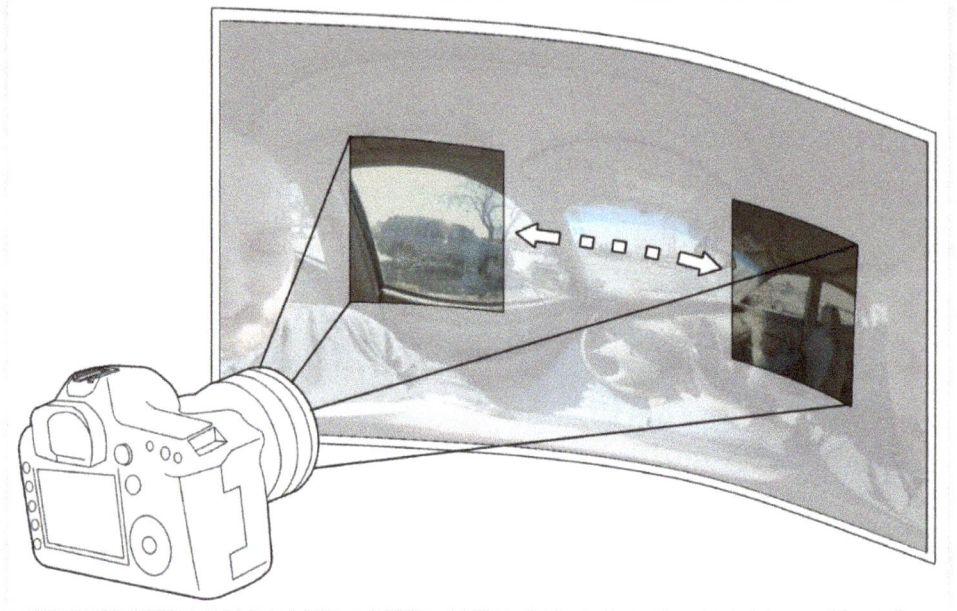

FIGURE 13.12 Using 360° video to mimic a panning view.

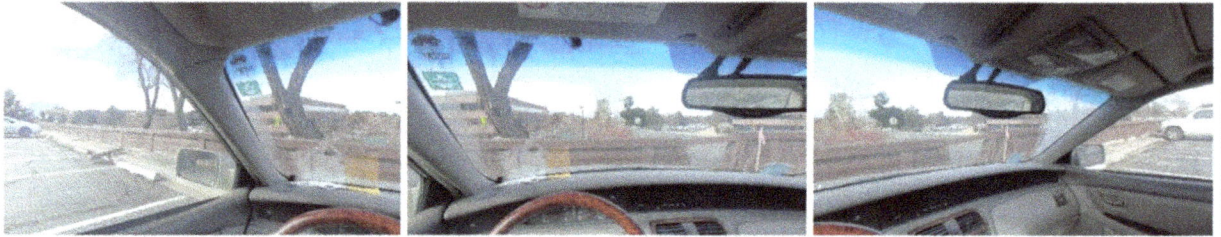

FIGURE 13.13 Cropped image to show view to the left.

13.3 Camera Setup and Representing a Driver's View

When capturing images that represent a vehicle operator's point of view, there are several variables to consider, including the height of the camera, what field of view to use, what settings best capture the view available to the operator, and how to represent the captured video to others. These considerations are addressed in this section.

13.3.1 Camera Height

Driver eye heights can vary. Seats can be adjusted, and drivers can be different heights. Even drivers of the same height can have differences in the length of their legs or torso that are significant enough to change the eye height by several inches. Seated posture can also make a difference. When representing driver views, the question would be: To what degree would these changes in height matter? The answer is that it depends on the location of the objects being viewed. A change in eye height of 6 in. makes very little difference for objects in the distance. For objects near the vehicle though, the eye height

FIGURE 13.14 Diagram showing viewing height differences for near and far objects.

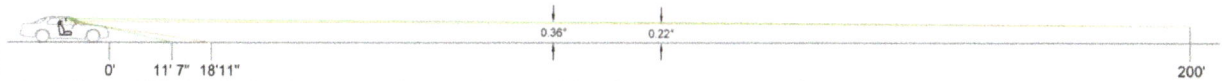

can influence how far in front of the vehicle a driver can see. For an overall view down the road, though, the eye height could be varied by a foot or more, and the camera would still capture a very similar view.

Figure 13.14 illustrates this graphically. This figure shows a scaled diagram with a cross section of a vehicle on a flat roadway with a 3 ft tall object placed 200 ft from the front of the vehicle. Two viewing positions are depicted. The one depicted with the green lines is 6 in. higher than the other. From each viewpoint, a line was drawn to the top of the 3 ft object 200 ft away. Lines of sight were also drawn from the top and bottom of the 6 in. range to the ground level immediately in front of the vehicle. This line was drawn to a point as close to the front of the vehicle as possible without having an intersection with the vehicle geometry, giving us a near range for the driver's line of sight.

For the view of the far object, there is negligible difference between the two viewpoints. One way to demonstrate this is to measure the difference in viewing angle that each viewpoint produces of the far target object. The difference in angle was only 0.14°. The angle of incidence from the top position driver's line of sight was 0.36°, and the angle from the bottom viewing position is 0.22°. However, the lines of sight for the nearer distances produce a larger difference. From the higher viewing position, the driver would be able to see the bottom of an object 11 ft, 7 in. in front of the vehicle. From the lower viewing position, the driver would be able to see the bottom of an object that was 18 ft, 11 in. from the front of the vehicle. For most accident situations, the view out ahead of the vehicle is the relevant one, and a difference in eye height of 6 in. will be insignificant.

Figure 13.15 is another illustration of the influence of different viewing heights. These photographs have 6 in. differences in camera height. The photograph on the left was taken with the lowest viewpoint—6 in. lower than the middle photograph—and the photograph on the right had the highest viewpoint, 6 in. higher than the middle photograph. The photographs were taken looking toward the center of a wall that had a height of approximately 4 ft and was approximately 200 ft in the distance. The viewing height changes what is depicted in the immediate foreground, and the view of up close objects like the steering wheel and sun visor changes. The overall view of the objects and scenery down the road is not significantly different, though.

To further demonstrate how the difference in 1 ft of height is insignificant in terms of changing the view of the distant object, these three photographs were cropped to not include the interior roof and steering wheel. The results of this cropping are shown in

FIGURE 13.15 Diagram showing viewing height differences for near and far objects.

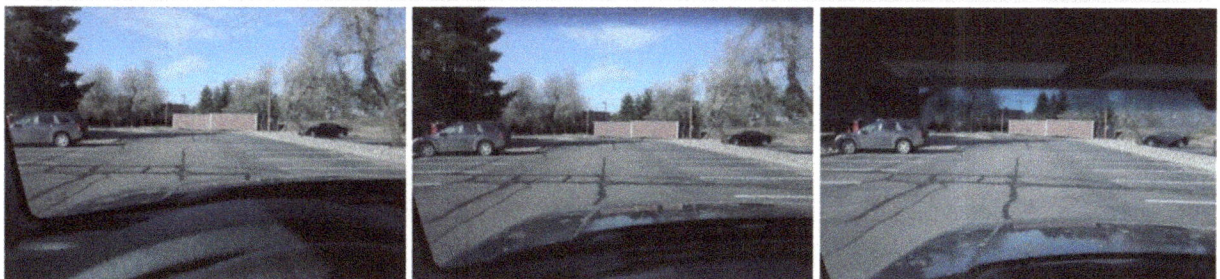

FIGURE 13.16 Diagram showing viewing height differences for near and far objects.

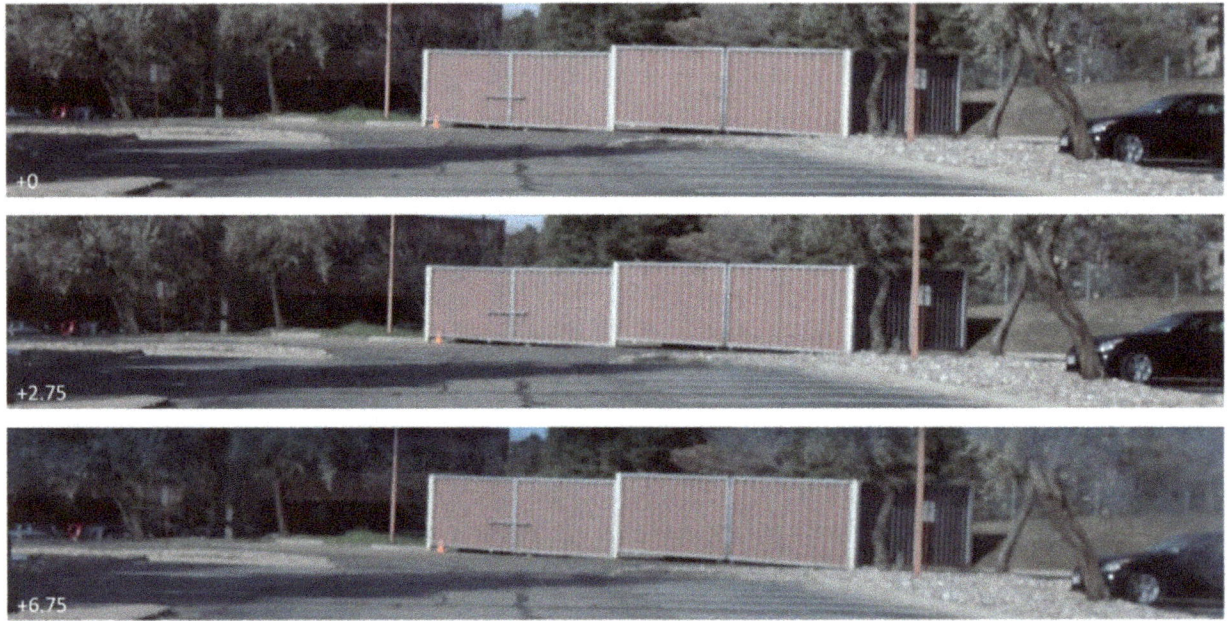

Figure 13.16. Visually, there is no difference between these images, and when comparing each cropped image within Adobe Photoshop, all three images aligned almost perfectly, thus confirming that the view was virtually the same regardless of the differences in camera height within the vehicle.

13.3.2 Field of View

The field of view is defined by the focal length of a camera lens, which is usually measured in millimeters (mm). The focal length determines the angular extents of the view that will be captured. Higher focal lengths will make the angular extents of the image smaller (zoom), while lower focal lengths will provide an image with wider angular extents. The focal length is a physical property of a lens. It describes the numerical relationship of the optical distance between the center of the lens and where light converges to form an image on the sensor or film. When adjusting the focal length of the camera, it is important to recognize the physical fact that <u>changing the focal length does not change the perspective</u>. This means that zooming is the same as cropping.

A camera lens functions the same in analog and digital cameras. The film is what captures the image in an analog camera; the sensor captures the image in a digital camera. Figure 13.17 illustrates the basic geometry of a camera and illustrates how the field of view changes for several different focal lengths. In this figure, l_{focal} is the focal length, w_{sensor} is the width of the camera sensor, and θ_{fov} is the angular field of view. As the lens moves further away from the sensor plane, the angle θ_{fov} becomes smaller, creating a narrower field of view. As the lens moves closer to the sensor plane, this angle becomes larger, creating a larger field of view. Since the sensor size is not changing, however, there will be more detail included in the image when zooming into an area. Adjusting the zoom, which changes the focal length and field of view, will not affect the perspective of the image. To change perspectives, the photographer would have to change their position.

These concepts are illustrated with actual photographs in Figure 13.18. This image is an overlay of three different photographs taken from the same position but at different

FIGURE 13.17   Basic geometry of a camera and illustration of the influence of focal length on the field of view.

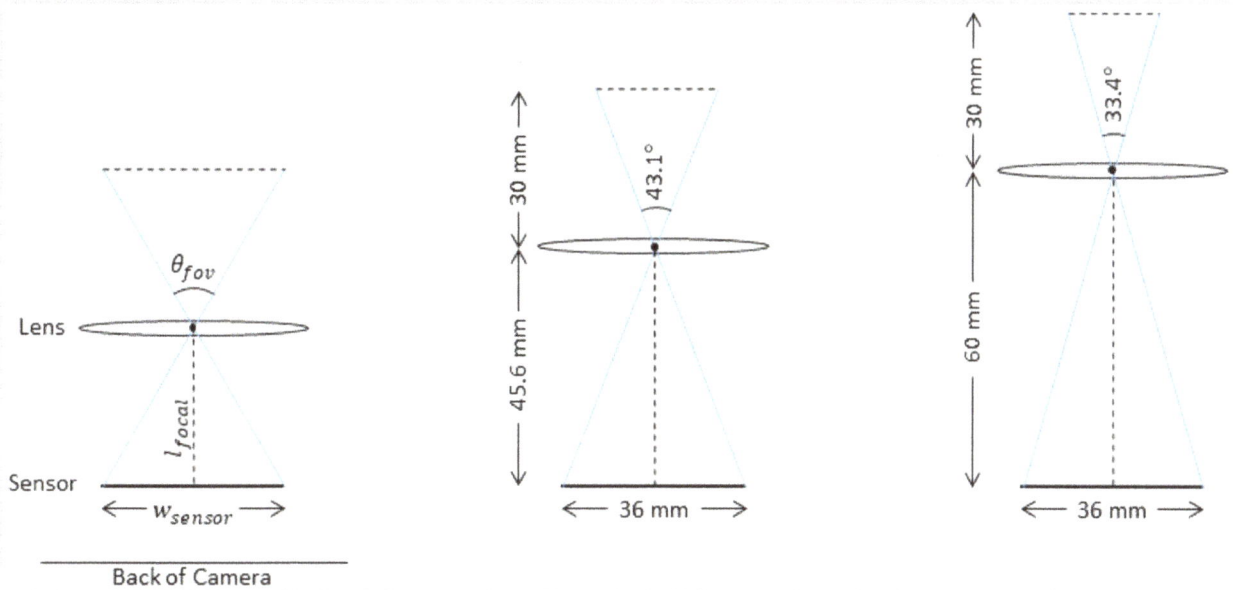

FIGURE 13.18   Illustration of the influence of focal length on the field of view (cropping).

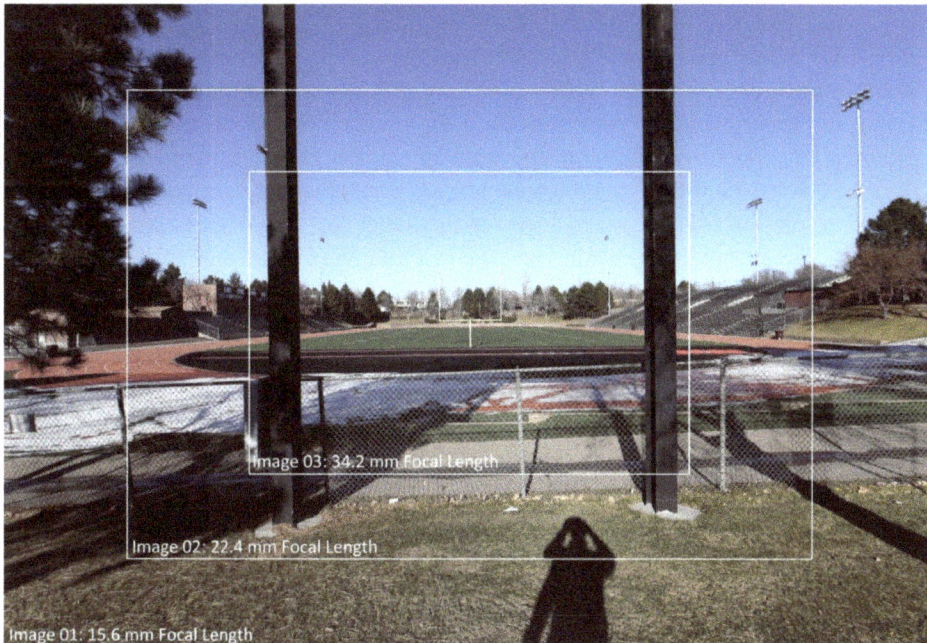

Image 03: 34.2 mm Focal Length

Image 02: 22.4 mm Focal Length

Image 01: 15.6 mm Focal Length

focal lengths. The images captured at longer focal lengths have been scaled to fit the overlaying image, demonstrating how zooming in or out on a scene from the same point of view is the same as cropping the amount of data that is captured. When zoomed in on an object, there will be a higher resolution of image data captured of the object, when zoomed out there will be a lower resolution of data captured of the same object, but the perspective will not change.

FIGURE 13.19   Graphical depiction for determining playback scale.

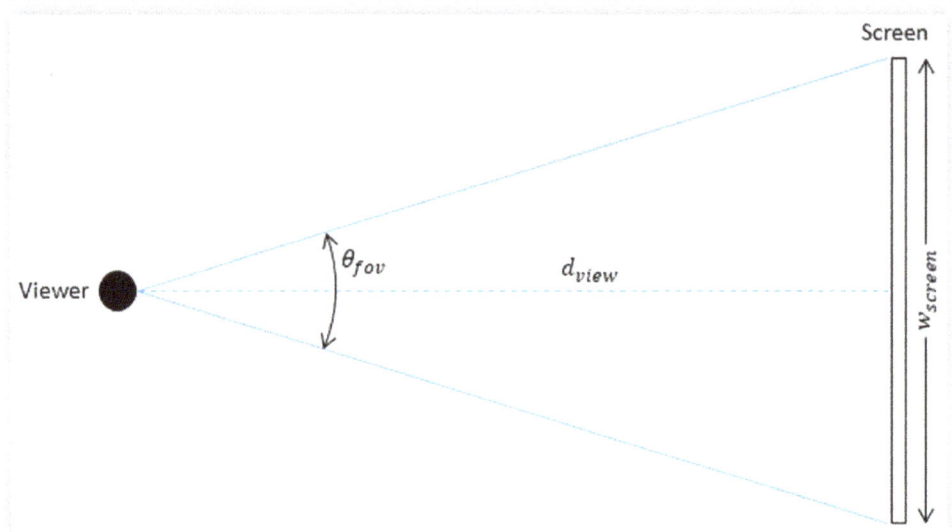

13.3.3 Scaling the Images for Playback

In some instances, video will need to be played back or photographs shown on a screen that is sized and positioned to give the audience a correct depiction of the size of objects as a driver would have (or could have) seen them. Figure 13.19 shows the geometry relevant to determining the correct display size and positioning. In this figure, d_{view} is the distance between the viewer and the screen, w_{screen} is the width of the screen, and θ_{fov} is the field of view for this viewing geometry. This assumes that the image will fill the entire width of the screen. Thus, the field of view could be the field of view of the original image that is going to be displayed. Alternatively, if the width of the screen and distance to the viewer cannot be controlled, the image could be cropped down to the field of view that will generate objects of the correct size, assuming of course that the image will still have adequate resolution to display the objects in the image in a crisp, clear manner.

The following equation would yield the distance the screen should be placed from the viewer for a specified screen width and field of view:

$$d_{view} = \frac{w_{screen}}{2 \cdot \tan\left(\dfrac{\theta_{fov}}{2}\right)} \tag{13.1}$$

13.4 Computer Visualization of a Motorcycle Crash

When visually depicting a motorcycle crash or the view available to a driver or motorcycle operator, there are several types of visualizations and methods available. In general, these can be categorized into computer-generated (CG) visualizations, photo- or video-realistic visualizations, or a hybrid between the two. Technically, these are all generated in the computer to some degree and hence could be classified as CG visualizations. However, there is a significant difference in the way the two types of visualizations are produced, how they look, how geometry that is visible in the visualization is created and rendered, and the flexibility to change views or interact within the environment.

FIGURE 13.20 Still images from a computer-generated animation of a motorcycle crash.

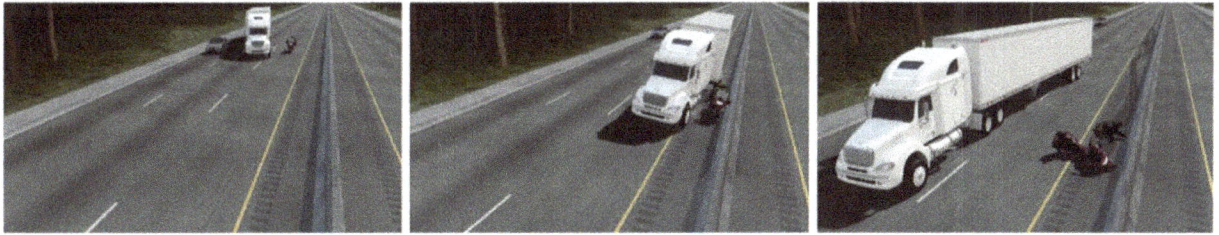

In CG visualizations, all the components are contained in a three-dimensional modeling and animating environment. The vehicles, the scenery, the motion, and the lighting are computer-generated and controlled or modified through the software's tools and algorithms. Figure 13.20 shows still images from a CG animation of a crash involving a motorcycle. In these images, the geometry of the vehicles, the trees, the roadway, and other geometry were textured and modeled within the computer software's environment. The underlying animation could be played back at any rate, including slow motion. The lighting of the environment and the textures and colors of the objects are also generated within the computer environment, and cameras can be placed anywhere in the environment without changing the underlying animation.

Another type of visualization utilizes video or photographs in addition to CG objects. Methodologies have been established for recording and representing photographic of video views of a scene, environment, or available view of the drivers and operators. If the camera settings and setup are done correctly, then the resulting images can be fair and accurate representations of the view they intended to capture. Unlike a CG animation, these renderings get the size, shape, color, and lighting from the actual environment, recording it in a digital medium. Figure 13.21 shows frames from an example of this type of visualization. In this example, video was obtained to record the view available to a motorcyclist. Live vehicles were used and recorded at the actual accident scene. However, since recreating the accident is not feasible or safe, portions of the visualization were generated in the computer. The CG portions of this visualization rely on the photographic and video-realistic source recordings to determine how the textures, colors, and lighting should appear.

This type of video visualization can also be created for nighttime scenarios. Neale and his colleagues presented a methodology for generating photo-realistic computer simulation environments of nighttime driving scenarios by combining nighttime photography and videography with video tracking and projection mapping technologies [2016]. Nighttime driving environments contain complex lighting conditions such as forward and signal lighting systems of vehicles, street lighting, and retroreflective markers and signage. The high dynamic range of nighttime lighting conditions make modeling of

FIGURE 13.21 Still images from a video-based motorcycle crash visualization.

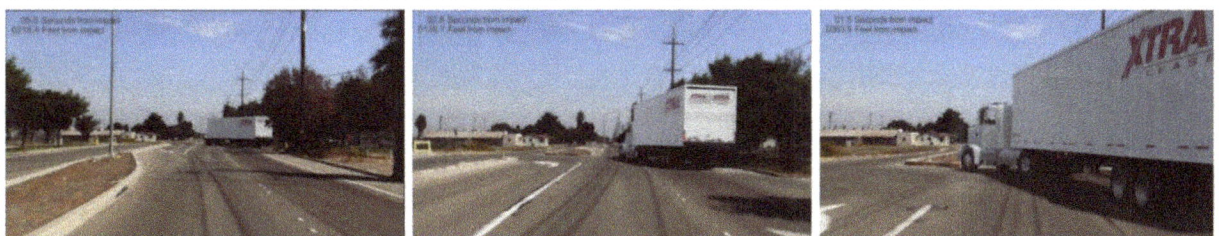

these systems difficult to render realistically through CG techniques alone. Photography and video, especially when using high dynamic range imaging (HDR), can produce realistic representations of the lighting environments. But because the video is only two-dimensional and lacks the flexibility of a three-dimensional, CG environment, the scenarios that can be represented are limited to the specific scenario recorded with video.

However, by combining the realistic imagery from video and photographs with the flexibility of a CG environment, it is possible to vary any number of factors such as the speed of vehicles and the driver lane position and to vary the types of vehicles and lighting conditions involved in the scenario. The combination of projection mapping, video tracking, and nighttime video and photography methodologies allows this flexibility. In addition to presenting the methodology and the resulting computer simulation environment, the final simulation is compared to actual video recordings of the same driving scenario to evaluate how similar they are in value, tone, color, and visibility. The realistic simulation environment helps the user visualize the driving environment in a manner that more closely resembles the actual environment one would experience in the real world. Another advantage of the simulated environment is that, because it is completely computer-generated, variables such as the roadway conditions, vehicle speeds and positions, and lighting conditions can all be changed, and a variety of factors that potentially contribute to accident causation can be visually represented for use in analysis, studies, or demonstrations. Some environments are more difficult to model than others, particularly low light level and nighttime environments where reflected light and artificial lighting sources create complex lighting situations. However, advances in digital photography and videography have made imaging these environments easier and more realistic.

While it is technically feasible to collect video-realistic recordings of real-world driving situations and even play back the recordings in high definition and in a calibrated manner where it represents what a driver would see, there are clear limitations. First, the video captured is linear in the sense that it can only be played forward or backward, but always in a prescribed sequence of images. Second, the conditions in which the video was captured represents the only set of conditions that can be played back. Without editing, compositing, or computer visualization, modifying the conditions of the driving situation that was recorded such as a driver's lane position, speed, or other traffic is limited. A third problem is that situations where accident conditions are of interest, such as driving through low lit areas, or testing a driver's perception-response to unexpected situations, may be dangerous to conduct in a live setting. The methodology discussed here avoids these limitations without sacrificing the quality and visual realism that high-definition and high dynamic range video recording possess. This methodology sets forth steps that allow video-realistic footage of driving situations to be obtained in a manner that maximizes both safety and controllability of the driving variables that are of interest in the testing. Primarily this is accomplished by separating the vehicles from the driving environment when collecting video footage and then combining the separate data using computer modeling and visualization techniques. Since the data collected is maintained throughout the process as video-realistic imagery, the ending quality is also video-realistic. Further, since the environment is eventually a CG environment, controlling and varying the driving parameters are safe and feasible.

Following is a general list of the steps involved in this methodology:

a. Collect video footage of the driving environment.

b. Collect geometry data of the driving environment.

c. Collect video footage of the vehicles under a variety of lighting conditions in a controlled area.

d. Collect geometrical data of the vehicles involved.

e. Use projection mapping techniques to create a video-realistic computer environment.

f. Use computer visualization techniques for creating vehicles with varying parameters.

g. Combine the environment and vehicle modeling systems into one system.

h. Vary the parameters of the vehicle and scene to generate any number of video-realistic simulation scenarios.

13.4.1 Case Study: Visualization of a Nighttime Scenario

To demonstrate this methodology, a baseline driving scenario was captured on video. This scenario involves a vehicle that is stopped at night on a roadway. Another vehicle is approaching that vehicle from behind. The view represented through video in this scenario is from the approaching driver's perspective. Figure 13.22 shows a diagram of this scenario, and Figure 13.23 shows a daytime photo of the area where the baseline scenario was performed.

The baseline footage will be used to compare and evaluate the results of a CG version of the same scenario produced through the outlined methodology. The live baseline recording is a linear, unaltered video recording of the vehicle and environment together, while its comparison counterpart produced through the methodology is a computer-generated, customizable, video-realistic version of the same scenario. After a comparison between the live baseline footage and the CG version is performed, the driving conditions of the CG scenario are then changed to include different vehicle lighting systems and a different lane position to demonstrate the ability to alter the scenario being represented while still maintaining photographic realism.

To obtain the baseline video, an area was selected, and a sequence of events determined that would represent a generic but relevant set of testing conditions. The site included a hill and a curve that act as visual obstructions for the driver, who is approaching a vehicle stopped in their lane of travel. The video is captured from the driver's view to represent the view available to the driver cresting the hill and rounding the curve. This driving scenario is just one example of a situation where evaluating the roadway lighting conditions, vehicle conspicuity, site lines, visibility, and driver perception and reaction would be of interest in a study or demonstration. The equipment used to calibrate the video footage and obtain the recording is depicted in Figure 13.24.

FIGURE 13.22 Layout of baseline scenario.

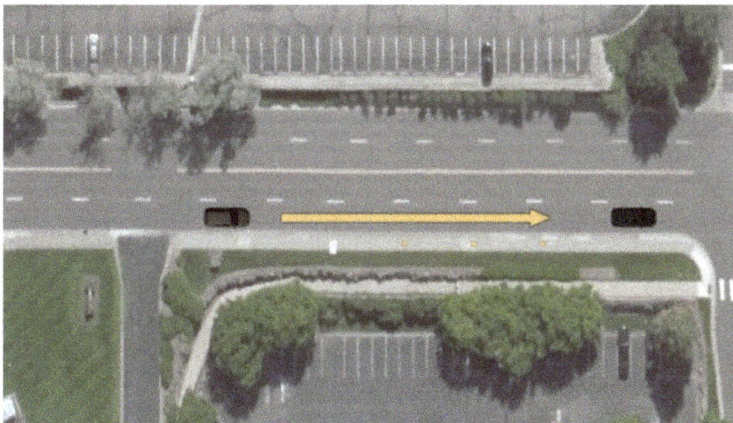

FIGURE 13.23 Daytime photo of baseline video setup.

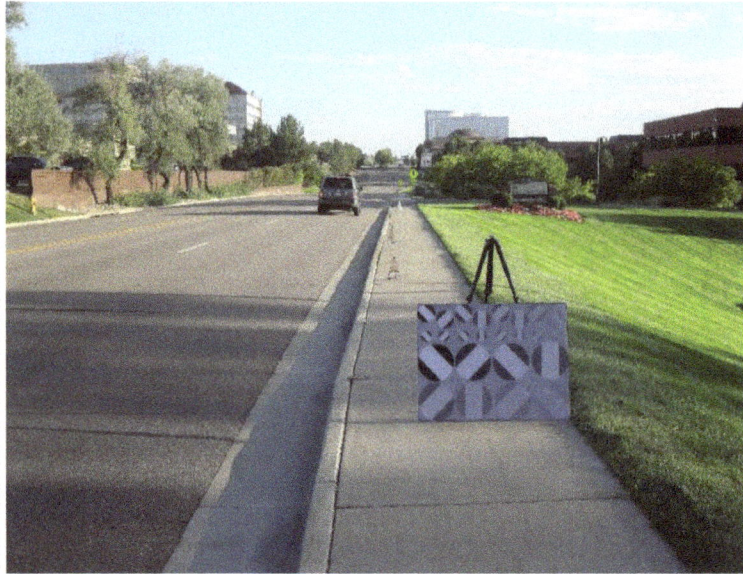

FIGURE 13.24 Video capture and calibration equipment.

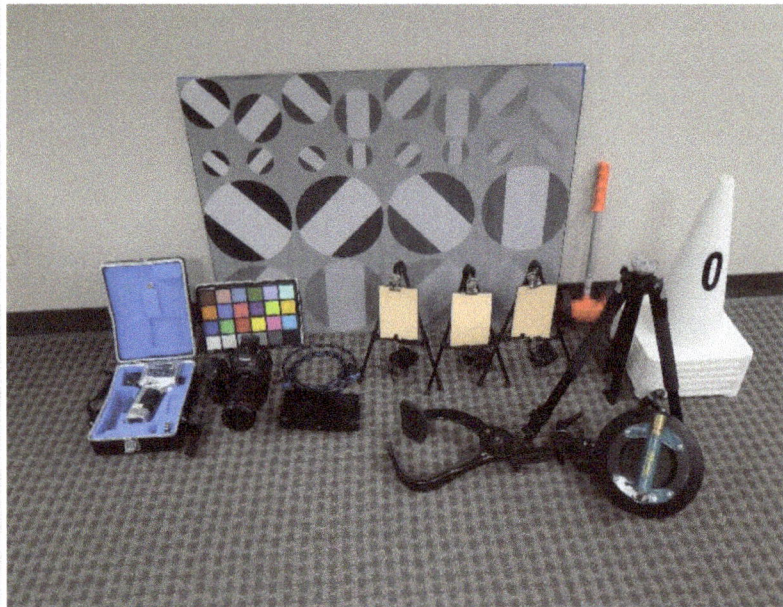

To obtain the highest quality footage and record a view where the lighting, colors, and values of the recording are representative of the actual scene when viewed live with the naked eye, a Canon C100 HD video camera and Atomos Shogun field monitor were used in conjunction with devices that enable calibration of the video image prior to recording. The calibration process relies on techniques from previously published literature [1, 2, 3, 4, 5, 6]. Augmenting these techniques is a quantified approach where light values are measured at the scene using a Konica Minolta LS-100 luminance meter. These luminance values are compared to the corresponding luminance values of pixels of the recorded footage to measure how the distribution of light values across the recorded field of view

FIGURE 13.25 Calibration equipment at the testing area.

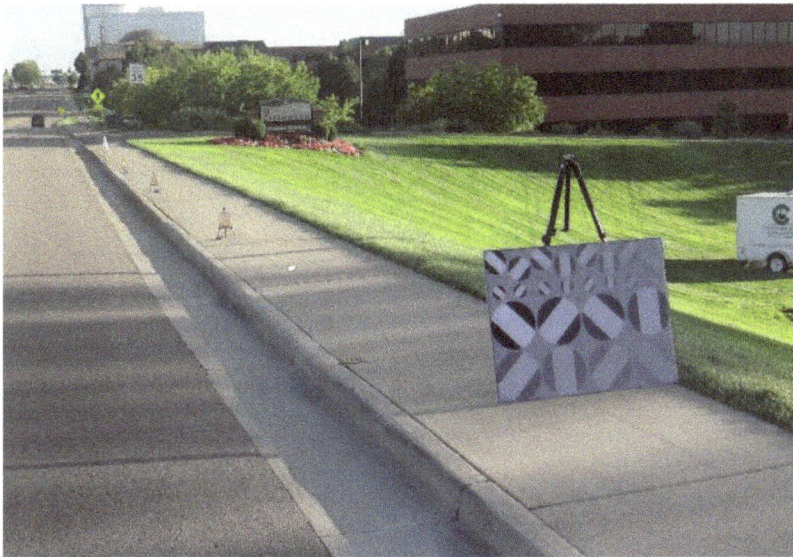

compare to the same light recordings at the actual scene. In general, the calibration process involves using a field monitor, which is held in the hand and used as a visual comparison to what is observed with the naked eye. An observer looks into the monitor that is showing a live view of what the camera sees. The observer can oscillate between viewing the monitor and viewing the real world and adjust settings on the camera such as the aperture, shutter speed, and ISO settings until a comparable match between what the monitor represents and what one observes in the actual world scene are the same.

To calibrate the camera at night and at the scene using the field monitor, a calibration chart with varying values and spatial frequencies was utilized along with three LED markers. These devices are shown setup at the testing site in Figure 13.25. The calibration chart uses a series of values from light to dark so that, when viewed in the monitor, adjustments can be made to the camera settings, so the values and spatial frequencies observed with the naked eye are commensurate with what is represented in the monitor. In addition to the chart, LED lights are placed at varying distances to further add markers that allow calibration of the field monitor to what is observed with the naked eye. These LED markers are also used in obtaining luminance measurements for quantifying the difference in light values across the entire digital image. By using the calibration method described above, and with the addition of LED markers that allow quantifying the comparison of the digital image to real-world measurements, a calibrated image can be captured.

To evaluate and quantify the real-world light measurements with the digital representation of those light values, an image is captured at the scene, and from this same vantage point, light values are recorded using the luminance meter. These measurements are recorded in cd/m^2 and represent a range of the darkest and lightest values in the scene. Figure 13.26 shows two photographic images. On the left is a digital image captured at the testing site. On the right is the same image, but this time with notations showing the luminance measurements taken during the calibration process. Figure 13.27 shows the results of the later comparison between the real-world light values and light values measured digitally using Photoshop CC. Several photographs are included in Figure 13.28 to show the camera setup, camera mount, and the Atomos field monitor used in the calibration process.

Nighttime digital image and luminance measurements.

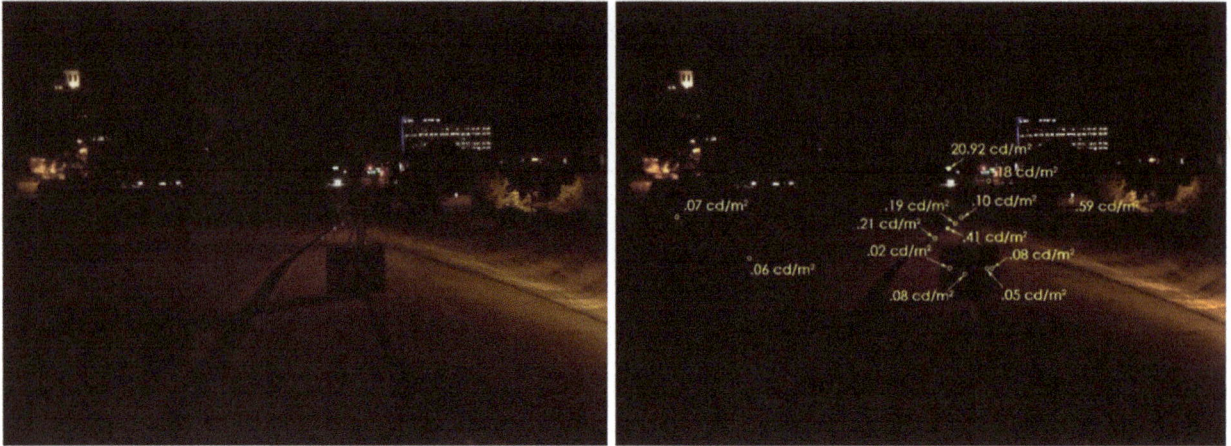

Comparison between actual and digitally measured luminance.

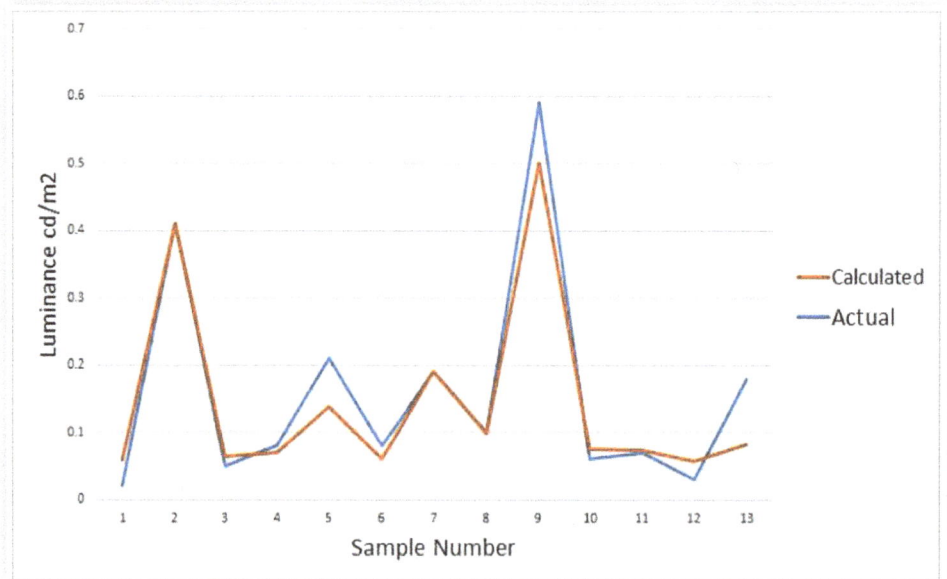

With the camera and field monitor calibrated to represent the lighting conditions and visibility similar to the naked eye, the driving sequence was captured on video, using a frame rate of 60 fps and HD resolution of 1920 × 1080. Figure 13.29 is a series of still images from this calibrated nighttime video showing a view available to the driver approaching the stopped vehicle. After obtaining video of the baseline sequence, a CG version of the same driving scenario was then created.

The first step of the methodology, collecting footage of the environment, is relatively easy in this case since the camera was already calibrated to record the driving scenario when the vehicle is stopped in the lane. Hence, the same camera settings and setup are used for recording the environment without the vehicle present. This footage will be used as a projection map for the CG scene of the geometry such that a user can then change variables such as the vehicle's location, vehicle parameters or vehicle type, or driving conditions. Figure 13.30 shows still images from the calibrated video footage of the environment with the vehicle no longer present.

FIGURE 13.28 Camera setup and calibration.

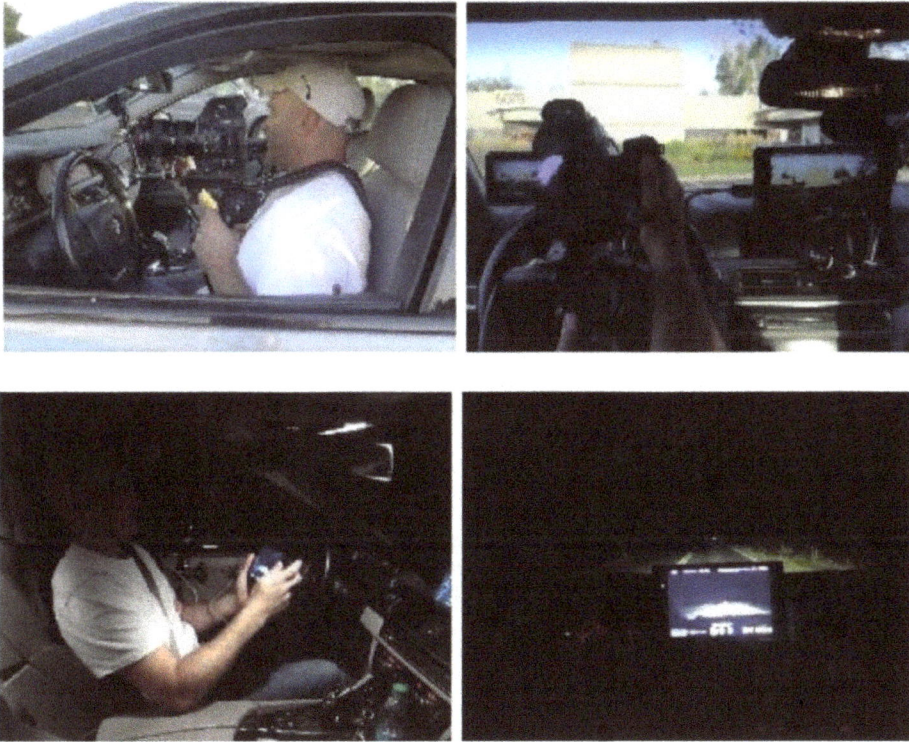

FIGURE 13.29 Video stills from baseline footage.

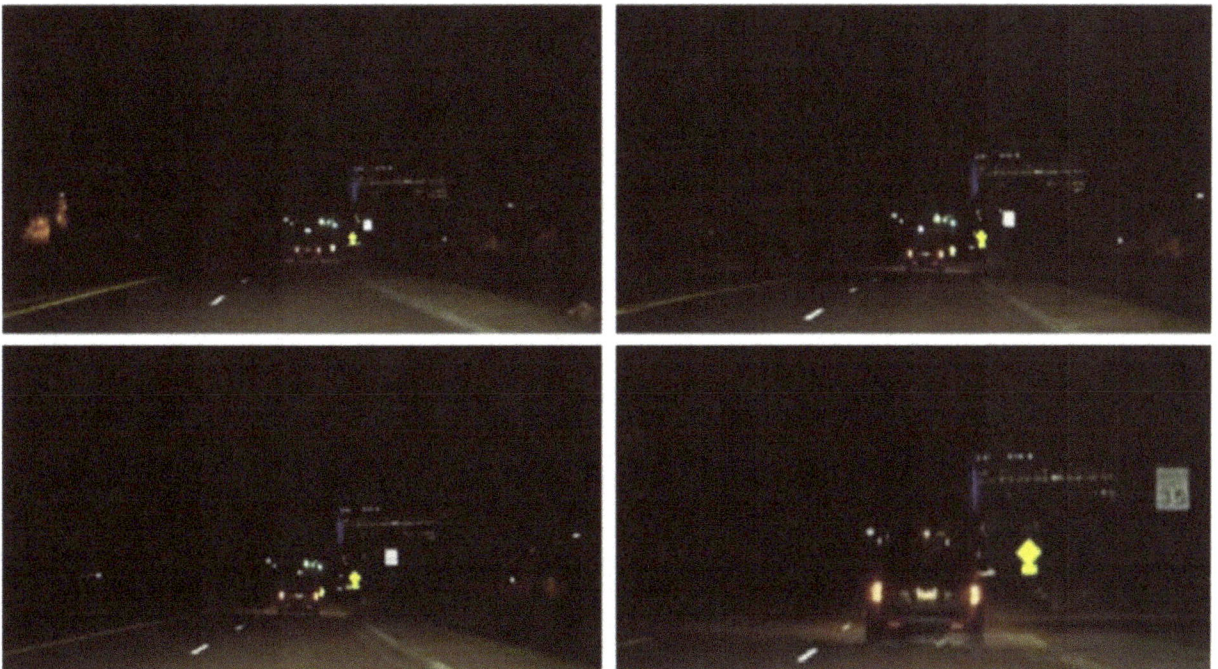

FIGURE 13.30 Video without vehicles.

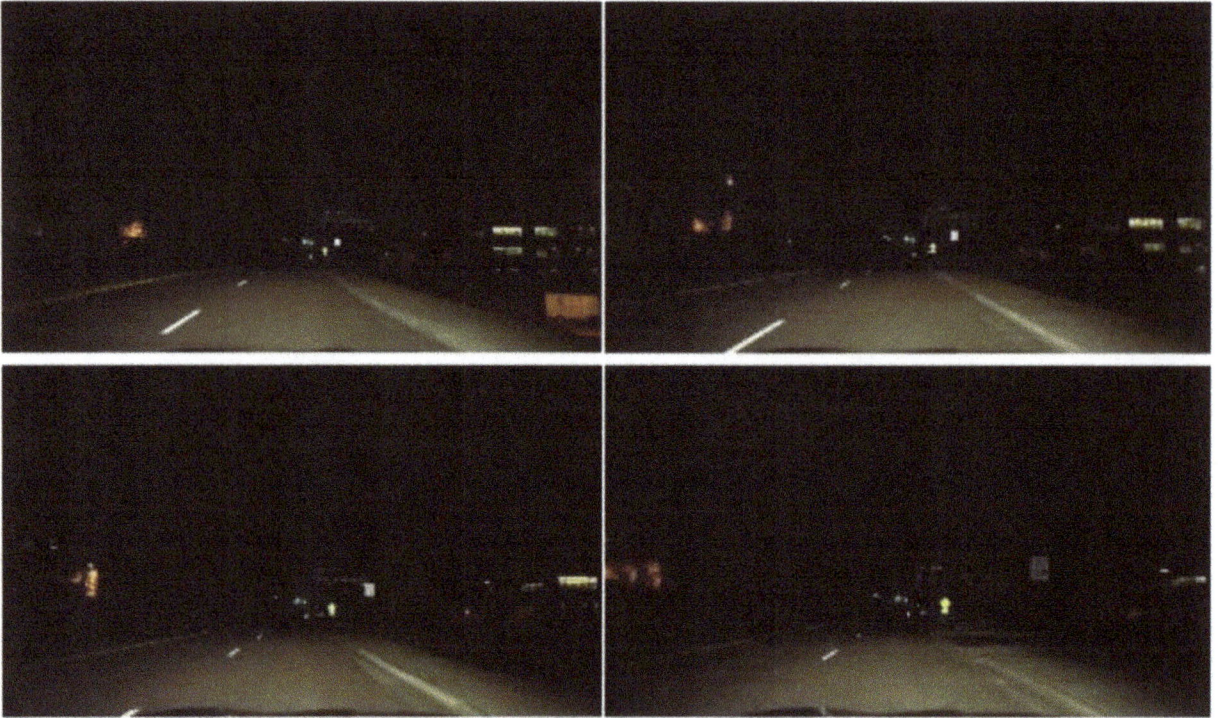

For the second step, mapping data must be collected for the environment in which the video was collected. Using scan data, the entire scene, including roadway geometry, trees, curbs, and surrounding buildings, can quickly and accurately be collected. Other methods for collecting geometry can also be used; though scanning is one of the quicker and encompassing methods. For some scenes, the video footage itself can be used to build geometry of the scene, through tracking technologies previously published. In the current example, a Faro laser scanner Focus 3D X330 was used to scan the entire scene, as well as a Sokkia Series 30R total station. Figure 13.31 shows the resulting computer scan geometry of the scene. This data was then imported into computer modeling programs,

FIGURE 13.31 Scan data of the site.

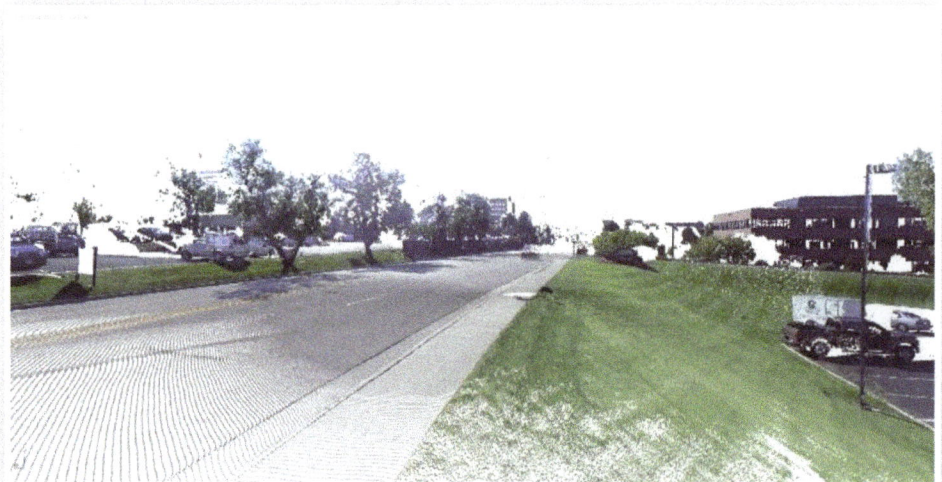

FIGURE 13.32 Calibration step setup.

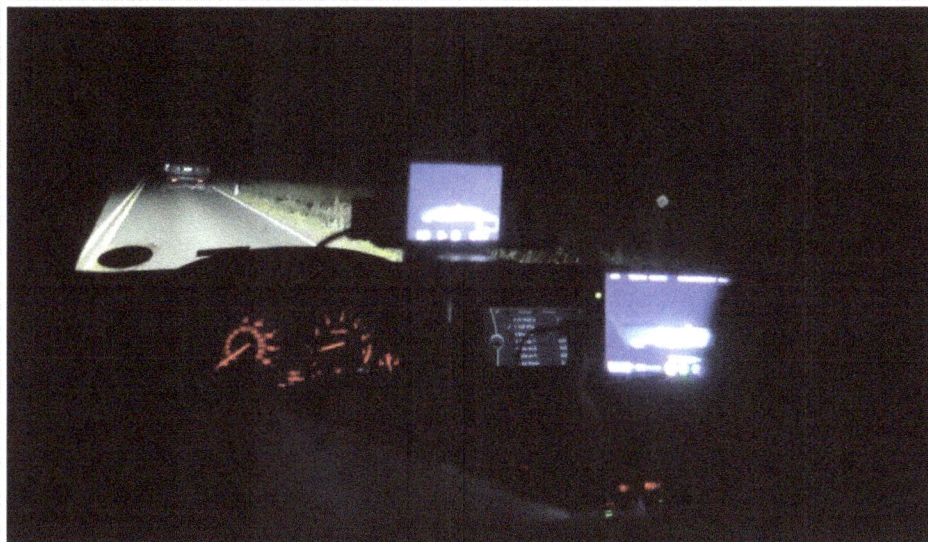

in this case Autodesk's 3D Max 2015 and The Foundry's Nuke 9, to further develop the modeling components.

The third step of the methodology involves collecting video and photographic footage of the vehicles by themselves, in a controlled environment. For this step, another area was used where the lighting and traffic can be controlled, so that safe and feasible footage of the vehicle could be obtained with light conditions of the vehicle being varied (i.e., with headlamp and tail lamps activated, without any lights activated, and with all lamps and hazards activated). Recording these variables during this step allows the use of these varying conditions to be utilized when producing the final computer simulations. This step of the methodology used the same calibration techniques that were employed when calibrating the monitor in the previous section where environment footage was obtained. The setup for this study is shown in Figure 13.32, and digital images of the vehicle the driver is approaching is shown in Figure 13.33, where different lighting configurations are shown. This series shows the vehicle at a distance of 100 ft with no lights activated, with running and headlamps activated, and with all lights activated including the hazard lamps.

Like the second step, where scene geometry was collected, three-dimensional geometry of the vehicles that would appear in the video was also collected, using the same geometry data collecting tools such as scanners and survey equipment. The purpose of having CG vehicles is to enable varying the position, conditions, speed, and appearance of the vehicle in the final computer simulation. When the vehicle is digitized,

FIGURE 13.33 No lights (left), running and headlamps only (middle), and all lights activated.

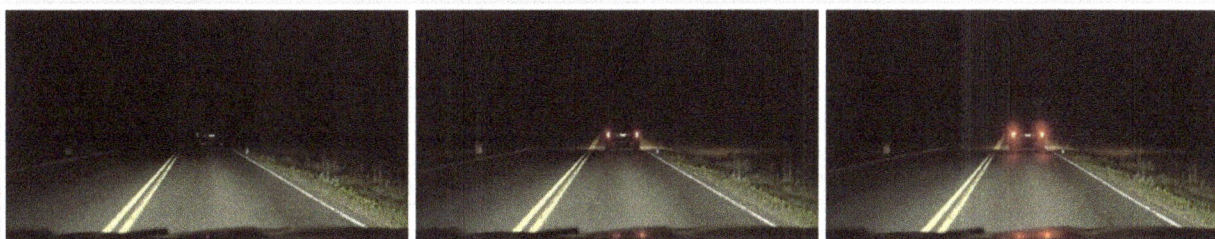

FIGURE 13.34   Photograph and computer model of vehicle.

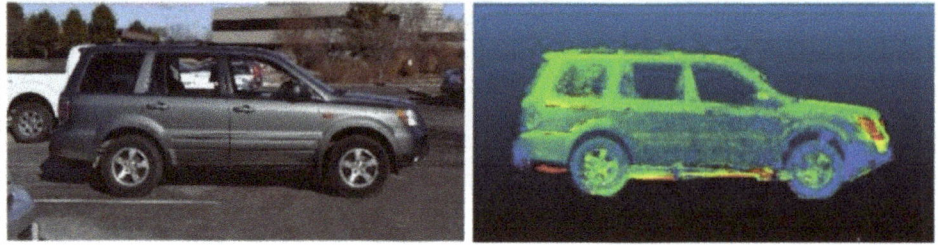

it becomes feasible to change variables such as color and reflectivity and lighting configuration and to add or remove items such as signal indicators and markings. Figure 13.34 shows the vehicle used in the live study and the digital reproduction of the vehicle.

The use of projection mapping technologies to take video sequences and map them to the surface of computer geometry has been described and published in previous literature [7]. In this case, nighttime video footage is used to project texture maps onto the scanned scene geometry that was obtained during the second step of the methodology. This method first tracks the position of the camera relative to the scanned scene geometry through video tracking and camera-matching photogrammetry. Then, for the sequence of frames in the video, individual frames are projected and mapped to the surface of the computer geometry, such that the geometry, when viewed from a CG camera, will show photo-realistic textures and lighting, since they are directly obtained from the video frames themselves. It is this projection of video frames that maintains the video-realistic quality of the scene environment in the final simulation. Figure 13.35 shows the process of projecting video frames on to the scanned geometry, and Figure 13.36 shows the resulting video-realistic simulation of this environment from a driver's perspective.

The computer models of the vehicles are also mapped with video and photographic footage obtained from step three where video and photographs were used to document the vehicle in varying lighting conditions. This mapping process essentially creates several variations of the computer model vehicle, each with a different lighting parameter. Color, size, and other appearances could also be modified, since the vehicle is in an editable computer model format. The series of images in Figure 13.37 shows the mapping

FIGURE 13.35   Projection mapping sequence on the terrain.

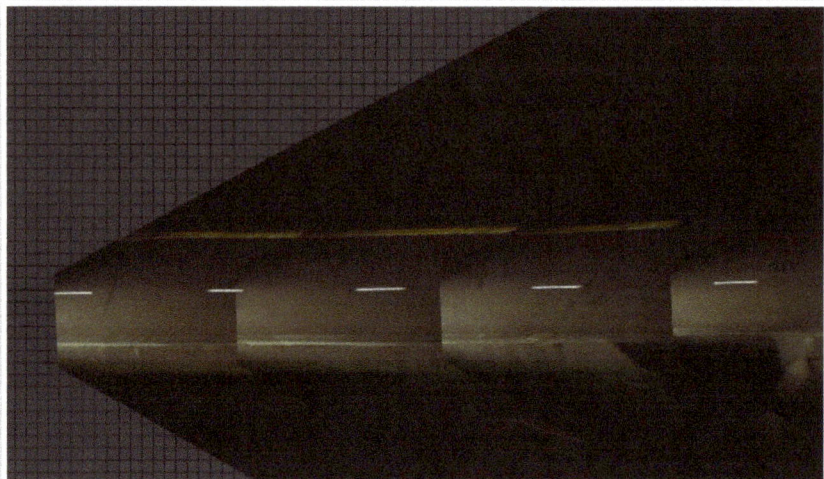

Computer projection mapping of the site.

Mapping process of vehicle computer geometry.

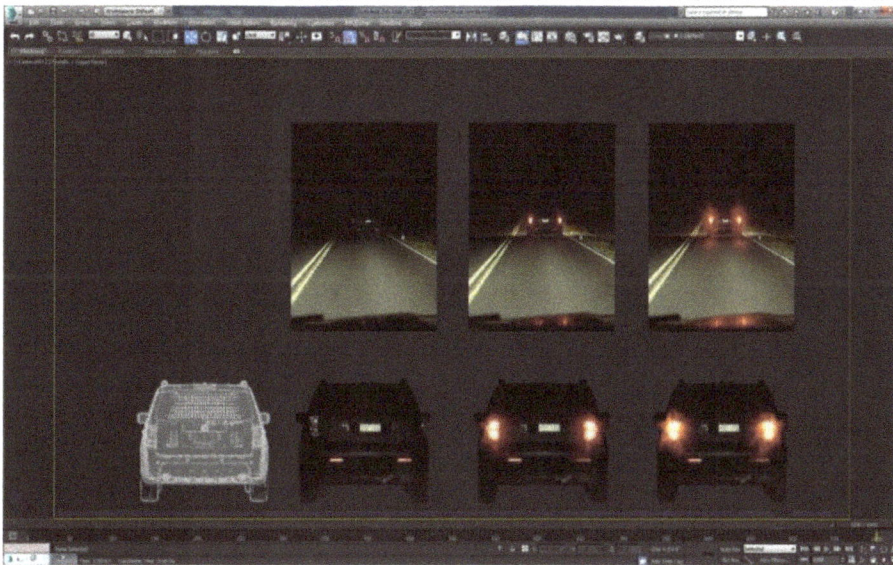

process, where digital imagery of the vehicle in different lighting configurations is transferred to the computer geometry of the vehicle. Figure 13.38 shows the vehicle in its simulated environment, and Figure 13.39 shows the vehicle rendered in the computer environment. This image shows that the CG environment and vehicle maintain their photo-realism just like the original baseline video footage.

Since both the scene and vehicle environments are scaled the same, and both contain photo-mapped geometry, a CG environment can be created incorporating both the vehicle and scene together in the same environment. This environment, because it is a simulated environment, can have any number of variables adjusted digitally. Figure 13.40 is a series of images showing the computer-simulated version of the original baseline video sequence. In this series, the vehicle has been shifted to pass the stopped vehicle on the left side.

FIGURE 13.38 Computer environment with computer-generated vehicle.

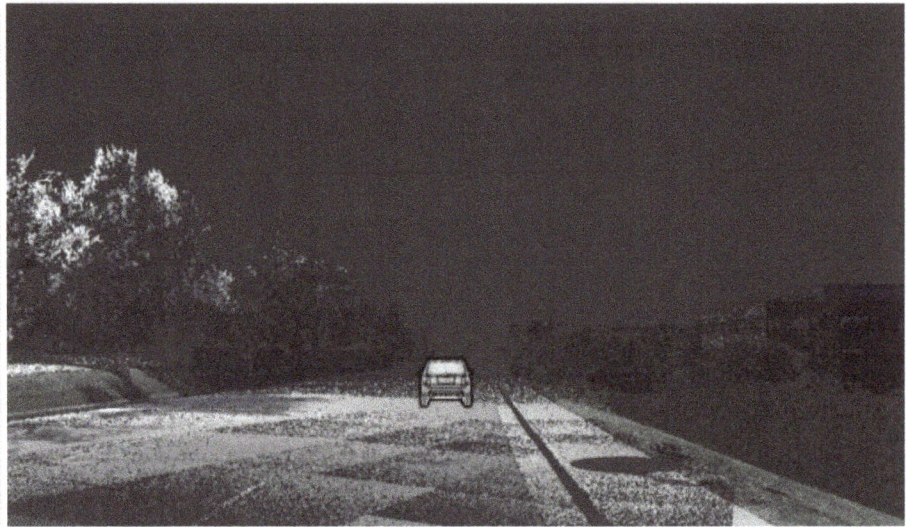

FIGURE 13.39 Rendered computer environment composite.

FIGURE 13.40 Moving through the video-realistic computer environment.

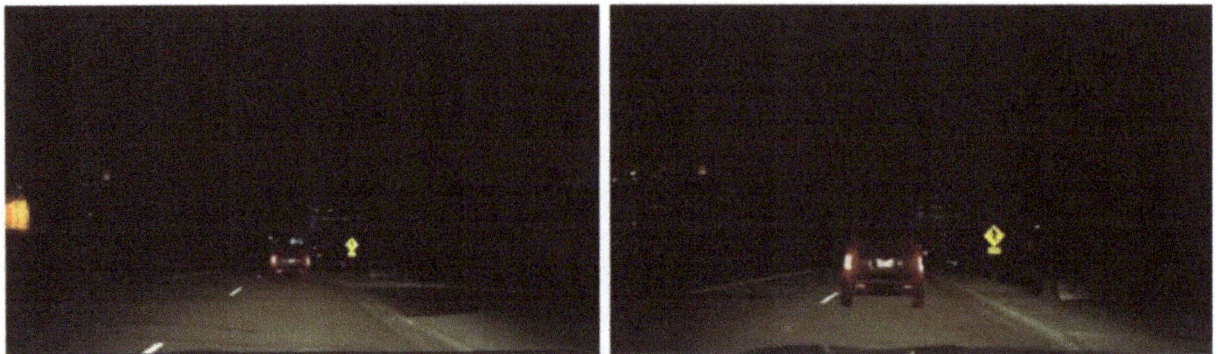

FIGURE 13.41 Computer environment with driving conditions changed.

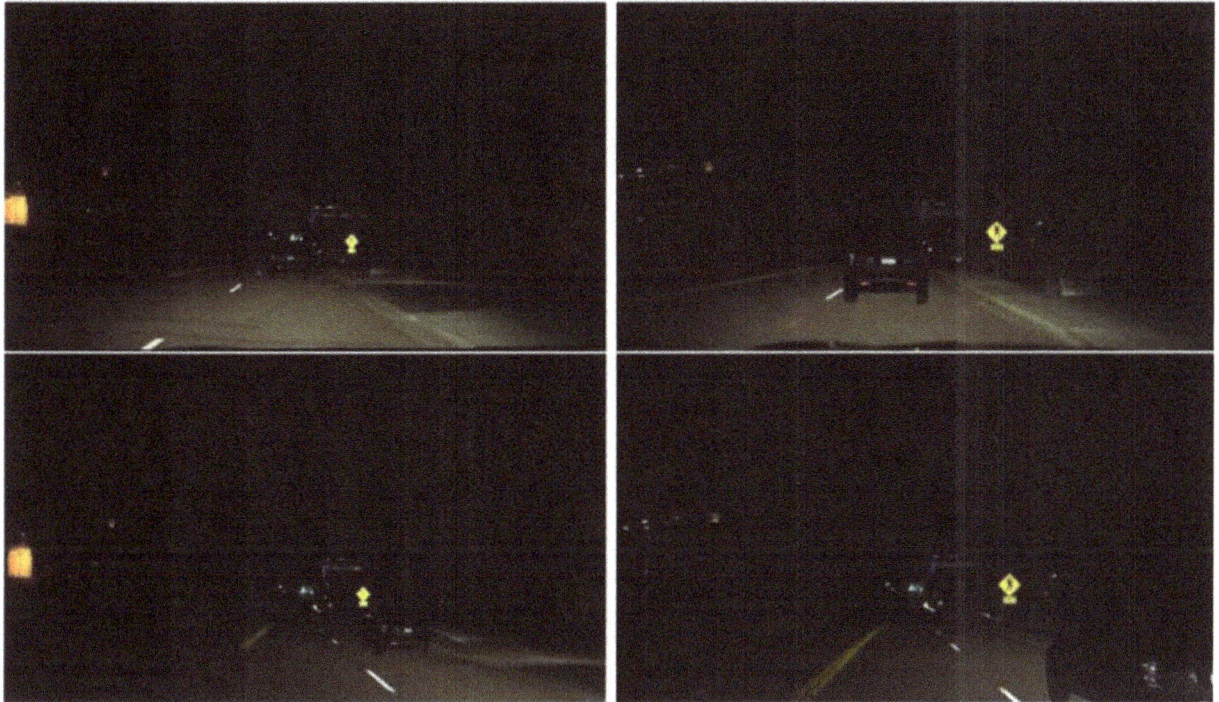

To illustrate the usefulness of having a computer-generated, video-realistic environment, a series of images are included in Figure 13.41 that include some driving scenario variables changed. The top row has the vehicle presented with all the lights off. The second row has the approaching vehicle in a different lane. Since these changes were made by simply swapping out the images of the vehicle or shifting the camera location in the computer environment, additional time-consuming testing was not needed. The following sections show other tests performed using the same methodology, where other vehicles and driving environments were documented with video and then the geometry of the scene and vehicles scanned and modeled in the computer.

In these additional scenarios, several driving conditions and different vehicles, including a tractor-trailer, were used to run a larger gamut of possible driving scenarios. This was to demonstrate that the methodology would be applicable for numerous driving environments and vehicle models and types. The two scenarios presented in this section include variances such as tractor-trailers, left-turning vehicles with side lights, and highway environments. Figure 13.42 shows diagrams of the two scenarios that were tested. From left to right, these are described as the following:

1. Tractor-trailer stopped on the side of a highway
2. Left-turning tractor-trailer

Each of these tests was conducted using the same equipment and calibration methodologies described in this paper. Images from the baseline video for these tests are shown in Figure 13.43 and are in the same order of scenarios listed above, starting with the tractor-trailer on the side of the roadway.

Computer models were created of the scenes and of the vehicles involved, and the vehicles were tested under several lighting conditions. The computer models and scene geometry were projection-mapped, the resulting computer environment was created,

FIGURE 13.42   Additional scenarios with a tractor-trailer.

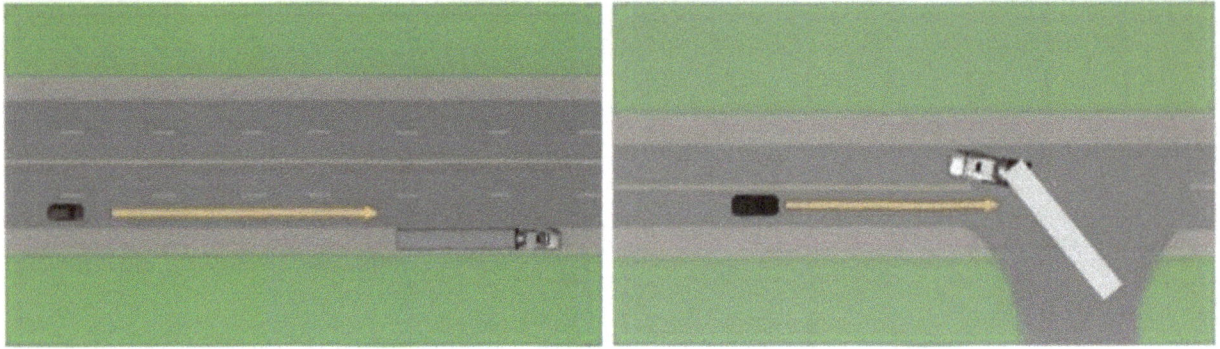

FIGURE 13.43   Baseline footage from additional scenarios.

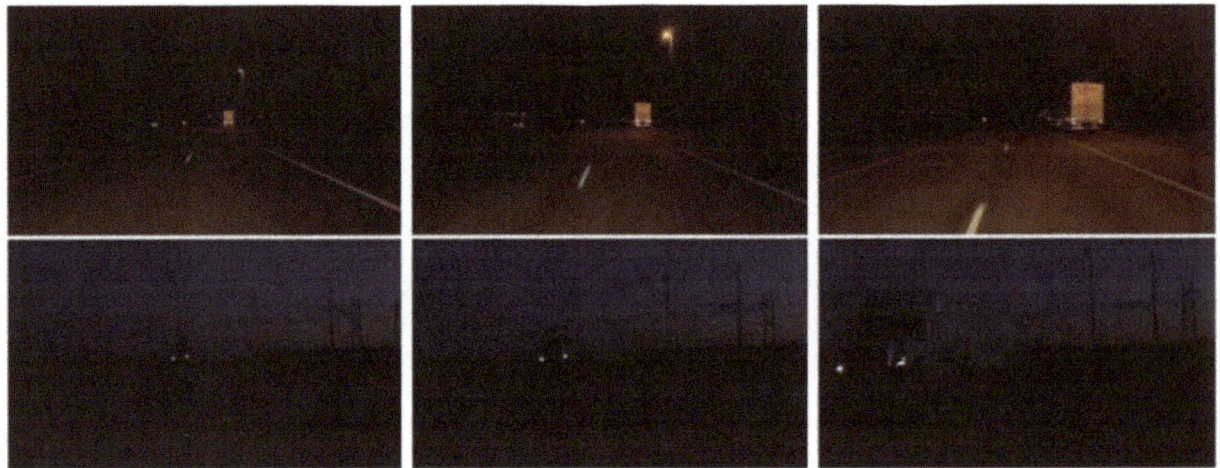

and video-realistic simulations produced to demonstrate how the variable of the driving scenario could be changed without additional testing. Figure 13.44 shows images from the simulated environments of these two additional scenarios, each following the same methodology described in this report. Shown in this figure are images from the final composited, simulated videos for both the stopped tractor-trailer scenario and the left-turning tractor-trailer scenario. The top row, based on the scenario of the stopped tractor-trailer, has a repositioned tractor-trailer in the direct lane of travel up to impact. The second row, based on the scenario of a left-turning tractor-trailer, has repositioned the approaching vehicle such that impact occurs with the side of the trailer.

This process results in a CG environment that is fully flexible but stills maintains a video-realistic quality. This same methodology, though presented for nighttime driving environments, would be applicable to daytime environments as well. In fact, the daytime environment would be easier to calibrate and track, since the features in the video would be more pronounced and the techniques for tracking and projection mapping are easier when there is higher contrast. Likewise, this methodology is not limited to just vehicles and roadway environments. If other non-vehicle features were needed in a study or demonstration, these features could be added using a similar process. Barricades, roadway signage, or construction conditions could be added by obtaining reference

FIGURE 13.44 Computer environment of modified sequence.

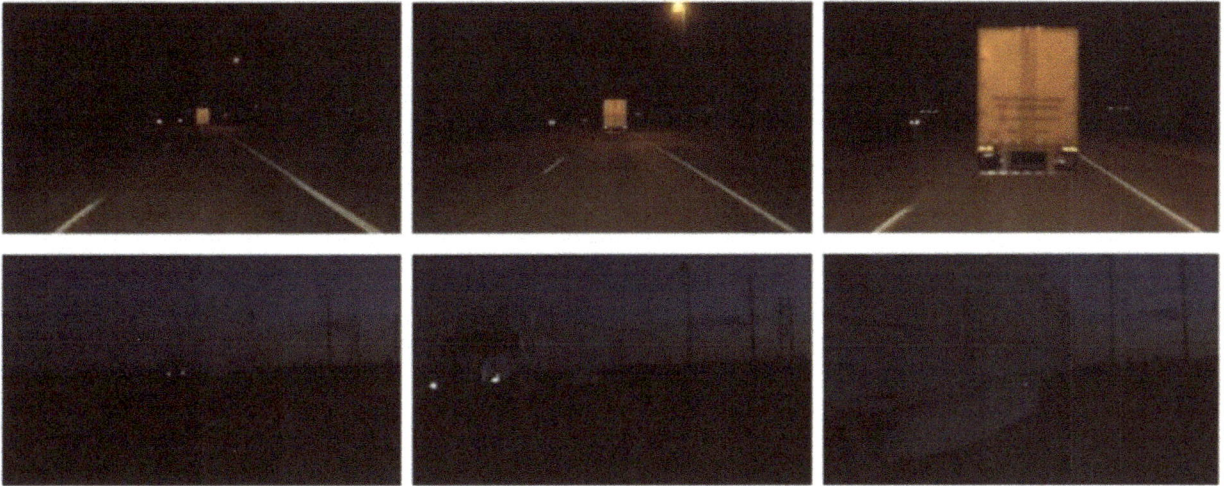

footage and geometry for each feature that is needed. These scaled models could be added to the environment and be represented under similar lighting, color, and contrast conditions, as if these features were present during the original study. Adding pedestrians in varying clothing, for instance, could be performed through the same method to evaluate conspicuity and visibility issues related to pedestrian accidents.

13.4.2 Case Study: Computer-Generated Visualization of a Truck Versus Motorcycle Crash

This section illustrates a process for producing a physics-based animation of a collision between a heavy truck and a motorcycle. The subject collision occurred on an interstate highway with three lanes in each direction. The eastbound and westbound lanes were divided by a concrete center median barrier. According to the police, the crash occurred when the truck driver swerved from the right lane to avoid a slow-moving car that had experienced a blowout on its left rear tire. The truck driver swerved his tractor-trailer to the left, across the center and left lanes, onto the left shoulder, and then back to right, eventually bringing his vehicle to a stop straddling the left and center lanes. While swerving through the left lane, the tractor collided with the motorcyclist. The speed limit in the area was 70 mph. According to witnesses and involved parties, the tractor-trailer and the motorcycle were initially traveling approximately 70 mph, and the slow-moving vehicle was traveling approximately 15 mph.

The tractor involved in this crash was towing an empty, 53 ft Wabash National van trailer, which also had antilock brakes. According to testimony by the truck driver, the semitrailer was empty at the time of the crash. The collision damaged components on the tractor, including the driver's side fuel tank, the driver's side steps, and the hardware and tank bands that attached the steps to the fuel tank. There was black, brown, and red material transfer to the fuel tank that came either from the motorcyclist's clothing or from his motorcycle.

The electronic control module (ECM) on the tractor's engine was equipped with an event data recorder (EDR) capable of recording data from hard braking events. The recorded data from these systems includes the vehicle-indicated speed, engine speed,

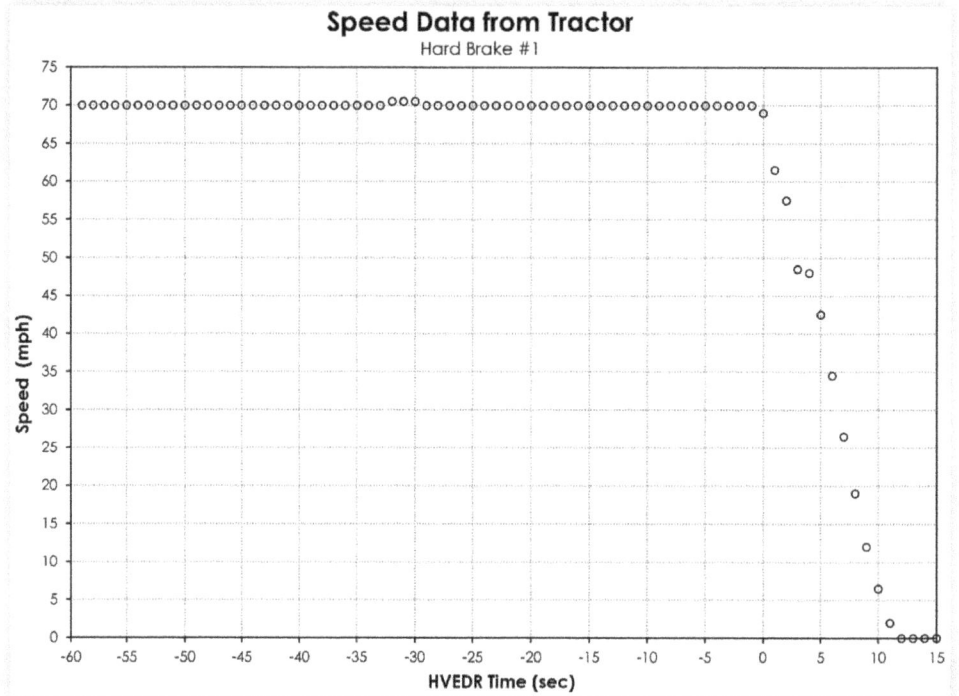

FIGURE 13.45   EDR speed data from the freightliner.

engine load, throttle, brake status, clutch status, and cruise control status reported at 1-s intervals for 59 s preceding and 15 s following the triggering event. An event is triggered when the system detects a change in wheel speed of 7 mph in a 1-s interval. Data was imaged from the tractor's ECM 19 days after the subject crash. The obtained data included two hard brake events and a last stop record. The event designated by the ECM as "Hard Brake #1" was determined to be from the subject crash.

Figure 13.45 is a graph showing the vehicle-indicated speeds reported in Hard Brake #1 at 1-s intervals for 59 s prior to and 15 s after the triggering deceleration event. The individual speed readings are designated on the graph with open black circles. This graph has time, in seconds, plotted on the horizontal axis, and the triggering event occurs at a time of 0 s. Times prior to this event are shown as negative, and times after this event are shown as positive. The tractor's vehicle-indicated speeds, in miles per hour, are plotted on the vertical axis. This data shows that the tractor-trailer was driving a speed of approximately 70 mph for the minute prior to this crash. The driver then applied his brakes with sufficient severity to trigger the recording of this data, ultimately coming to a stop around 12 s later.

Figure 13.46 is similar with the exception that it focuses on the time from 5 s before to 15 seconds after the triggering brake event. Again, time is plotted on the horizontal axis, and vehicle-indicated speeds are plotted on the vertical axis. On this graph, filled red circles designate times when the ECM indicated the driver was applying the brakes, and filled blue circles designate times when the ECM indicated the driver was applying the throttle. This data indicated that the driver had the throttled applied up until 1 s prior to the braking. The system indicated that sometime between time −1 s and time 0 s, the driver released the throttle. The system then indicated that the brakes were not applied at time 0, but they were applied by time 1 s. Thus, the system indicated that the driver applied the brakes sometime in this 1-s interval between 0 and 1 s.

In the absence of heavy braking or swerving, the EDR on a heavy truck will capture the actual speed of the vehicle. This speed is typically accurate to within 1 mph.

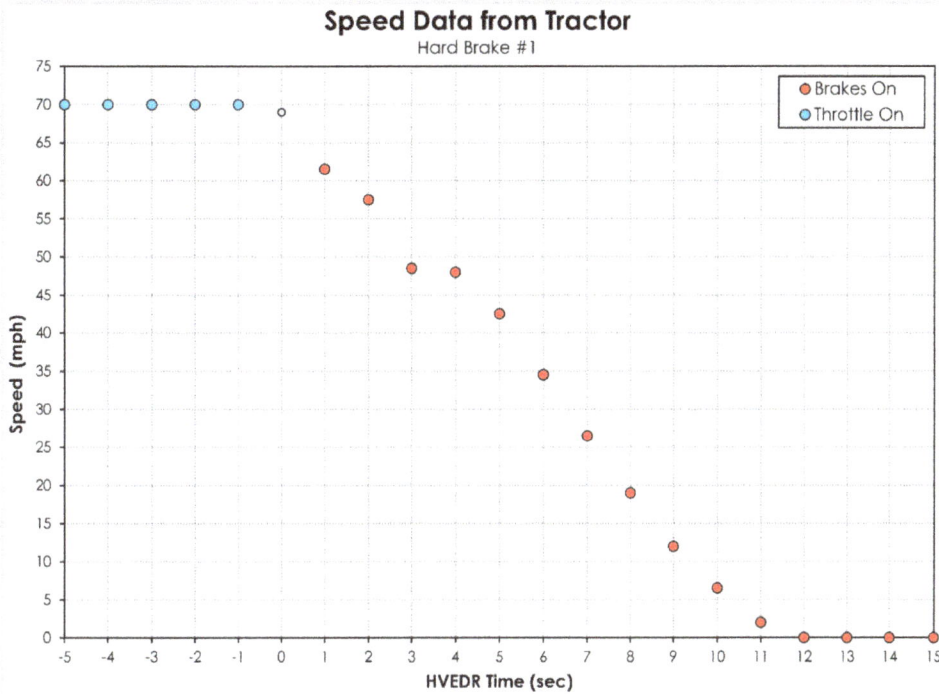

However, in the presence of heavy braking or swerving, the vehicle wheels can be traveling more slowly than the vehicle itself, and this can cause the vehicle-indicated speeds to be lower than the actual vehicle speed. The speed data during the hard brake event was analyzed in accordance with techniques that take this into account [8, 9, 10, 11, 12, 13, 14, 15]. The next graph (Figure 13.47) adds a black line indicating the probable speed of the tractor based on this analysis. This analysis showed that the driver of the tractor-trailer initially applied his brakes at a level sufficient to decelerate his vehicle at approximately 0.26 g. At an EDR time of 5 s, the driver increased the level of his brake application, producing a deceleration of approximately 0.32 g.

The motorcycle involved in the subject crash weighed approximately 800 lb. The motorcycle was inspected, photographed, and mapped with a Faro laser scanner. The colorized scan data is depicted in Figure 13.48.

Damaged components on the motorcycle included the windshield, gauge cluster shade, both side mirrors, handlebars with associated hand control levers, front wheel cowling, and both turn signal indicators. Both radiators, which reside inward of the front tire, were also damaged. The front tire exhibited scuff marks aligned radially over the circumference of the treaded surface. The left side of the motorcycle showed damage that included the upper and lower faring, shifter pedal, passenger foot board, side luggage case, rear speaker cover, and elbow rest. The left side of the vehicle also had scratches aligned horizontally, spanning from approximately the front headlight to the left rear luggage case. The tip-over-bar on this side has also been displaced in an upward direction with scratches deposited on its underside. The right side of the motorcycle exhibited damage that included the side luggage case, speaker cover, upper and lower cowling, gas tank, brake pedal, tip-over-bar, and foot peg which was no longer attached to the vehicle. Both the tip-over-bar and shifter pedal had been displaced upward and exhibited scratching. Multiple scratch patterns were deposited on this side of the vehicle.

FIGURE 13.47   EDR speed data plotted with reconstructed speeds.

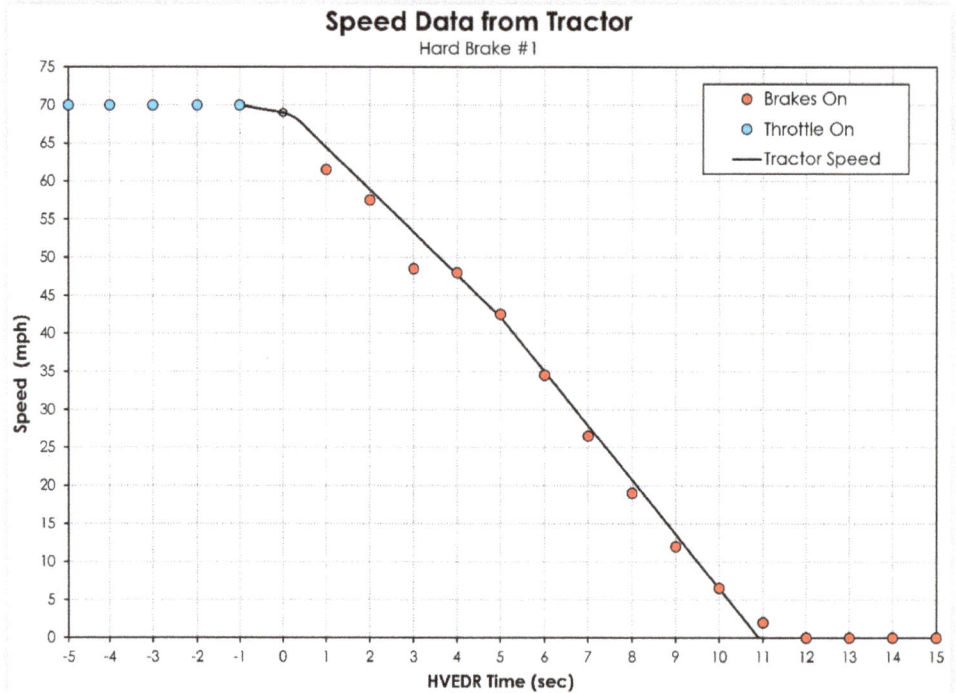

Speed Data from Tractor
Hard Brake #1

- Brakes On
- Throttle On
- Tractor Speed

FIGURE 13.48   Faro scan data for the motorcycle.

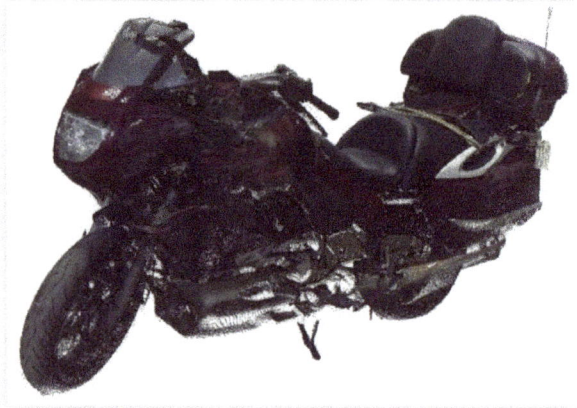

The accident site, which is shown in Figure 13.49, was inspected, documented, photographed, digitally mapped, and videoed. As the photograph shows, the roadway around this crash had three asphalt-paved travel lanes separated by dashed white lines. There was a paved shoulder on the left side of the travel lanes, separated from the travel lanes by a solid yellow edge line and bordered on the left by a concrete center median barrier. There was a wider paved shoulder on the right side of the travel lanes, separated from the travel lanes by a solid white edge line. The roadway in this area had a slight downgrade of around 1 percent. This accident occurred in a straightaway. A Sokkia total station was used to map the site.

Investigating officers took 40 photographs at the scene of this crash, which depicted physical evidence. The physical evidence included tire marks deposited by the tractor-trailer in the left lane and shoulder, paint transfer and scraping on the concrete center median that was deposited by the motorcyclist and his motorcycle, and scraping and debris on the roadway from the motorcycle. The rest positions of the motorcycle, the rider, and the tractor-trailer were also documented. Camera-matching photogrammetric analysis was used to locate the evidence depicted in the police photographs. Figure 13.50 shows one of the accident scene photographs that I analyzed. Figure 13.51 shows this same photograph aligned with the mapping of the accident site. Figure 13.52 shows the evidence in the photograph traced, along with the vehicle rest positions. Several of the police photographs were analyzed using the same technique. Figure 13.53 shows portions of the physical evidence diagram that resulted from this photogrammetric analysis.

FIGURE 13.49 Photograph of accident area.

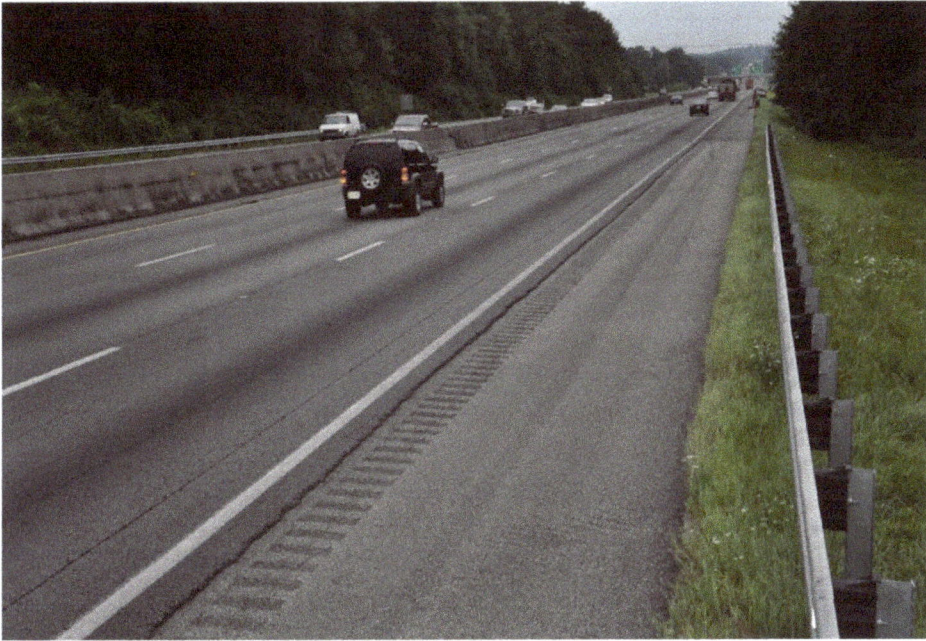

FIGURE 13.50 Accident scene photograph.

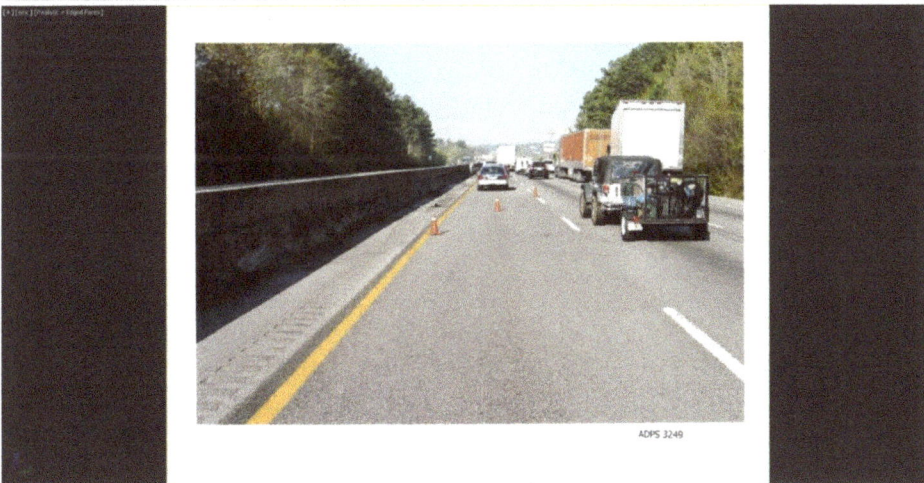

The motion of the vehicles during this crash was next analyzed based on the ECM data, the physical evidence, and the descriptions by the witnesses and involved drivers. To conduct this analysis, the accident analysis software called PC-Crash was used [16]. This software employs physics-based equations to calculate the motion of vehicles that result from steering, braking, and acceleration inputs of the drivers and from impacts. In addition to driver inputs, PC-Crash allows the analyst to specify the vehicle and scene geometries and the roadway surface conditions. This analysis resulted in a reconstruction that included the timing of the truck driver's steering and brake inputs, the timing of the collision, the speeds of the vehicles at the time the collision, and the motion of the vehicles.

FIGURE 13.51 Mapping data overlaid on accident scene photograph.

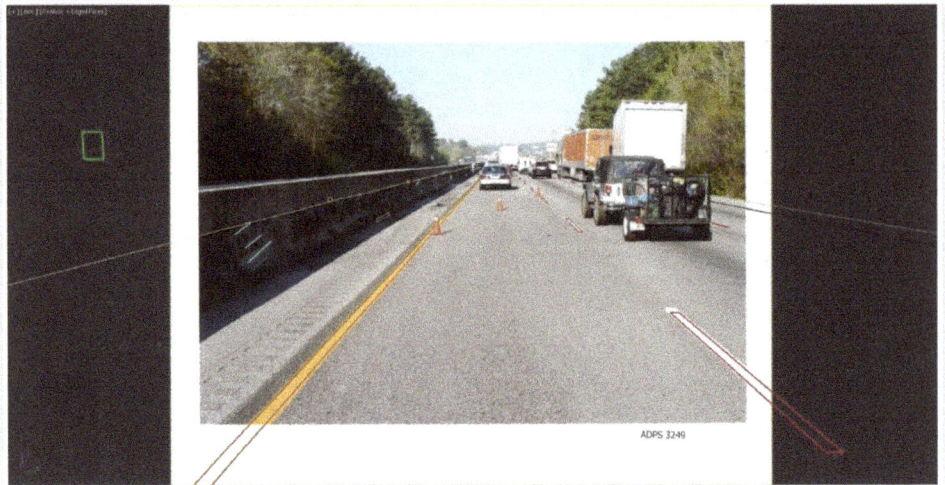

FIGURE 13.52 Physical evidence traced from camera-matching.

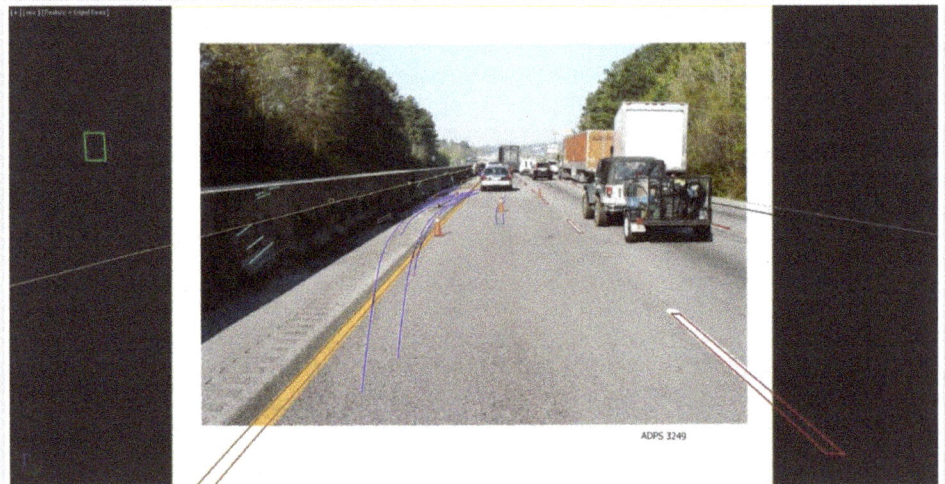

FIGURE 13.53 Portions of the physical evidence diagram from the photogrammetric analysis.

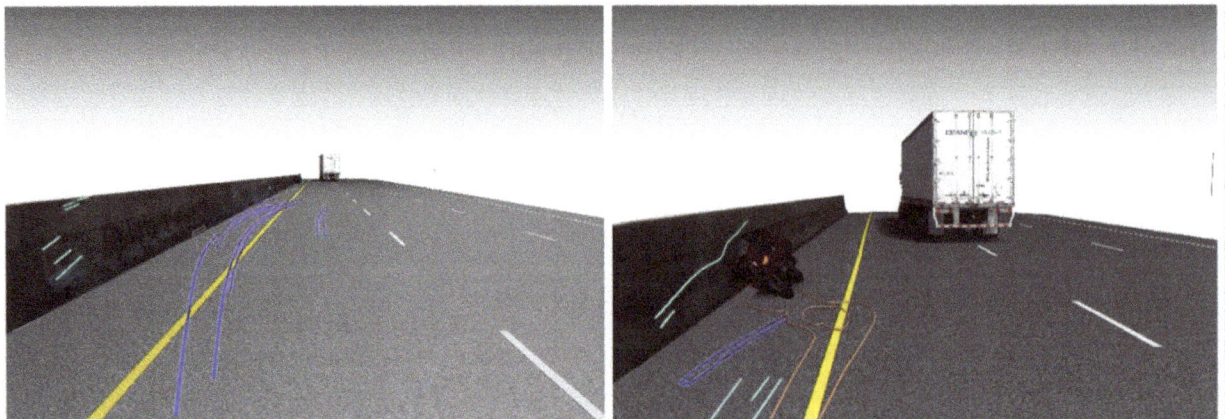

FIGURE 13.54 Comparison between the EDR data, the reconstructed speeds, and the PC-Crash simulation for the tractor-trailer.

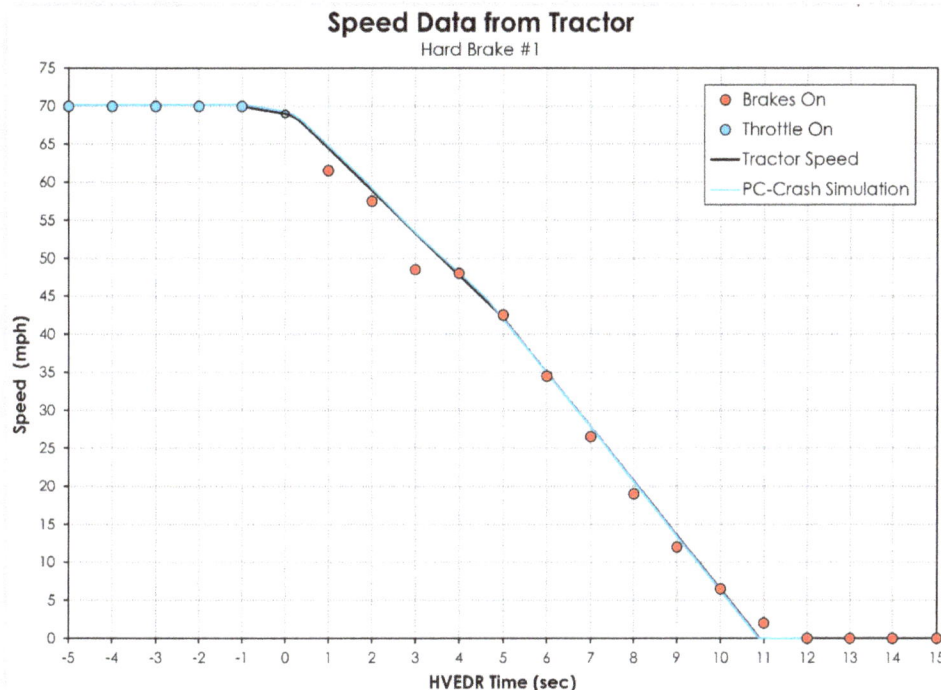

FIGURE 13.54 Comparison between the EDR data, the reconstructed speeds, and the PC-Crash simulation for the tractor-trailer.

Figure 13.54 is a graph that shows the speed of the tractor in the simulation compared to the speed data from the tractor's event data recorder. This graph has time plotted on the horizontal axis and the tractor's speed on the vertical axis. The black curve depicts the tractor's actual speed, as determined from the reported speeds of the EDR, and the blue curve depicts the tractor's speed in the simulation. This graph shows that the simulation exhibited excellent agreement with the speed data from the Freightliner EDR. The alignment of the simulation data with the EDR data also enabled identification of when within the EDR data certain events during the accident sequence took place. Based on this alignment, the tractor impacted the motorcyclist at a time of approximately 1.5 s in the EDR data. The truck driver applied the brakes of his vehicle approximately 1.3 s after he swerved.

The postimpact motion of the motorcycle was not simulated with PC-Crash. However, the physical evidence and principles of physics were used to analyze and model this motion of the motorcycle and of the rider. As the tractor-trailer swerved into and through the left lane, the tractor struck the motorcycle. This impact occurred between the front of the motorcycle and the left side of the tractor. The collision forced the motorcyclist and his motorcycle into the center median barrier. The front left of the motorcycle shows direct impact damage to the upper portions of the vehicle consistent with impacting the center barrier. The evidence on the center median barrier from this impact (scratches and paint transfer) indicated that the motorcycle impacted the barrier in a near upright orientation. At this impact location, yellow paint markings were visible on the upper edge of the barrier from the motorcyclist's helmet. The height of this material transfer was indicative of the rider also being upright on the motorcycle during this impact. This first impact with the barrier also bent the tip-over-bar upward against the motorcycle and caused scratching to its underside.

The left side of the motorcycle impacted the barrier again approximately 75 ft east of the first impact. This impact deposited evidence on the barrier indicative of the left handlebar grip and clutch lever contacting the barrier surface. These marks are visible as a black scuff mark and white scrape mark jointly traveling along the wall. Both surfaces on the motorcycle show contact damage consistent with this interaction with the barrier. A fluid trail began on the ground beyond the location of this impact with the barrier. The fluid trail ended near the motorcycle's rest position against the barrier. This fluid trail demonstrates that the motorcycle was rotating as it traveled to rest. The right side of the motorcycle exhibited several scratch patterns in multiple orientations consistent with such rotation. A breach in the gas tank as well as a disconnected lower radiator hose was also found on the right side of the motorcycle. The damage evident on the right side of the motorcycle is consistent with the motorcycle impacting the ground on its right side and rotating while sliding to rest.

In the area where the fluid trail began, there were also yellow and orange streaks of material deposited on the barrier. The streak marks match the color of the helmet and orange shirt worn by the motorcyclist. The left side of the helmet exhibited scratch marks consistent with contacting the barrier at this point. Additionally, the upper left portion of the rider's chest showed abrasions. The distance from the rider's helmet to the upper left chest abrasions was consistent with the gap between the yellow and orange streaks on the barrier and suggested the rider's head and chest were in contact with the barrier at that location. Due to the difference in rider and motorcycle motion after the second barrier impact, the rider and motorcycle likely began to separate at this location, with the motorcycle leaning to the right and the rider leaning to the left.

The motorcycle was photographed at the scene with its right side leaning against the barrier facing west. Within the photographs, fluid is seen covering the center of the front tire around the circumference of its treaded area. This area of the tire would not encounter the fluid trail the motorcycle was depositing while coming to rest due to the motorcycle sliding on its side. Additionally, the fluid trail terminates a few feet southwest of the motorcycle leaning against the barrier. The fluid trail ending abruptly in addition to the wetted center of the tire indicated that the motorcycle was likely moved from its initial position of rest to the location at which it was ultimately photographed.

Using the motion from the PC-Crash and application of principles of physics to model the postimpact motion of the motorcycle and rider, animations were produced. Because these animations utilized the physics-based motion of the vehicles directly from PC-Crash, they depict motion that is physically realistic and determined directly from the physical evidence. Frames from this animation are included in Figure 13.55.

The process described here illustrates several principles that can be used to produce physics-based animations that are likely to be admissible in a trial. **First, create properly scaled computer models of the scene and vehicles**. In a litigation context, animations like this one are often intended to be a demonstrative exhibit to help an expert explain their opinions. Modern jurors are sophisticated and accustomed to high-quality television, video, and animation production. They are accustomed to a high level of physical realism, and so, physical realism will help to build credibility for an animation. Physical realism begins with having objects in the animation that are correctly sized relative to one another. Jurors will perceive errors in scale, and this will give them cause to doubt the credibility of the animation.

Beyond the benefit to the jury, the process of putting together an animation in an accurately scaled computer environment can help the expert to develop their opinions by helping them to understand how objects fit together and interact [17, 18]. An example would be analysis of how two vehicles collided by creating accurately scaled models of the vehicles and their damage in a computer animation software package. Another

FIGURE 13.55 Frames from the physics-based animation.

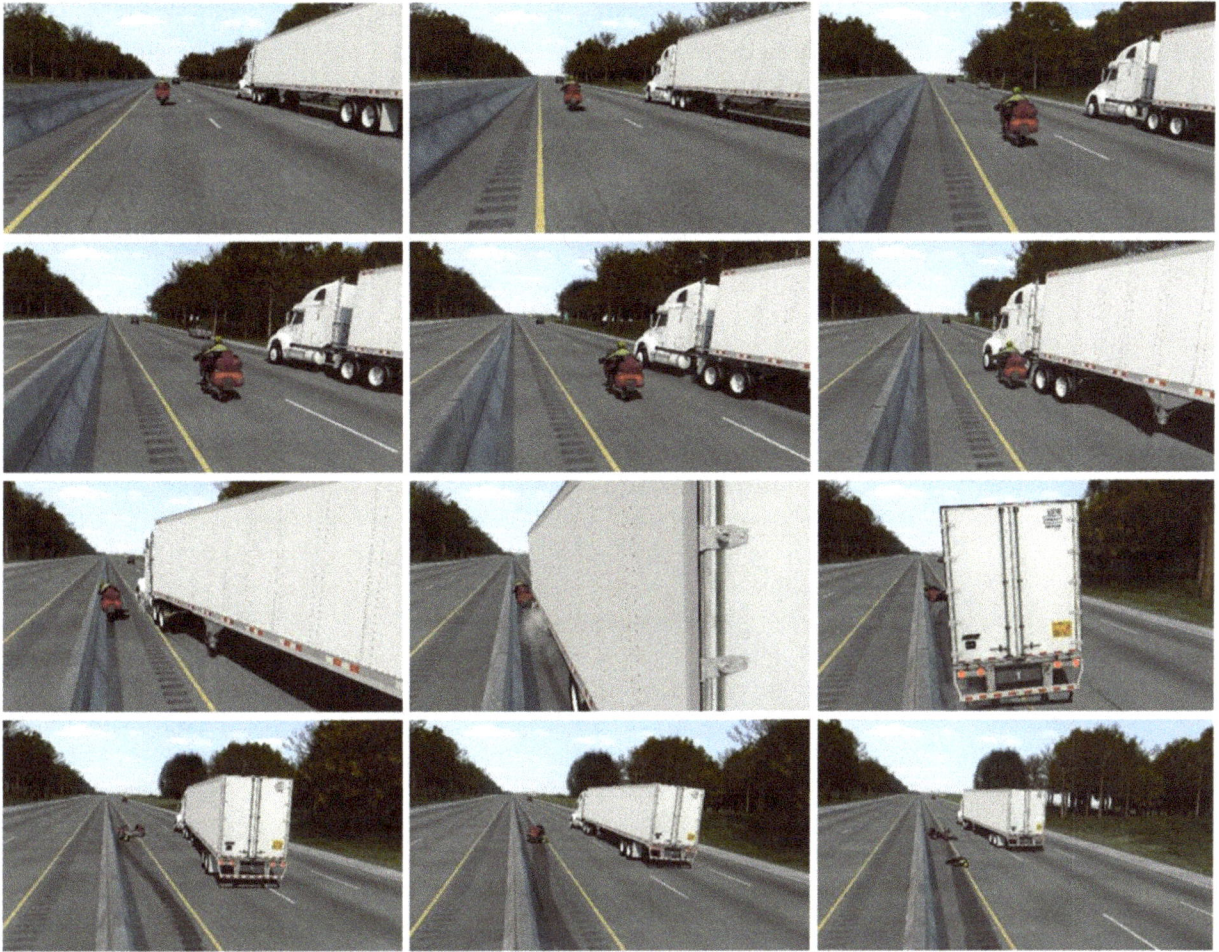

example would be using correctly scaled objects to evaluate geometric visibility for a driver in an accident.

Second, connect the animation to the physical evidence. Car crashes typically leave physical evidence-tire marks, gouges, debris, and vehicle damage. The vehicle rest positions are also typically known. The vehicle motion in an animation will be credible to the extent that it is consistent with the physical evidence and explains how that evidence was created. The animation should reveal to the jury how that evidence was created and help them understand the case better. If an animation helps jurors understand the physical evidence better, then it will provide them with value. The value an animation provides to a jury is one of the criteria for its admissibility [19, 20].

Third, reconcile eye-witness accounts of the crash to the animation. Accident reconstructionists generally agree that eye-witnesses may not be good at estimating times, speeds, and distances. However, this should not discount the general account of a witness, or description of the event, as the overall story being and experience being described by a witness could be very credible. An accident reconstructionist should not dismiss the story that a witness tells without some systematic examination of that story. In certain situations, physical evidence and physical principles would compel an accident reconstructionist to dismiss what a witness says. In other situations when the only facts related to how a crash occurred come from the eye-witness, what is represented in the animation should reflect that testimony within the confines of physical evidence and physical principles.

Fourth, build the animation based on principles of physics. In an animation of a vehicular crash, the motion of the vehicles is going to be perceived as more realistic if that motion is grounded in physics. Physics-based motion gives the animation credibility because the motion of the vehicles looks and feels right. As Grimes [21] has noted: "Unfortunately, the word 'animation' is often associated with cartoons, where objects are not bound to the laws of physics. In contrast, an accurate depiction of a collision requires the animation to be consistent with the physical laws-of-motion. Computer animation requires sufficient data to produce all the images of the vehicle traveling through the collision scene. Therefore, credible animations must be based upon a detailed reconstruction of the collision sequence." In another article, Grimes proposed the term "scientific animation" to describe an animation in which the objects are properly scaled and the depicted motion obeys the laws of physics [22]. Day used the term "scientific visualization" to refer to animations in which the underlying vehicle motion is generated by a physics-based simulation software package [23]. Grimes defined scientific visualization as "a computer animation in which the motion of the primary objects is based on scientific analysis or scientifically accurate equations" [24]. Martin presented applications of this principle of building animations with principles of physics [25]. Massa demonstrated techniques for evaluating and critiquing the physical realism of an animation [26].

Fifth, incorporate the electronic evidence. Many vehicles now record electronic crash-related data, and analysis of this data is usually a part of an accident reconstruction. The engine control module on the semi-tractor in this case study recorded crash-related data (speed, for instance), and this data was analyzed when producing the motion of the tractor-trailer for the animation. This relates back to the principle of tying the animation to the physical and testimonial evidence. The electronic data on modern vehicles is another source of evidence about the crash, and an animation that is consistent with the known evidence will be more credible than one that is not.

Sixth, incorporate relevant secondary details. Car crashes occur at a particular time and place. Including accurate secondary details about the scene, such as road signs, vegetation, correct lighting, and logos on vehicles can add credibility to an animation. In the animation discussed here, several secondary details have been removed so that the case is not identifiable. However, if this animation was going to be shown to a jury, these details would be included. It is important to distinguish between primary and secondary details—or essential and nonessential details [20]. Animations can be reliable and admissible without the secondary (nonessential) details. However, including these secondary details will help orient the jury and will give the jury a sense that you understand the context in which a crash occurred [21, 22]. Grimes distinguishes between primary and secondary details as follows: "The basic difference is that primary objects are important to the purpose of the presentation and secondary objects are only for helping orient the audience" [24]. Sound is another example of a secondary detail that can help to orient jurors and increase their understanding of what is happening in the animation. Neale covered methods for scientifically incorporating sound into an animation [27, 28].

Seventh, present the animation production process in a transparent way. While physical realism can add credibility to an animation, a jury should not be left with the impression that they are watching the real event. Animations are often a demonstrative exhibit illustrating an expert's opinions. A transparent presentation of the process through which the animation was created will help the jury understand the accident better but will not leave them with a misunderstanding of what they are watching. Present the physical evidence, present the analysis of the physical evidence, present how principles of physics were brought to bear on the physical evidence, and then present how physical evidence and physics flow directly into the animation. Transparent presentation of the process also helps lay the foundation for an animation, making it more likely to be admitted. Along these lines, Grimes [24] argues that "any presentation that is presumed to be based on scientific principles should be thoroughly documented such that a similarly qualified person can reproduce the findings." McLay, Kiely, and Sheehan discussed the process of laying the foundation for an animation [29]. Fay covered several examples of cases in which animations were either admitted and excluded [30].

References

1. Holohan, R.D., Billing, A.M., and Murray, S.D., "Nighttime Photography – Show It Like It Is," SAE Technical Paper 890730, 1989, doi:10.4271/890730.
2. Klein, E. and Stephens, G., "Visibility Study – Methodologies and Reconstruction," SAE Technical Paper 921575, 1992, doi:10.4271/921575.
3. Ayres, T.J., "Psychophysical Validation of Photographic Representations, Safety Engineering and Risk Analysis (SERA-Vol. 6), *1996 American Society of Mechanical Engineers (ASME) International Mechanical Engineering Congress and Exposition*, Atlanta, GA, November 17-22, 1996.
4. Krauss, D.A., "Validation of Digital Image Representations of Low-Illumination Scenes," SAE Technical Paper 2006-01-1288, 2006, doi:10.4271/2006-01-1288.
5. Allin, B.D., "Digital Camera Calibration for Luminance Estimation in Nighttime Visibility Studies," SAE Technical Paper 2007-01-0718, 2007, doi:10.4271/2007-01-0718.
6. Ayres, T.J. and Kayfetz, P., *Calibration and Validation of Videographic Visibility Presentations*, (Seattle, WA: American Academy of Forensic Sciences, 2010).
7. Neale, W.T.C., Marr, J., and Hessel, D., "Nighttime Videographic Projection Mapping to Generate Photo-Realistic Simulation Environments," SAE Technical Paper 2016-01-1415, 2016, doi:10.4271/2016-01-1415.
8. Bedsworth, K., Butler, R., Rogers, G., Breen, K. et al., "Commercial Vehicle Skid Distance Testing and Analysis," SAE Technical Paper 2013-01-0771, 2013, doi:10.4271/2013-01-0771.
9. Bayan, F., Cornetto, A., Dunn, A., Tanner, C. et al., "Comparison of Heavy Truck Engine Control Unit Hard Stop Data with Higher-Resolution On-Vehicle Data," *SAE Int. J. Commer. Veh.* 2, no. 1 (2009): 29-38, doi:10.4271/2009-01-0879.
10. Plant, D., Cheek, T., Austin, T., Steiner, J. et al., "Timing and Synchronization of the Event Data Recorded by the Electronic Control Modules of Commercial Motor Vehicles – DDEC V," *SAE Int. J. Commer. Veh.* 6, no. 1, (2013), doi:10.4271/2013-01-1267.
11. Reust, T., "The Accuracy of Speed Captured by Commercial Vehicle Event Data Recorders," SAE Technical Paper 2004-01-1199, 2004, doi:10.4271/2004-01-1199.
12. Reust, T. and Morgan, J., "Commercial Vehicle Event Data Recorders and the Effect of ABS Brakes During Maximum Brake Application," SAE Technical Paper 2006-01-1129, 2006, doi:10.4271/2006-01-1129.
13. Reust, T., Morgan, J., and Smith, P., "Method to Determine Vehicle Speed During ABS Brake Events Using Heavy Vehicle Event Data Recorder Speed," *SAE Int. J. Passeng. Cars – Mech. Sys.* 3, no. 1 (2010): 644-652, doi:10.4271/2010-01-0999.
14. Ruhl, R., Senalik, C., and Southcombe, E., "Numerical Methods for Evaluating ECM Data in Accident Reconstruction and Vehicle Dynamics," SAE Technical Paper 2003-01-3393, 2003, doi:10.4271/2003-01-3393.

15. van Nooten, S. and Hrycay, J., "The Application and Reliability of Commercial Vehicle Event Data Recorders for Accident Investigation and Analysis," SAE Technical Paper 2005-01-1177, 2005, doi:10.4271/2005-01-1177.

16. Rose, N. and Carter, N., "An Analytical Review and Extension of Two Decades of Research Related to PC-Crash Simulation Software," SAE Technical Paper 2018-01-0523, 2018, doi:10.4271/2018-01-0523.

17. Hull, W. and Newton, B., "The Animation Computer as a 3-D Reconstruction Tool," SAE Technical Paper 920754, 1992, doi:10.4271/920754.

18. Fay, R. and Gardner, J., "Analytical Applications of 3-D imaging in Vehicle Accident Studies," SAE Technical Paper 960648, 1996, doi:10.4271/960648.

19. Jones, I., Muir, D., and Groo, S., "Computer Animation - Admissibility in the Courtroom," SAE Technical Paper 910366, 1991, doi:10.4271/910366.

20. Hull, W., Newton, B., Macaw, C., and Miller, R., "Functional Classifications and Critique Methods for Litigation Support Forensic1 Accident Reconstruction Animations," SAE Technical Paper 960651, 1996, doi:10.4271/960651.

21. Grimes, W., "Computer Animation Techniques for Use in Collision Reconstruction," SAE Technical Paper 920755, 1992, doi:10.4271/920755.

22. Grimes, W., "Classifying the Elements in a Scientific Animation," SAE Technical Paper 940919, 1994, doi:10.4271/940919.

23. Day, T., "The Scientific Visualization of Motor Vehicle Accidents," SAE Technical Paper 940922, 1994, doi:10.4271/940922.

24. Grimes, W., Dickerson, C., and Smith, C., "Documenting Scientific Visualizations and Computer Animations Used in Collision Reconstruction Presentations," SAE Technical Paper 980018, 1998, doi:10.4271/980018.

25. Martin, K., Banister, J., and Piziali, R., "Engineering Visualization of Vehicle Accidents: Data Sources and Methods of Production," SAE Technical Paper 910369, 1991, doi:10.4271/910369.

26. Massa, D., "Using Computer Reverse Projection Photogrammetry to Analyze an Animation," SAE Technical Paper 1999-01-0093, 1999, doi:10.4271/1999-01-0093.

27. Neale, W.T.C., Terpstra, T., and Bortles, W.M., "Evaluation of Discrete Vehicle Accident Sounds for use in Accident Reconstruction," *Proceedings of Meetings on Acoustics*, 2008, Vol. 5.

28. Neale, W.T.C. and Terpstra, T., "Methodology for Physics-Based Sound Composition in Forensic Visualization," *Proceedings of Meetings on Acoustics*, 2007, Vol. 1.

29. McLay, R., Kiely, S., and Sheehan, M., "Case Studies in Animation Foundation," SAE Technical Paper 940920, 1994, doi:10.4271/940920.

30. Fay, R., "Computer Images and Animations in Court," SAE Technical Paper 970965, 1997, doi:10.4271/970965.

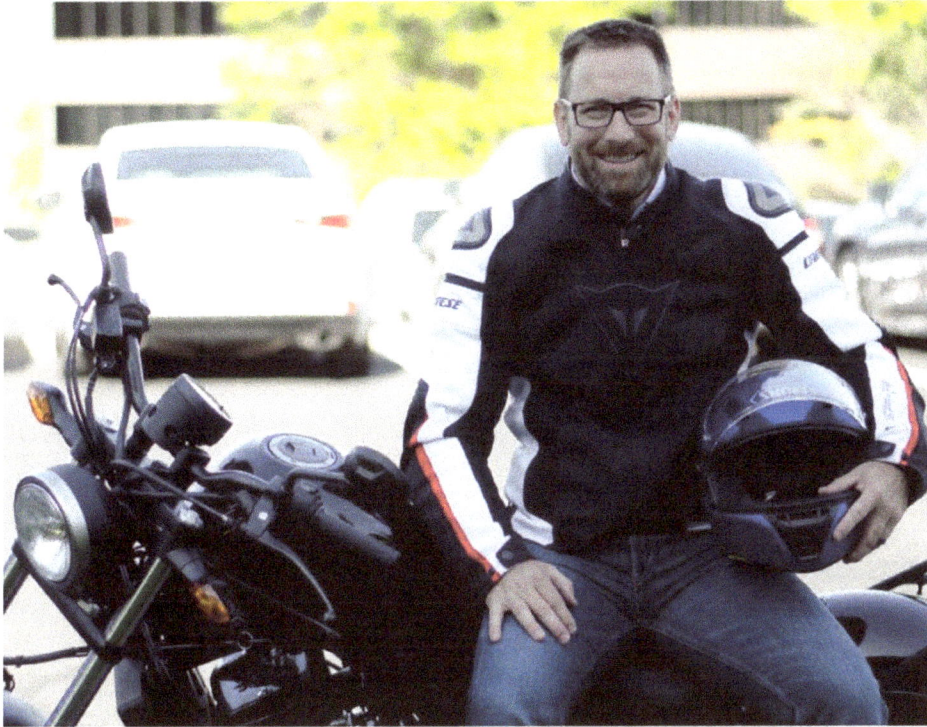

Nathan A. Rose laid his first motorcycle down back in 1976, when as an 18-month-old he pulled the bike down on himself while trying to climb on while the adults weren't paying attention. He only recently recovered from this experience and took up motorcycling at the ripe old age of 43. He now rides his 300cc Honda Rebel—what his friends refer to as his "badass moped"—wherever and whenever he can while he ponders what bike he's going to buy next and where he's going to store it. His wife has other plans for the money. Nathan has completed the Motorcycle Safety Foundation's Basic and Advanced Rider Courses, and he now fancies himself the safest rider on the road.

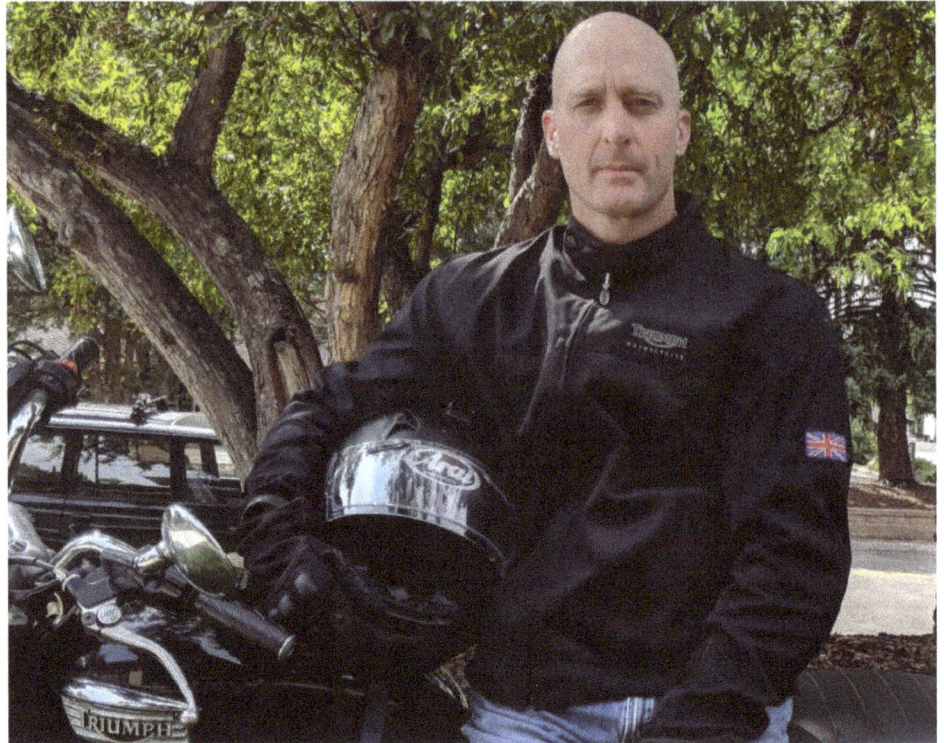

William T.C. Neale: The open-air experience and unique physical interaction a rider has with a motorcycle is what first sparked William T.C. Neale's fascination. The thrill of riding grew to the point where Mr. Neale had to share it with others. In fact, the majority of hours he spends around motorcycles is not riding through Colorado's notoriously beautiful mountain roads but rather navigating repeated ovals in a small, painted parking lot. But here he gets to witness that unforgettable expression of a student's first encounter with the bikes potential to throttle, shift, and weave. He also has shared the thrill of riding with his wife and two children, Maximus and Madeline, who occupied the rear seat of his "Bonnie Black" the moment their little legs reach the foot pegs. Ride Safe and Ride Wise!

www.ingramcontent.com/pod-product-compliance
Lightning Source LLC
Chambersburg PA
CBHW040140200326
41458CB00025B/6326